Handbook of Teaching
for Physical Therapists

Handbook of Teaching for Physical Therapists

Second Edition

Edited by

Katherine F. Shepard, Ph.D., P.T., F.A.P.T.A.

Professor and Director of the Ph.D. Program in Physical Therapy, Department of Physical Therapy, College of Allied Health Professions, Temple University, Philadelphia

Gail M. Jensen, Ph.D., P.T.

Professor and Director, Transitional Doctor of Physical Therapy Program, Department of Physical Therapy, School of Pharmacy and Allied Health Professions, Creighton University, Omaha, Nebraska

With 12 Contributing Authors

Foreword by
Joseph P. H. Black, Ph.D.
Senior Vice President for Education, American Physical Therapy Association, Alexandria, Virginia

BUTTERWORTH
HEINEMANN

An Imprint of Elsevier

Boston   Oxford   Auckland   Johannesburg   Melbourne   New Delhi

Every effort has been made to ensure that the drug dosage schedules within this text are accurate and conform to standards accepted at time of publication. However, as treatment recommendations vary in the light of continuing research and clinical experience, the reader is advised to verify drug dosage schedules herein with information found on product information sheets. This is especially true in cases of new or infrequently used drugs.

Recognizing the importance of preserving what has been written, Butterworth–Heinemann prints its books on acid-free paper whenever possible.

Library of Congress Cataloging-in-Publication Data

Handbook of teaching for physical therapists / edited by Katherine F. Shepard, Gail M. Jensen ; with 12 contributing authors.—2nd ed.
    p. ; cm.
  Includes bibliographical references and index.
  ISBN-13: 978-0-7506-7309-9 ISBN-10: 0-7506-7309-5
   1. Physical therapy—Study and teaching—Handbooks, manuals, etc. 2. Patient education—Handbooks, manuals, etc. I. Shepard, Katherine. II. Jensen, Gail M.
  [DNLM: 1. Physical Therapy—education. 2. Teaching—methods. WB 18 H236 2002]
  RM706 .H36 2002
  615.8'2'071—dc21

                                                                          2001052648

ISBN-13: 978-0-7506-7309-9
ISBN-10: 0-7506-7309-5

British Library Cataloguing-in-Publication Data
A catalogue record for this book is available from the British Library.

The publisher offers special discounts on bulk orders of this book.
For information, please contact:

Manager of Special Sales
Butterworth–Heinemann
225 Wildwood Avenue
Woburn, MA 01801-2041
Tel: 781-904-2500
Fax: 781-904-2620

For information on all Butterworth–Heinemann publications available,
contact our World Wide Web home page at: http://www.bh.com

10 9 8

Printed in the United States of America

Contents

Contributing Authors

Katherine F. Shepard, Ph.D., P.T., F.A.P.T.A., is Professor and Director of the Ph.D. Program in Physical Therapy, Department of Physical Therapy, College of Allied Health Professions at Temple University in Philadelphia. She received a bachelor of arts degree in psychology from Hood College, a bachelor of science degree in physical therapy from Ithaca College, and master's degrees in physical therapy and sociology, as well as a doctor of philosophy degree in sociology of education from Stanford University. She is the recipient of the Temple University Lindback Award for Distinguished Teaching, the American Physical Therapy Association (APTA) Section for Education Award for Leadership in Education, the APTA Baethke-Carlin Award for Teaching Excellence, and the APTA Golden Pen Award for outstanding contributions to the journal *Physical Therapy*. She is a Catherine Worthingham Fellow of the APTA. She has written and lectured extensively on academic and clinical education, the behavioral sciences, and qualitative research design.

Gail M. Jensen, Ph.D., P.T., is Professor in the Departments of Physical Therapy and Occupational Therapy, Director of the Transitional Doctor of Physical Therapy Program, and Faculty Associate, Center for Health Policy and Ethics at Creighton University, Omaha, Nebraska. She holds a bachelor of science degree from the University of Minnesota and a master of arts in physical therapy and a doctor of philosophy degree in educational evaluation from Stanford University. She has previously served on the editorial boards of *Physical Therapy* and the *Journal of Physical Therapy Education* and is currently deputy editor for *Physiotherapy Research International*. Dr. Jensen serves as a reader-consultant and on-site reviewer team leader for the Commission on Accreditation in Physical Therapy Education and is on the academic faculty of the Kaiser-Hayward Physical Therapy Residency Program in Advanced Orthopedic Manual Therapy. She has been involved in federally funded interdisciplinary education grant activity, working with Native Americans in rural Nebraska since 1997, and serves as Co-Director of the Office of Interprofessional Scholarship and Service at Creighton University. A recipient of the American Physical Therapy Association's Golden Pen Award, she has publications and presentations in the area of professional education, reflective practice, interdisciplinary education, clinical reasoning, and qualitative research.

Tracy Chapman, M.Ed., serves as Assistant Director of the Office of Information Technology and Learning Resources for the School of Pharmacy and Allied Health Professions at Creighton University in Omaha, Nebraska. She received a bachelor of science degree in business from the University of South Carolina, an elementary teaching certification from Southwest Texas State University, certification in special education from the University of Nebraska at Omaha, and a master's degree in instructional technology from West Texas A&M University. She is the lead instructional designer for more than 30 online courses for the School of Pharmacy and Allied Health Professions and coordinator of computing technology faculty development for the school across the disciplines of physical therapy, occupational therapy, and pharmacy. She has presented numerous school and university workshops, with the purpose of preparing faculty for moving their teaching and learning to the online environment, including the best practices for using Web-based resources for teaching and learning and effective use of hardware and software tools to enhance teaching and learning.

Jeanne M. Davidson, P.T., O.C.S., serves as Senior Physical Therapist at York Hospital in York, Maine. She received a bachelor of science degree in physical therapy in 1979 from Russell Sage College and completed the Kaiser Permanente Physical Therapy Residency Program in Advanced Orthopedic Manual Therapy in 1985. For more than 8 years, she was a clinical specialist at St. Mary's Spine Center in San Francisco. She was on the faculty at the Kaiser Permanente Physical Therapy Residency Program from 1991 to 1994 and continues to be an active faculty alumna. She has taught continuing education courses in orthopedics and manual therapy for the past 15 years.

Julie Gahimer, H.S.D., P.T., is Associate Professor of Physical Therapy at the Krannert School of Physical Therapy at the University of Indianapolis. She received a bachelor of science degree in physical therapy from St. Louis University, a master's degree in physical therapy from the University of Indianapolis, and a doctor of health science from Indiana University. Her doctoral degree focused on the areas of college and school health education and patient education. She currently serves on the editorial board of the *Journal of Physical Therapy Education*.

Judith R. Gale, P.T., M.A., M.P.H., O.C.S., is Assistant Professor in the Department of Physical Therapy at the School of Pharmacy and Allied Health Professions at Creighton University in Omaha, Nebraska. She received her bachelor of arts degree in psychology from San Francisco State University, her master's degree in physical therapy from Stanford University, and her master of public health degree in epidemiology from the University of Alabama at Birmingham. She is currently pursuing a clinical doctorate in physical therapy at Creighton University. She is a board-certified specialist in orthopedics. She teaches in the areas of physical assessment, differential diagnosis, orthopedics, and human immunodeficiency virus/acquired immunodeficiency syndrome.

Jody S. Gandy, Ph.D., P.T., has served on the American Physical Therapy Association staff since 1990 and currently is Director of the Department of Physical Therapy Education. Her primary responsibilities include planning and facilitating academic and clinical education initiatives for physical therapists and physical therapist assistants. She received her bachelor of science degree in physical therapy in 1975 from Ithaca College, a master's degree in counseling and personnel studies in 1983 from Glassboro State College, and a doctor of philosophy degree in psychoeducation processes in 1993 from Temple University. She has provided numerous presentations on clinical education, teaching and learning, conflict management, and mentoring and has published in several of these areas. Before her current position, she was actively involved in clinical education as Assistant Professor, Associate Chair, and Academic Coordinator of Clinical Education at Temple University, and as Director and Center Coordinator of Clinical Education at Children's Seashore House in Atlantic City. She was the recipient of the 1989 Mary McMillan Scholarship (Doctoral) Award, 1991 Mohonasen High School Hall of Fame Award, 1995 Excellence in Clinical Teaching Award from the New York State Physical Therapy Clinical Education Consortium, and 1998 Temple University Hyman Dervitz Lectureship.

Christopher D. Lorish, Ph.D., is Associate Professor of Education in Medicine at the University of Alabama School of Medicine. He received his doctor of philosophy in education in 1980 from Ohio State University. His research interests include patient and community education, treatment adherence, and psychosocial issues in chronic disease. A focus of his recent work is developing methods for applying concepts from behavior theory to health promotion and disease prevention issues faced by health professionals as they work with patients.

David M. Morris, P.T., M.S., is Associate Professor and Co-Academic Coordinator of Clinical Education in the Department of Physical Therapy at the University of Alabama at Birmingham (UAB). He received a bachelor of science degree in physical therapy from the University of North Carolina–Chapel Hill and a master's degree in physical therapy education from UAB. He is currently completing his doctorate in health education/promotion at UAB. He is also Director of Training for the UAB Constraint-Induced Movement Therapy Research Project. He has written and lectured extensively on the topics of clinical education, aquatic rehabilitation, and constraint-induced movement therapy.

Elizabeth Mostrom, Ph.D., P.T., is Professor and Director of Clinical Education, Program in Physical Therapy, School of Rehabilitation and Medical Sciences at Central Michigan University in Mt. Pleasant, Michigan. She received a bachelor of science degree in health education from West Chester State College, a master of science degree in physical therapy from Duke University, and a doctor of philosophy degree in educational psychology from Michigan State University. She has served on the editorial advisory boards of several professional journals and is currently the editor of the *Journal of Physical Therapy Education*. She is a past recipient of the American Physical Therapy Association's Mary MacMillan Scholarship for doctoral students and a Foundation for Physical Therapy doctoral research grant. Her research interests, publications, and professional presentations span the areas of student and professional learning and development, clinical education, and qualitative research.

Diane E. Nicholson, Ph.D., P.T., N.C.S., is Associate Professor of Physical Therapy at the University of Utah, Salt Lake City, and the Research Coordinator in the Movement Analysis Laboratory at the Intermountain Shriners Hospital for Children in Salt Lake City. She received her bachelor of science degree in physical therapy in 1979 from the University of Delaware, her master's degree in physical therapy in 1984 from the University of North Carolina–Chapel Hill, and her doctor of philosophy degree in kinesiology in 1992 from the University of California, Los Angeles. She is a board-certified neurologic clinical specialist. Her principal areas of teaching and research focus on motor control and learning to optimize physical function in persons with neurologic disorders.

Paul Ogbonna, Ed.D., P.T., is Founder and Director of PEN Physical Therapy and Rehab Services in Ewing, New Jersey, and the Consultant Physical

Therapist for the Physical Therapy Department at Hagedorn Psychiatric Hospital in Glen Gardner, New Jersey. He received his first degree in physical therapy from the College of Medicine, University of Lagos, Nigeria, his master's degree in pediatric physical therapy from Sargent College of Health and Rehabilitation Sciences, Boston University, and his doctor of education in special education with specialization in early intervention and rehabilitation of children with developmental disabilities at the School of Education of Boston University. He designed and developed the Preparatory Review Educational Course Program for foreign-educated physical therapists preparing to take the physical therapy license examination in the United States. He belongs to numerous professional organizations and is a member of the American Physical Therapy Association. He is a member of Phi Beta Delta, the Honor Society for International Scholars, and a member of the Board of Mid-Jersey CARES for Special Children Regional Early Intervention Collaborative. He is a book reviewer for *Advance for Physical Therapists and PT Assistants* magazine.

Karen A. Paschal, P.T., M.S., is Assistant Professor and Director of Clinical Education in the Department of Physical Therapy at Creighton University in Omaha, Nebraska. She received her bachelor of arts degree in biology from the University of South Dakota and her master's degree in physical therapy from Duke University, and she is currently completing her doctoral dissertation in development psychology at the University of Pittsburgh. She is a member of the Commission on Accreditation in Physical Therapy Education and serves as a manuscript reviewer for *Physical Therapy* and the *Journal of Physical Therapy Education*. She is a credentialed trainer for the American Physical Therapy Association's Clinical Instructor Education and Credentialing Program. She has a broad background in clinical education, with a focus on clinical learning, authentic assessment, and professional development.

Carol Jo Tichenor, P.T., M.A, is Director of the Kaiser Permanente Physical Therapy Residency Program in Advanced Orthopedic Manual Therapy— a postprofessional residency program that combines intensive clinical mentoring and coursework in advanced orthopedic manual physical therapy—in Hayward, California. She received her bachelor of arts degree in psychology in 1971 and her master's degree in physical therapy in 1973 from Stanford University. Her professional focus is on the design, development, and evaluation of postprofessional physical therapy residency education. She has been very involved in the development of curriculum standards and guidelines related to residency education for more than 10 years.

Foreword

The physical therapy profession, no less than others, seems always to be in transition. From dependence on the judgment and decisions of other health care professionals to full partnership in the health care delivery system, the profession has proved its ability to meet the challenges posed by a volatile, uncertain future and changing expectations in practice, education, and research. Throughout its remarkable history, the profession has always pinned its hopes and aspirations on the kind of educational experiences that would lead to the preparation of the most knowledgeable, competent, and caring practitioners whose self-confidence, clinical skills, adaptability, and service orientation would serve the interests of the patient. It is readily apparent that the requisite transitions have been well managed, because physical therapists (PTs), in partnership with physical therapist assistants (PTAs), have moved into positions of greater responsibility requiring more complex decision-making and reasoning skills. As the focus of care broadens from a matter of the patient's disease or physical impairment to wider considerations of prevention, wellness, and the patient's quality of life, including differences of race, culture, outlook, and learning, PTs will likely discover that yesterday's achievements rarely suffice as a guarantor of tomorrow's successful transition.

Consistent with a vision for a terminal clinical doctorate (D.P.T.) for all graduates of PT professional education programs by 2020, the profession must now focus on the transition to a doctoring profession. Physical therapy is hardly the first to adopt a vision for a doctoring profession (e.g., medicine, osteopathy, dentistry, veterinary medicine, optometry, pharmacy, podiatry, law, and psychology); we will certainly not be the last. But a word of caution is in order: Although the long-term benefits of such a transition are rather transparent, the associated obligations are considerably less so. Contrary to conventional wisdom, the D.P.T. will not be the sole criterion of a doctoring profession. In addition to the D.P.T. degree, the profession must ultimately exhibit the critical indicators that have become the hallmark of a doctoring profession. For physical therapy, these will include an *enduring* commitment to the following:

- Uniform and systematic approach to patient and client management
- Evidence-based practice
- Continuous progress from novice to expert practitioner
- Refinement and expansion of the clinical science of physical therapy through active engagement in clinical research
- Interdependence and collaboration in practice, education, and research
- Ethical, legal, and professional behaviors
- Lifelong learning shaped by ongoing personal and professional self- and peer-assessment that is self-initiated, rigorous, and honest

If these indicators are to be achieved within the next decade, it is imperative that the academic and clinical education communities embrace new teaching and learning paradigms. Proven and innovative teaching theories combined with fresh approaches to the practical application of those theories can serve as an intentional and forward-looking curricular framework for the preparation of practitioners who can deliver physical therapy services based on historical precedent, sound research, proven treatment outcomes, and a mastery of communication and relational skills.

The profession's readiness to manage this extraordinary transition depends on its willingness to shift attention away from narrow regional or institutional interests to those larger interests represented by (1) the rapidly changing expectations of patients and their families for high-quality, cost-effective health care; (2) the professional and postprofessional education needs of all students, PTs, and PTAs; and (3) the global needs of the profession, including the expansion and refinement of the clinical science known as physical therapy. The larger the view, the greater the possibility for constructive change, adaptation, and innovation and the lesser the risk that the profession will be characterized by confusion, uncertainty, or unresponsiveness.

Cultivating that larger view requires continuous improvement in the quality and efficacy of teaching and learning. For that reason alone, the publication of the *Handbook of Teaching for Physical Therapists* could not come at a more opportune time. The demand for high-quality care at a reasonable price, the high cost of professional preparation, increased competition among health care providers, the inevitable boundary disputes, and the expanding role of patients in achieving and maintaining optimum health—all of these factors place enormous burdens on the processes of teaching and learning. This Handbook offers a wealth of resources, not only for those who are engaged in teaching entry-level students, but also for every PT and PTA who, in the course of providing physical therapy services, is charged with teaching a patient or learning from a colleague or mentor.

The authors' approach is unique and delightfully utilitarian. From the specific learning objectives and profoundly relevant life incidents at the beginning of each chapter to the substantive theoretical concepts and practical applications, this Handbook offers an understandable and useful resource for transforming the reader into a more mature, confident, and effective teacher and learner. This Handbook is for the educator and practitioner who recognize that a successful transition to a doctoring profession requires the preparation of active, interdependent, and self-directed practitioners by teachers who possess a continuously expanding realm of academic and clinical theory and the all-too-rare proclivity for admitting to a certain amount of ignorance as a prerequisite for learning.

Every physical therapy educator and practitioner holds the key to the successful management of the profession's developmental transitions. This Handbook will provide the eager and expectant reader with new and provocative insights into how teaching and learning can radically transform and benefit the physical therapy student, the practitioner of any age or setting, and the patient or client. Perhaps more important, this Handbook will offer the entire physical therapy profession an exciting, reflective, and experience-based resource for managing the promise and peril of the exceedingly complex, but thoroughly attainable, transition to a doctoring profession.

Joseph P. H. Black, Ph.D.

Preface

Every day, physical therapists (PTs) and physical therapist assistants (PTAs) are engaged in teaching. They identify strategies to facilitate change in patients' health behaviors, demonstrate lifting techniques to family members, guide students through clinical internships, present in-service programs to their health care colleagues, deliver professional presentations at local and national meetings, serve on curricular committees, plan health promotion programs for the community, and consult with teachers in the local school system. Perhaps no process other than teaching so permeates the professional contributions made by members of the physical therapy profession.

Teaching is a skill that PTs often take for granted. We have all experienced many years of being taught. During these years, we have observed ineffective teaching that leaves teachers and students frustrated and alienated from learning more about teaching—or learning more altogether. Few PTs and even fewer PTAs have been exposed to the substantial body of knowledge and theory that exists in education. From observing expert teachers at work, we know that skill in teaching requires much more than knowing the material, illustrating lectures with PowerPoint, or learning how to construct a valid examination. Effective learning experiences are crafted by expert teachers, suffused with practical and theoretical knowledge, compellingly delivered with accurate insight into the needs of the learner, and constantly assessed and improved.

This Handbook has emerged from an ongoing dialogue of our own experiences as PTs, educators, and researchers. Our interest and background in educational theory are tied to a specific belief and value about the central importance of teaching and learning to those practicing physical therapy. Our philosophy of education provides the philosophical foundation for the Handbook. Essentially, we embrace William Butler Yeats' observation that "education is not the filling of a pail, but the lighting of a fire." Students who have teachers who understand and engage in the pedagogic process of lighting fires become clinicians and educators who are delighted by the acquisition of knowledge and the development of new skills, are perceptive and sensitive to the world around them, give themselves permission to allow their joyful creative abilities to surface, and embrace the challenge and excitement of continual professional growth.

Consistent with lifelong learning, we ourselves are committed to providing the reader with a text that is driven by inquiry and reflection. We believe that one is always a teacher *and* student in physical therapy practice. These roles are constantly interchanging. The PT and PTA must initiate and engage in both roles to do either one well. We also believe that teaching within the clinic or classroom is always more chaotic and complicated than what theory may account for, and constant inquiry and adaptation are essential skills. Theory does provide a framework for understanding practice, and practice yields ever more useful theory. Thus, a dedicated state of inquiry or reflection—that is, becoming a reflective practitioner—is needed to teach and learn in chaotic settings and to maintain the dialogue between theory and practice.

In an effort to link theory and practice in this text, we have invited expert contributors known for their practical experience in "the real world" as well as their theoretical understanding and expertise. By including these expert contributors, we are celebrating the learning community of scholars in physical therapy education who are reflective and responsible stewards of their work.

Finally, as qualitative researchers, we are committed to understanding teaching from the inside—that is, from the individual and collective experiences of learners and teachers. You will read stories from the "trenches" of practice in each chapter. We hope these examples of your colleagues at work as teachers will facilitate your intuitive understanding of some of the broader conceptual issues proposed.

Teaching and learning are perhaps the most important skills a PT and a PTA can acquire. Development of sound, practically relevant, theoretically based educational strategies can result in significant reform of our ability to perceive, understand, and deliver knowledge, insight, and skills to students, patients, colleagues, and the public.

We have many people to thank for this book. First, thanks to our mentors at Stanford University in the Department of Physical Therapy and School of Education. Our experiences at Stanford are embodied in the Stanford motto "Die Luft der Freiheit Weht" ("the winds of freedom blow"). We were urged to question, grapple with new ideas, and be intrigued with failures. These experiences set our course as teachers and scholars. Our thanks to the Ph.D. students at Temple University and the D.P.T. students at Creighton University who gracefully provided excellent feedback to the first edition. Our heartfelt gratitude to Judith R. Gale, P.T., M.A., M.P.H., O.C.S., and Rosalie Lopopolo, Ph.D., P.T., M.B.A., who were more involved in this book than they wanted to be—creating tables and figures, formatting text, reviewing drafts, and proofreading. Additional thanks to our colleagues, friends (human and animal), and family members who unconditionally accept us and our life journeys. You each know who you are. Thanks to Barbara Murphy and Leslie Kramer, formerly at Butterworth–Heinemann, as well as Mary Drabot—all of whom steadfastly shared in our excitement about this Handbook and smoothed the way with their perceptive and skillful interventions. Thanks, also, to Holly L. Hoe of Silverchair Science + Communications, Inc., who, with kindness, persistence, and skill, put this book together.

Finally, thanks to all those to whom this book is dedicated—the many students who have taught us so profoundly for so many years.

K.F.S.
G.M.J.

Introduction

Katherine F. Shepard and Gail M. Jensen

Good teaching comes in many flavors and colors. It occurs when a teacher leads you to a vista that changes forever the way you see. It happens when someone introduces you to a delicious idea that you can chew on for the rest of your life. It occurs when somebody helps you discover possibilities in yourself you didn't know were there. Good teaching is many things. It has no essential quality. It takes place through books, it occurs in classrooms, [in health care clinics], it emerges in conversations and in the presence of those who give us a vision of how life in its large and small moments might be lived.

—Eliot Eisner, Professor of Education and Art, Stanford University (Stanford *Educator*, Spring 1995;3.)

Purpose of the Handbook

For many students who learn in physical therapy academic settings, the experience is one of struggling to understand and remember an endless array of ill-connected knowledge bits. Many of these knowledge bits have a half-life of 3–5 years, and others already are outdated for physical therapy practice in today's health care system. Certainly, the strain of teaching and learning in academic settings is due in part to the knowledge explosion in the sciences as well as in the guiding principles and techniques of physical therapy practice, especially in clinical specialty areas.

For many patients who learn in clinical settings, the experience is one of attempting to focus attention and grasp information under the most difficult of circumstances—that is, while ill or in pain or experiencing devastating loss.

Typically, patients are exposed to rapidly delivered sound bites of important, perhaps even lifesaving, information delivered by a multitude of fleeting health care professionals who are strangers (and who may not even understand or speak the patient's native language). Certainly, some of this strain of teaching and learning in health care settings is due to the realities of health care delivery systems in which everyone labors under time restrictions that limit access to clinicians and shorten contact with patients and families.

The fragmented learning and embarrassingly limited outcomes that often occur with such experiences in academic and clinical settings are perplexing and sad. However, crises also present us with opportunities to use our ingenuity and strengths as health care providers and teachers. When we find ourselves competing with time and costs to deliver the most effective health care possible, do we find ourselves teaching more? Are we involving the patient as well as family and caretakers much earlier in learning to assume health care tasks? Are we thinking about what we as physical therapists (PTs) and physical therapist assistants (PTAs) can do to facilitate healthy practices in the community? And have we figured out what is essential for novice practitioners to know and how we can prepare them to acquire knowledge throughout their professional lives?

The primary purpose of this book is to stimulate the growth of the reader in teaching and learning by presenting theoretical concepts and related practical applications that will improve skills in the educational processes used in academic and clinical settings.

What Is Teaching? What Is Learning?

From the perspective of many experienced educators, effective teaching involves the following: (1) deeply *comprehending* the information to be taught, (2) being able to *transform* and present that information in such a way that students "get it," (3) engaging the student in *active collaborative* learning experiences, and (4) teaching the student how to learn by constant *inquiry and reflection*, which lead the student to acquire her or his own new knowledge and comprehensions. (This teaching process is discussed more thoroughly in Chapter 3.) Similarly, for students to learn, they must comprehend and transform ideas, information, and beliefs through inquiry and reflection during learning experiences in which they, the students, are active participants and collaborators. Such learning results in a change in students' store of information, behaviors, perceptions, feelings, and interactions.

Because this process of teaching and learning is two inseparable sides of the same coin, designating one person as the teacher and another person as the learner is an artificial distinction, much like saying kinesthetic perceptions and functional movement should be considered as two separate and distinct entities. For either process to work well, both processes must work in concert. At any given moment, anyone can be the learner or the teacher— patients and families, students participating in formal academic programs, health care colleagues, community neighbors, and one's self.

Characteristics of Good Teachers and Learners

As Eliot Eisner stated, good teaching is many things and comes in many colors and flavors. We think, however, that there are three major components that must be present for good teaching and learning to occur:

1. Teachers must understand deeply the topics that they are teaching and ceaselessly engage in adding to their knowledge stores. To be continually learning requires curiosity, initiative, and intellectual excitement about uncovering more and more about a specific topic or field. Learning means seeking out and engaging in experiences that foster learning—reading, clinical practice, conferences, research, talking with colleagues over coffee, and, of course, being stimulated by one's students. Reflecting on these experiences results in transformation of the knowledge so that it becomes an integral part of what and how one teaches. Where there is no passion for the topic or for teaching, there is no thinking about what and how one is doing and how it might be done better; there is only the repetitive transmission of dusty, uninspired information from yellowed notes.

2. Teachers must know about the students whom they are teaching. This awareness and knowledge comes from listening to students speak—learning what they understand as well as how they think and reason, through watching students' faces, postures, and gestures; observing students perform manual skills; reading student papers; and noting how students interact with people around them. The ability to effectively transform and transmit knowledge rests on understanding students. This understanding undergirds the teacher's ability to figure out ways to capture the students' curiosity and interest, to create experiences that challenge students to think and risk, and to persistently support students for the discipline, patience, and sometimes tedium it takes for learning to occur.

The effective teacher remembers well what it is like to be a student. From this memory comes empathy for students in academic settings who must sit through hours of writing down new and often perplexing information, sitting in uncomfortable chairs, and not being allowed to move or to speak without permission. From this memory also comes sensitivity to a student's anxiety about undersupervision and frustration with oversupervision by the clinical instructor. Similarly, practitioners in clinical settings who have encountered physical disabilities of their own have a greater tacit understanding of how to teach patients to achieve maximum recovery.

Knowing the student is not only easier but a highly pleasurable activity if the student is the only individual being taught, is verbal about his or her educational needs, is motivated by the need to know, and is graciously responsive to the PT or teacher's interest and assistance. However, this situation is rare. The task of knowing a student is clearly daunting when faced with a classroom of 50 students or a minimally verbal patient who has no family advocate and is scheduled for discharge tomorrow. However daunting, without knowing something about one's students and how they think, what their values and goals are, and what anxieties or concerns they have about the information or skill to be learned, one cannot teach well. Simply put, if the information being delivered is inflexible to the proclivities of the learner, little or no learning occurs.

3. Teachers must be acquainted with a number of different theoretical approaches and techniques (pedagogy) that can facilitate learning for richly diverse groups of students. The more one knows about these approaches and techniques, the more innovative and flexible one can be in providing learning experiences that match the student's quest. The military model of teaching often prevails in academic and clinical settings. The military model involves the rigid, repetitive sequence of demonstrating a task to be accomplished, breaking the task into component parts, teaching the component parts, having the student master the component parts, and then putting the components together. This method is certainly effective in teaching a well-known task for which a right and wrong way is clearly demarcated (e.g., learning how to assemble and disassemble a rifle). However, it is highly questionable whether this method is responsive to most individual learning in academic or clinical settings, which inherently involves perceptions, attitudes, beliefs, prior learned behaviors, and building-block information that the learner may or may not hold.

There are many intriguing methods that one can use to teach and to assess teaching—problem-solving cases, journals, peer teaching, virtual classrooms, portfolios, interactive laboratories with experts, stories, community activities, and so forth. By presenting these techniques, we hope to engage readers in learning more about them and thus expand their teaching, learning, and assessment repertoires.

Overview of the Handbook

This edition of the Handbook is generally divided into two main sections. In the first section (Chapters 1–7), the focus is on designing academic and clinical education programs and on teaching and assessing the performance of PTs and PTAs in academic and clinical settings. In the second section (Chapters 8–13), the focus is on teaching patients and families in clinical and community settings. A final chapter (Chapter 14) presents information on postprofessional clinical residency education for the skilled practitioner.

All chapters included in the first edition have been updated, and five new chapters have been added, including use of computer technology in teaching and learning (Chapter 4), assessment of the teaching-learning process (Chapter 5), teaching and learning about patient education (Chapter 6), facilitating adherence to healthy lifestyle behavioral changes (Chapter 10), and using computer materials in home education programs (Chapter 12).

Although each chapter is designed to be read independently of all other chapters, in some cases understanding will be greatly enhanced if several chapters are read together. For example, the reader would benefit from reading the chapter on preparation for teaching in the academic setting (Chapter 2) before reading about techniques for teaching in academic settings (Chapter 3). Likewise, preparation for teaching in clinical settings (Chapter 6) will greatly add to one's understanding of teaching techniques used in the clinical setting (Chapter 7). In the second section, understanding of how to assess the patient's receptivity for learning (Chapter 9) and facilitating patients' adherence to healthy lifestyle behaviors (Chapter 10) are designed to be read concurrently.

The Scholarship of Teaching

Teachers need to find ways to bring teaching and learning, which are primarily private and hidden activities, into the arena of public and community property. The visible scholarship of teaching needs to continue to grow and flourish in physical therapy. Shulman* argues that this scholarship of teaching and learning should be motivated by a spirit of faithfulness or fidelity. This fidelity should include integrity of the discipline; the learning of students; the society, community, and institution where one works; and the teacher's sense of self as scholar, teacher, and valued colleague.

Our hope is that this *Handbook of Teaching for Physical Therapists* will continue to evolve over time with the sharing of educational research, intuitive ideas, and practical experiences that are part of the community property of physical therapy education. The work of the educational community in physical therapy transcends the ability of any one person and rests with all the members of the community as the work and ideas are critically examined and shared. If the readers of this book grapple with, enjoy, debate, and muse over the concepts presented in this Handbook and then share the ongoing development and assessment of their own educational endeavors, we will have come a long way toward creating a true community of educational scholars.

---

*Shulman L. Inventing the Future. In P Hutchings (ed). Opening Lines: Approaches to the Scholarship of Teaching and Learning. Menlo Park, CA: Carnegie Foundation for the Advancement of Teaching, 2000;95–105.

1

Curriculum Design for Physical Therapy Educational Programs

Katherine F. Shepard and
Gail M. Jensen

The physical therapy program at Stanford University had been in existence since 1940. As a young faculty member in the early 1970s I assumed we belonged at Stanford just as much as any other department in the university. I never realized how changing the philosophy, mission, and expectations in other parts of the university could affect the very existence of our program. In 1982, the School of Medicine changed its mission from developing physicians to developing physician-researchers (MD-PhDs) and covertly designated the land on which the physical therapy building was located as the new center of Molecular Genetic Engineering. Subsequently, an all-physician review committee informed us that we didn't belong in the School of Medicine because we didn't have a PhD program and weren't producing "scholars." While meeting with the university president on an early spring evening to plead our case, he informed us that if we were to be considered scholars we should be publishing in the *Journal of Physiology* (his field was physiology) and not *Physical Therapy* (a technical journal by his standards). It was devastating to belatedly realize how the pieces were being put in place to discontinue our program. Our own mission statement, philosophy, and program goals were essentially ignored as they were now incongruent with the new university sanctioned "direction" of the medical school. The Stanford University Board of Trustees acted to close the program with the graduating class of 1985. (Shepard)

The moral of this story is that the philosophy and goals of any physical therapist or physical therapist assistant program must be in concert with the philosophy and goals of the program's institution or the program will not survive.

Chapter Objectives

After completing this chapter, the reader will be able to

1. State the four questions posed by Ralph Tyler[1] to guide curriculum design and describe the three-phase process of how faculty engage in curriculum development, as suggested by Decker Walker.[2]
2. Defend the need for a clearly stated program philosophy and goals to guide curriculum planning. Demonstrate how program philosophy and goals can be articulated with university philosophy, societal needs, and professional functions.
3. Define implicit, explicit, and null curricula and identify components of each type.
4. Discuss five areas of perennial conflict between the curricular needs of health care professional programs and the academic traditions that undergird liberal arts education.
5. State the purpose of professional accreditation and outline the process of accreditation used by the American Physical Therapy Association (APTA).

Curriculum Design

Everything depends upon the *quality* of the experience which is had. The quality of any experience has two aspects. There is an immediate aspect of agreeableness or disagreeableness, and there is its influence upon later experiences. The first is obvious and easy to judge. The *effect* of an experience is not borne on its face. It sets a problem to the educator. It is his business to arrange for the kind of experiences which, while they do not repel the student, but rather engage his activities are, nevertheless, more than immediately enjoyable since they promote having desirable future experiences. . . . Hence the central problem of an education based upon experience is to select the kind of present experiences that live fruitfully and creatively in subsequent experiences.[3]

For educational experiences to be coherent and enjoyable to the individual student, as well as relevant to the desired performance of the program graduate, an all-embracing framework for educational experiences—a curriculum design—must be in place. *Curriculum design* refers to the content and organization of the curricular elements of philosophy, goals, coursework, clinical experiences, and evaluation processes. There is a rational assumption that what drives the curriculum designed for the education of physical therapists and physical therapist assistants is preparation for practice in the health care arena, which involves the development of knowledge, skills, attitudes, and values that undergird competent physical therapy practice.

A curriculum design reflects input, directly or indirectly, from literally thousands of people. People with health care needs, regulatory bodies, such as regional and professional accreditation groups and state board licensing agencies, members of the APTA who establish and act on professional standards, physical therapy clinicians, faculty and administrators in the college or university in which the program is located, and each generation of students have an impact on curriculum design. A curriculum design must be steadfastly relevant to the current tasks and standards of physical therapy practice, and dynamically responsive to rapidly changing practice environments and human health care needs.

Developing a Curriculum

Eliot Eisner noted that the word *curriculum* originally came from the Latin word *currere*, which means "the course to be run." He states, "This notion implies a track, a set of obstacles or tasks that an individual is to overcome, something that has a beginning and an end, something that one aims at completing."[4]

Tyler's Four Fundamental Questions

Four fundamental questions identified by Ralph Tyler in 1949 are useful in deciding how to develop a "racecourse."[1] These four questions are rediscovered by each generation of faculty seeking to develop a physical therapy curriculum.

1. What educational purposes or goals should the school seek to attain?
2. What educational experiences can be provided that are likely to attain these purposes?

3. How can these educational experiences be effectively organized?
4. How can it be determined whether these purposes or goals are being attained?

These questions and the answers to these questions should be inter-related, with each question and answer building on the preceding question(s) and answer(s). The easiest, and often first place for a group of novice faculty to begin, however, is with the second and third questions. Faculty can confidently produce and organize educational experiences based on their own personal experiences in physical therapy education and practice. However, if curricula are designed in such a way that the answers to questions 2 and 3 are not directly related to question 1, it is like setting sail without plotting a course. That is, despite knowing everything about sailing a ship, sailing with no clear destination may be disastrous. The result of an analogous educational program is haphazard curricular growth, which, at the least, is perplexing to faculty, students, and clinical educators and, at most, can produce graduates who are ill-focused and perplexed about their roles in the health care system.

In designing a curriculum, the elements must be logically ordered. This logic can be obtained by thinking about how each level is directly responsive to the levels above and below. As illustrated in the curricular design column in Figure 1-1, the content of a physical therapy educational program (i.e., coursework, learning experiences, and evaluation processes) is based on meeting program objectives designed to fulfill the program's goals. The program goals reflect the philosophy of the program and the institution. Evaluation of the program graduate therefore demonstrates the success or lack of success of the program's ability to build a curriculum that meets its stated goals.

Tyler's Question 1: Program Philosophy and Goals
Macro Environment

Figure 1-2 demonstrates how the philosophy and goals of any physical therapy curriculum are imbedded in a global (macro) environment that includes society, the health care environment, the higher education system, and the knowledge related to physical therapy.[5]

It should be evident to the reader that when any component of this macro environment changes, it is necessary to consider changing the physical therapy curriculum. Historical changes outside the profession (e.g., medical discoveries such as the Sabin polio vaccine), and inside the profession (e.g., the creation of the physical therapist assistant), have lead to curricular changes.[6] The aging of post–World War II "baby boomers" has decreased patient care stays in acute care and rehabilitation hospital settings, and physical therapy direct-access state laws have spawned curricular changes in

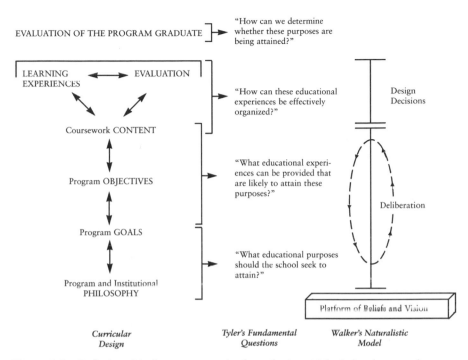

Figure 1-1 Relationship between curriculum design, Tyler's fundamental questions, and Walker's naturalistic model.

entry level and advanced coursework for physical therapists and physical therapist assistants. Other changes include the federal government movement in support of health and health promotion/prevention activities. For example, Healthy People 2010 goals and objectives must be considered and included when submitting all federal grants and other health initiatives. This focus on health rather than disease is captured in Chapter 13. Read this chapter as well as the Pew Health Professions Commission Reports[7] and other recent literature[8] to consider ways to include an emphasis on prevention and community health as well as interprofessional collaboration in physical therapy curricula work.

David Rogers proposed a set of goals for medical educators and students broad enough to be responsive to this global environment (Table 1-1).[9] Note that what the student is to know (i.e., the language of the discipline and the ways of science) is only part of what people who engage in curriculum design must be concerned with. Students must also be prepared to reason, to become sensitive and responsive to cultural diversity and society's needs, to undergird decisions and actions with empathy, and to begin a quest for knowledge that will last throughout their professional lives.

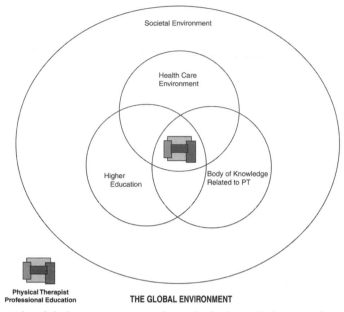

Societal Environment

Health Care Environment

Higher Education

Body of Knowledge Related to PT

Physical Therapist Professional Education

THE GLOBAL ENVIRONMENT

Figure 1-2 The global environment within which physical therapy education exists. (Reprinted with permission from American Physical Therapy Association Education Division. A Normative Model of Physical Therapist Professional Education: Version 2000, Alexandria, VA: American Physical Therapy Association, 2000.)

Authors such as Donald Schön[10]; David Kern, and his colleagues from the Johns Hopkins University School of Medicine[11]; Miller and Schmidt[12]; Cruess et al.[13]; as well as Threlkeld, Jensen, and Royeen[14] (when writing about the clinical doctorate degree in physical therapy) all write convincingly that health professionals must better organize professional education around what actually happens, as well as what *should* happen, in clinical practice. For example, students must be taught thinking and insight skills, such as reflection-in-action and reflection-on-action, and intellectual humility as well as social responsibility to prepare them for the complex, unique, uncertain, and challenging health care situations they will face. Clearly the knowledge, critical thinking, humanistic skills, and professional responsibility and obligations advocated by these authors could be incorporated into the goals of any physical therapist or physical therapist assistant program.

Macro Environment: Body of Knowledge
Related to Physical Therapy
The APTA monographs, *A Normative Model of Physical Therapist Professional Education: Version 2000*[5] and *A Guide to Physical Ther-*

Table 1-1   Proposed Educational Goals for Educators

Teach students the language of physical therapy and its underpinning disciplines (anatomy, physiology, kinesiology).
Introduce students to the ways of science. Teach them to understand and respect the nature of scientific evidence.
Teach students how to reason and manage ambiguities and gaps in knowledge.
Teach students how to communicate with people from different cultures, value systems, and backgrounds.
Expand students' capacity for constructive empathy. Teach students to help others by using their own compassion.
Introduce students to social concerns that exist beyond the issues of patients they treat. Foster a feeling of responsibility for those who are poor or isolated.
Inculcate a personal love of learning. Help students develop habits required for continual learning.

Source: Adapted from DE Rogers. The Education of Medical Students for Tomorrow. In Council on Graduate Medical Education. Reform in Medical Education and Medical Education in the Ambulatory Setting. Washington, DC: U.S. Department of Health and Human Services. HRSA-P-DM-91-4;5, 1991.

apy Practice,[15] have been a boon to physical therapy educators. These monographs help educators define the body of knowledge related to physical therapy.

One of the main functions of the *Normative Model* is to "provide a mechanism for existing, developing, and future professional education programs to evaluate and refine curricula and integrate aspects of the profession's vision for professional education into their vision."[5(p5)]

The *Normative Model* is based on 19 practice expectations that define the expected entry level performance of a physical therapist. Educators can use this monograph to review how their coursework in Foundational and Clinical Sciences relates to examples of content, terminal behavioral objectives, and related instructional objectives suggested by content experts. Although certainly not exhaustive, the suggestions can be extremely helpful, especially in guiding novice physical therapy instructors, as well as those program faculty who are not physical therapists. See Table 1-2 for an example.

A Guide to Physical Therapy Practice presents the current practice of physical therapy by outlining common practice roles and defining the types of tests, measures, and treatment interventions commonly used by physical therapists.[16] In addition, preferred practice patterns are offered for four body systems: musculoskeletal, neuromuscular, cardiopulmonary, and integumentary. Each of the sections on preferred practice patterns contains the patient/client diagnostic group being considered; *International Classi-*

Table 1-2   Example of Information in the Normative Model of
Physical Therapist Professional Education

Primary content	Examples of terminal behavioral objectives	Examples of instructional objectives
	After completion of the content, the student will be able to:	
Pathology: Differential diagnosis related to pathology	Define the signs and symptoms that distinguish/differentiate the common musculoskeletal and neuromuscular diagnoses in patients seen by physical therapists.	Compare the advantages and disadvantages of MRI and computer axial tomography (CAT) scan for diagnosing bone tumors or a lumbar disk problem.
	Explain the laboratory and imaging techniques (e.g., blood tests, chest films, MRI) used to differentiate these musculoskeletal and neuromuscular diagnoses.	Describe the signs and symptoms of a patient with brittle diabetes. Describe how nerve conduction studies can distinguish between neurapraxia, segmental demyelination, and axonal degeneration.
	Describe the "red flags" that require medical consultation or emergency attention.	Define positive MRI findings that support the diagnosis of multiple sclerosis.

MRI = magnetic resonance imaging.
Source: American Physical Therapy Association. A Normative Model of Physical Therapist Professional Education: Version 2000. Alexandria, VA: American Physical Therapy Association, 2000.

fication of Diseases, Ninth Revision, Clinical Modification (*ICD-9-CM*) codes; types of examinations, tests, and measures; anticipated prognosis; expected number of visits per episode of care; patient care goals and related physical therapy interventions and anticipated outcomes; as well as prevention and risk-factor reduction strategies. Thus, the guide is rich with information that can be used by educators teaching and students learning clinical course content.

Together, the *Normative Model* and *Guide to Physical Therapy Practice* are extremely useful resources for any physical therapist, clinical, or academic educator who carries the responsibility of transmitting the core knowledge of physical therapy to the next generation. In addition to these APTA-conceived documents, the *Journal of Physical Therapy Education* presents a steady stream of ideas and special issues directed toward physical therapist and physical therapist assistant educators. For example, in one

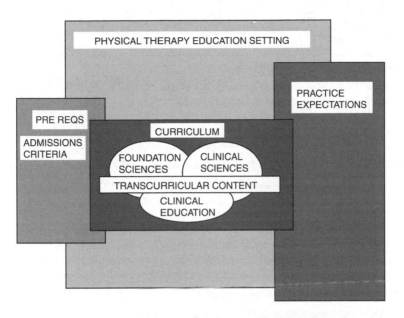

A CONTEXTUAL FRAMEWORK FOR THE CURRICULUM

Figure 1-3 The immediate (micro) environment within which physical therapy education exists. (Pre Reqs = prerequisites.) (Reprinted with permission from American Physical Therapy Association Education Division. A Normative Model of Physical Therapist Professional Education: Version 2000, Alexandria, VA: American Physical Therapy Association, 2000.)

recent issue devoted to moral and ethical development, guest editor Dr. Elizabeth Mostrom writes, "Taking both historical and contemporary views, all of the contributors to this special issue offer important insights and recommendations for the education of practitioners, grounded in strong moral character and commitments, who will be caring, competent, creative, and courageous physical therapists who are well prepared to meet the ethical challenges of the new millennium."[16]

Micro Environment

Figure 1-3 demonstrates how a particular physical therapy curriculum is imbedded in its micro environment or immediate educational institution and clinical practice settings. It is this micro environment that presses for uniqueness among the philosophies and goals of the physical therapist and physical therapist assistant educational programs. For example, Table 1-3 demonstrates how the philosophy of the physical therapy curriculum at Creighton University reflects the "inalienable worth of each individ-

Table 1-3 Example of Related University, School, and Program Mission Statements

From mission statement: Creighton University
Creighton exists for students and learning. Members of the Creighton community are challenged to reflect on transcendent values, including their relationship with God, in an atmosphere of freedom of inquiry, belief, and religious worship. Service to others, the importance of family life, the inalienable worth of each individual and appreciation of ethnic and cultural diversity are core values of Creighton.
From mission statement: School of Pharmacy and Allied Health at Creighton University
The Creighton University School of Pharmacy and Allied Health professions prepares men and women in their professional disciplines with an emphasis on moral values and service to develop competent graduates who demonstrate concern for human health. This mission is fulfilled by providing comprehensive professional instruction, engaging in basic science and clinical research, participating in community and professional service, and fostering a learning environment enhanced by faculty who encourage self-determination, self-respect, and compassion in students.
From program philosophy: Doctor of Physical Therapy Program at Creighton University
The faculty of the Department of Physical Therapy subscribe to the general tenets of Creighton University and the School of Pharmacy and Allied Health with an emphasis on affirming that each individual ultimately should assume responsibility for maintaining the quality and dignity of his or her own life.

Source: Department of Physical Therapy, School of Pharmacy and Allied Health, Creighton University, Omaha, NE.

ual." It also shows the emphasis on moral values in mission statements of the university and the college in which the physical therapy program is located.

More complete examples of how the philosophy and goals of the micro environment influence the program's philosophy, goals and outcomes, and curriculum are demonstrated in Tables 1-4 and 1-5. In Table 1-4, a Program in Physical Therapy's Mission Statement identifies the mission of the university as well as the program's mission (which applies to both the Doctor of Physical Therapy [DPT] and PhD programs). Table 1-5 is a DPT program philosophy, an explication of DPT goals and outcomes, and an overview of the curriculum themes that support attainment of these outcomes. Notice how the mission, philosophy, goals and outcomes, and curriculum themes fit together to provide a coherent framework for making this particular program operational.

Faculty time spent considering macro-level and micro-level philosophy and goals is time well spent. Developing program goals and outcomes and related curricular themes together encourages academic and clinical faculty

Table 1-4 Mission Statement, Department of Physical Therapy, Temple University

---

The Department of Physical Therapy is an integral part of the College of Allied Health Professions, which in turn is an integral part of Temple University, particularly the Health Sciences Center. Temple has had a unique mission, since its creation in 1884, to serve the needs of its working class community. Temple's founder, Rev. Russell Conwell, created Temple "to make an education possible for all young men and women who have good minds and the will to work."

The primary missions of the Department of Physical Therapy are:
1. To provide the opportunity for individuals from diverse cultural backgrounds to enter the physical therapy profession.
2. To prepare physical therapy practitioners to meet the health care needs of society.
3. To discover and convey knowledge related to physical therapy.
4. To provide services to the academic, professional, and public communities.

Source: Department of Physical Therapy, College of Allied Health Professions, Temple University, Philadelphia, PA.

to reflect on and explicate their own philosophy and goals and come to a common understanding of their profession's and college's or university's philosophy and goals. Such an activity unifies and grounds academic and clinical faculty in a focused endeavor.

Tyler's Question 2: Educational Experiences

Once goals and philosophy are understood, the next question to be answered is what educational experiences are needed to achieve these purposes. Coursework in physical therapist and physical therapist assistant programs consists of foundation sciences, such as anatomy and pathology; clinical sciences, such as therapeutic exercise and management of patients with specific clinical problems (e.g., orthopedics or cardiopulmonary); transcurricular content, such as ethics, administration, and research; and clinical education (see Figure 1-3). Of course, the actual coursework designed and offered depends on the program's practice expectations and the type and depth of prerequisite coursework.

Within each course, written objectives identify specific attitudes, behaviors, and skills that the instructor expects each student to develop. Included in these objectives are expectations that directly relate to the program's philosophy and goals. For example, if one of the program's goals is to develop critical thinking skills, each instructor should present objectives and related learning experiences to stimulate development of students' abilities to reflect, critically analyze, and make rational decisions. Figure 1-4 shows a logical connection between an element of a program's philosophy or mission and how a

Table 1-5 Doctor of Physical Therapy (DPT) Program Philosophy, Goals and Outcomes, and Overview of Curricular Themes, Temple University

---

DPT Philosophy

Students enter the program from diverse cultural, experiential, and educational backgrounds.

The program educates graduates to practice ethically in diverse health care settings to serve the present and future needs of a diverse society, and to engage in lifelong professional development.

Graduates are prepared with professional behavior skills, critical thinking skills, theoretical and practical knowledge, and psychomotor skills that will enable them to assume the multifaceted life-long roles of a health care professional: clinical practitioner, manager, teacher, learner, consultant, researcher, and advocate.

DPT Goals and Outcomes

The performance of a successful graduate of this program includes:

1. Examination, evaluation of, diagnosis of, prognosis of, and intervention for human movement dysfunction to produce defined outcomes.
2. Promotion of wellness and prevention of illness for individuals and communities.
3. Evidence-based practice, within a patient care management and disablement framework, which is based on scientific principles and critical inquiry, including the analysis of effective outcomes from the perspective of both the health care system and the person and family receiving services.
4. Practice that is responsive to the diverse psychological, sociocultural, and spiritual beliefs and needs of the person and family receiving services.
5. Ethical and effective patient care management of contemporary physical therapy services.
6. Professional behavior in all aspects of performance.
7. Lifelong learning directed at continually improving physical therapy care.
8. Engagement in the growth and development of the profession of physical therapy through service, including participation in the clinical and didactic education of future practitioners and colleagues.
9. Collaboration, coordination, and consultation with other health care professionals, government agencies, reimbursement sources, and care management organizations to facilitate clinically effective and cost-efficient services.
10. Scholarly contributions to the profession.

DPT Curricular Themes That Support the Philosophy and Goals and Outcomes

The DPT curriculum:

- Is based on the disablement model
- Emphasizes practice based on theory and evidence and their interactions
- Includes knowledge of the measurement properties of tests and measures used in examining patients
- Uses the patient care management model
- Includes attention to biological, social, and cultural differences over the lifespan and their influence on health and disease
- Emphasizes continuous ethical behavior
- Emphasizes lifelong professional development

Source: Department of Physical Therapy, College of Allied Health Professions, Temple University, Philadelphia, PA.

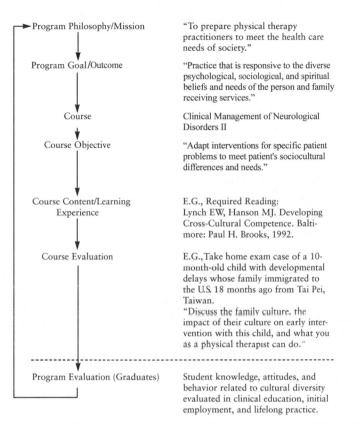

| Program Philosophy/Mission | "To prepare physical therapy practitioners to meet the health care needs of society." |

Program Philosophy/Mission — "To prepare physical therapy practitioners to meet the health care needs of society."

Program Goal/Outcome — "Practice that is responsive to the diverse psychological, sociological, and spiritual beliefs and needs of the person and family receiving services."

Course — Clinical Management of Neurological Disorders II

Course Objective — "Adapt interventions for specific patient problems to meet patient's sociocultural differences and needs."

Course Content/Learning Experience — E.G., Required Reading: Lynch EW, Hanson MJ. Developing Cross-Cultural Competence. Baltimore: Paul H. Brooks, 1992.

Course Evaluation — E.G., Take home exam case of a 10-month-old child with developmental delays whose family immigrated to the U.S. 18 months ago from Tai Pei, Taiwan. "Discuss the family culture, the impact of their culture on early intervention with this child, and what you as a physical therapist can do."

Program Evaluation (Graduates) — Student knowledge, attitudes, and behavior related to cultural diversity evaluated in clinical education, initial employment, and lifelong practice.

Figure 1-4   Example of the logical connection between program philosophy, program goal/outcome, course objective, course content and learning experience, and program evaluation. (From: Course designed by K Nixon-Cave. Department of Physical Therapy, Temple University.)

course in pediatrics presents this element in course objectives, required readings, and stimulation of student thought during an examination. Further information on designing coursework is provided in Chapters 2 and 3.

Tyler's Question 3: Organization

Tyler suggests three factors to consider in organizing educational experiences: continuity, sequence, and integration.[1] *Continuity* refers to the vertical reiteration of curricular elements—that is, providing continuing opportunities for students to practice and develop the cognitive, affective, or psychomotor skills they have learned. For example, teaching students good body mechanics in an early basic skills lab is followed by attention to, and reinforcement of, these same skills throughout clinical lab courses.

Sequence is related to continuity but moves beyond the reiteration and development of a single skill. Thus, sequence is the process of having each experience build on prior experience while moving increasingly broader and deeper into the material. For example, students assume greater and greater responsibility for patient care through each successive clinical internship. It would be considered poor sequencing to have a student spend the same amount of time observing the instructor during the last clinical internship as during the first internship.

Integration refers to the horizontal relationship of learning experiences. For example, a kinesiology and anatomy course might be placed together so that the same body segments are covered within similar time periods, and knowledge gained in one course could overlap and clarify knowledge gained in the other course.

Obviously, proper continuity, sequence, and integration can be extraordinarily helpful in assisting the student to master curricular content. However, there are many structural constraints to organizing a curriculum. The primary consideration is the academic calendar of the college or university in which the program is located (i.e., the length of each semester or quarter and how many units of work are normally expected of students within that institution within the given time frame). Consideration must also be given to availability of clinical sites—it would be impossible to expect clinical internships to occur only in the summer when the usual academic year is not in session (and clinics may have the greatest number of staff on vacation). In addition, faculty and clinical expertise must be juggled across classes in different years of the program, with available laboratory space factored in as a major structural constraint. One can see how easy it would be to organize a curriculum based on structural constraints alone!

In addition to these resource and structural constraints, the faculty who design physical therapy curricula are concerned about what students *must* know before their first clinical experience. Faculty often desire that students know at least a little about nearly everything before entering their clinical internships. This is strongly reinforced by clinical instructors who, faced with examining and treating patients within dwindling time periods, want students to know at least something about typical clinical problems they will be treating and common evaluation and treatment strategies that will enable them to be immediately useful. Due to the pressures of the clinical environment, most clinical administrators are understandably more receptive to accommodating students during their last clinical internship as compared with the students' first internship. This desire to have immediately useful patient-care skills even during an initial clinical assignment may result in a curricular organization that is antagonistic to the program's overall philosophy and goals. For example, a common strategy to "get it all in" is the presentation of foundation courses (i.e., biological and physical science courses) and clinical skill courses as early as possible in the curriculum. Courses deemed less relevant to hands-on patient care (e.g., the behavioral sciences, clinical management, and research courses) are taught late or last in the curriculum. In sacrificing long-term goals for short-term goals, faculty must realize they are also giving students a strong implicit message about what they consider most important in physical therapy practice.

Review once again the examples of general curriculum goals proposed by Dr. David Rogers in Table 1-1 and examples of more specific curricular outcomes set forth in Table 1-5. Is it possible that a student will attain these goals if the biological sciences exclusively predominate the initial thinking and subsequent structure of a physical therapy educational program? This concern was echoed in the document produced by the 1993 IMPACT conference:

> The word *transcurricular* was chosen to place emphasis on the need to interweave principles and applications from these content areas throughout the entire curriculum . . . to prepare students to assume the multiple roles required of them in clinical practice, such as provider of treatment, teacher, and supervisor.[18]

Table 1-6 illustrates how one physical therapy program explicated its view of the relatively equal importance of foundation sciences (Biological/Physical/Clinical Sciences; Behavioral Sciences), clinical management, research, and clinical practice by presenting all these educational components in almost every semester of a 3-year physical therapy program. The reader should be able to identify elements of continuity, sequence, and integration in this curricular organization.

In summary, the organization of educational experiences should relate directly to fulfilling the program's philosophy and expected outcomes for its graduates. Thus, it is more important for the faculty member to concentrate on how each student will perform after graduation than to concentrate on how many technical skills the student has before the first clinical internship.

Tyler's Question 4: Evaluation

If the objectives, content, and learning experiences of each course or clinical experience relate to the program's philosophy and goals, then student and instructor evaluation of each course and clinical component will give the faculty a good sense of whether the program's goals are being attained. Of course, the ultimate measure is how the graduates perform in clinical practice.

Table 1-6 Department of Physical Therapy Curriculum Matrix (130 credits), Temple University

Year/semester	Biological/physical/clinical sciences	SH	Behavioral sciences	SH	Clinical management	SH	Research	SH	Clinical practice	SH
DPT I/F (14 wks, 21 credits)	Anatomy lecture	3	Psychosocial Aspects of Wellness/Illness	3	Clinical Decision Making	3		—	8 hrs/mo Clinical Clerkship	—
	Anatomy lab	3			Clinical Examination and Intervention Skills I	3		—		—
	Bioscience I	3								
	Movement Science I	3								
DPT I/Sp (14 wks, 20 credits)	Neurosciences	3			Clinical Examination and Intervention Skills II	2	Critical Inquiry	2	8 hrs/mo Clinical Clerkship	—
	Bioscience II	3			Clinical Examination and Intervention Skills III	3				
	Movement Science II	4			Exercise and Exercise Physiology	3				
DPT II/F (13 wks, 18 credits, +9 clinic credits)	Movement Science III	3	Teaching, Learning, Group Dynamics	3	Clinical Management of Musculoskeletal Disorders I	3	Research Design	3	Clinical Internship I	9+
									(18 wks, Nov–Mar)	9

Term	Course	SH	Course	SH	Course	SH	Course	SH
DPT II/Sp (7 wks, 10 credits, +9 clinic credits)	Bioethics	3	Clinical Management of Cardiopulmonary Disorders	3	Clinical Management of Neuromuscular Disorders I	3	Research I	1
DPT III/F (14 wks, 20 credits)	Clinical Medicine and Pharmacy	3	Clinical Management of Musculoskeletal Disorders II	3	Clinical Management of Musculoskeletal Disorders III	3	Research II	2
	Medical Diagnostics	2	Health Care Systems	3				
			Management of Physical Therapy Practices	3				
DPT III/Sp (6 wks, 5 credits, +18 clinic credits)			Clinical Management of Neuromuscular Disorders II	4	Research Intensive	3	Clinical Internship II	18
			Orthotic and Prosthetic Devices	1			(18 wks, Feb–Jun)	
			Grand Rounds I	2				
			Grand Rounds II	2				

DPT = Department of Physical Therapy; F = fall; SH = semester hours; Sp = spring.

Program evaluation should cover all general and specific curricular goals. See Figure 1-4 for a specific example of how program evaluation provides a feedback loop so faculty can determine how successfully the student has been taught to achieve a program goal. Referring once again to Tables 1-1 and 1-5, do the graduates, for example, know how to reason and manage ambiguities and gaps in knowledge? Are they able to communicate with people from different cultures and backgrounds? Do they have a personal love of learning? Can they teach patients, families, colleagues, the public? Do they demonstrate professional ethical behaviors? Regular systematic evaluation of recent graduates by surveys, interviews, or focus groups will assist the program faculty in completing the curriculum design connections and answering the most important curricular question: Did the educational program achieve what it stated it would achieve in the program's philosophy and goals (outcomes)?

See Table 1-7 for examples of a variety of sources that might be tapped for meaningful program evaluative information. The data retrieved can be aligned with the philosophy and goals of any particular physical therapist or physical therapist assistant program.

Walker's Curricular Platform

Decker Walker proposed a naturalistic model of how faculty *really* go about developing a curriculum.[2] He suggests that faculty discussions that culminate in a shared vision for a program form the platform on which all deliberations and eventual decisions about the program rest (see Figure 1-1). Walker states, "the word *platform* is meant to suggest both a political platform and something to stand on. The platform includes an idea of what is and a vision of what ought to be, and these guide the curriculum developer in determining what he should do to realize his vision."

In addition, Walker suggests that curriculum development does not follow an orderly progression from goals to objectives to content and then to evaluation, as was suggested by Tyler, but instead faculty move back and forth between all of these elements in a process of deliberation. This deliberation informs the design decisions. We believe the Tyler and Walker models are useful in helping faculty understand the process of curriculum development. Tyler delineated the component parts of the process, and Walker described how faculty actually discuss, debate, and negotiate to arrive at a curriculum.

It is useful for all academic and clinical faculty members to have the agreed-on program philosophy and goals (a synthesis of the platform) in front of them when preparing their academic or clinical course objectives and related learning experiences. During this preparation time, faculty can use the philosophy and goals as a guide in their planning. For example, if the program

Table 1-7 Examples of Program Evaluation Data

Sources	Examples of types of data
Students	Recruitment activities
	Admissions (prerequisite coursework required, grade point averages, cultural diversity profile)
	Academic performance (timely feedback to students, remediation activities)
	Retention (assistance available)
Faculty	Resumes (preparation for teaching; scholarship [publication and grants]; service to department, university, and profession; practice and consultation activities; honors and awards)
	Faculty development plans
Academic curriculum	Course syllabi (content, types of learning experiences, level of evaluation)
	Minutes of faculty retreats and planning sessions
	Student evaluations
	Faculty and peer evaluations
Clinical curriculum	Development of clinical sites
	Types and lengths of clinical rotations
	Student evaluation of clinical instructors and learning opportunities
	Clinical instructor evaluation of student clinical performance
Environment	Support services (library holdings, computer labs, financial aid opportunities, health care services provided)
Graduates	Alumni surveys (clinical positions held; continuing education courses taken; specialist certifications awarded; participation in local, state, and national professional activities; participation in research and publications; community volunteer activities)
	Licensure examination scores
	Employer satisfaction surveys
	Patient satisfaction surveys

Source: Western Association of Schools and Colleges Accrediting Commission for Senior Colleges and Universities. Achieving Institutional Effectiveness through Assessment. Oakland, CA: Western Association of Schools and Colleges, 1992;31.

included macro-level goals articulated by Rogers, the instructor would think about how to set up learning experiences that "teach students to reason and manage ambiguities and gaps in knowledge" or "expand students' capacity for constructive empathy" (see Table 1-1). Similarly, if the program goals and outcomes included "evidence-based practice, within a patient care management and disablement framework, which is based on scientific principles and critical inquiry, including the analysis of effective outcomes from the perspective

Table 1-8 Physical Therapist Assistant Program Mission: Clarkson College

The Physical Therapist Assistant Program at Clarkson College is designed to give students a diverse educational experience rich in both basic and applied sciences. Students of the program will be prepared to work under the supervision of a licensed physical therapist and be expected to demonstrate good ethical judgment and compassion in the treatment of patients. The physical therapist assistant will adhere to all professional and ethical standards set forth by the American Physical Therapy Association.

The Physical Therapy Assistant Program will provide an optimal environment to help prepare students who can deliver quality health care in a variety of clinical settings. The College will offer a broad educational experience to enable the practitioner to transfer the theoretical learning into clinical practice. The student will be nurtured into becoming an integral member of the health care team demonstrating exemplary professional communication skills when dealing with other health care providers. Scholarly preparation of the physical therapist assistant will develop a highly motivated critical thinking individual concerned with the improvement of the quality of life as is consistent with the mission of the College.

Source: Clarkson College, Omaha, NE.

of both the health care system and the person and family receiving services" (see Table 1-5), the instructor would consider how course learning experiences and course materials could facilitate student learning in these areas.

The program philosophy and goals and outcomes that provide the platform on which the physical therapy program rests should be discussed and revised, if necessary, every year before curriculum planning for the following year. (That is, before Tyler's second and third questions are discussed and answered.) Furthermore, every student in the physical therapy or physical therapist assistant program could benefit from having a copy of the program's philosophy and goals and outcomes, and an opportunity to discuss these philosophy and goals and outcomes with the faculty early on as well as during her or his academic program. Such discussion and reflection on the intent of the program can be powerful tools in helping students understand the coursework and required educational experiences, as well as socializing them into the profession.

For an example related to physical therapist assistant education, see Table 1-8. In this mission statement, a physical therapist assistant program has clearly stated what the student will be prepared for consistent with the standards of the profession and the mission of the college.

Implicit, Explicit, and Null Curriculum

Throughout the design and implementation of a physical therapy curriculum, the faculty can gain insight about the program by considering the three types of curriculum that Eisner identified as being taught in all educational programs: the *implicit, explicit,* and *null* curriculum.[4,18] The explicit curriculum is publicly stated and is available to everyone. The implicit curriculum, which is more subtle and potentially more powerful, is known especially by students and graduates of the program. The null curriculum may be known to only a few or to no one because it includes the elements that are left out of the explicit curriculum, and it is a potential blind spot in planning.

Explicit Curriculum

The explicit curriculum includes those explicitly defined and publicly shared aspects of the curriculum that are found in university catalogues, program brochures, and course syllabi. Explicit curricular elements include, for example, the prerequisite courses, the program's stated philosophy and goals/outcomes, course objectives and required readings, the sequence and type of clinical affiliations, and the faculty's credentials.

Physical therapy students often identify the type of program they want to enter based on this explicit curriculum. Explicit elements, such as the location, length, and cost of the program, as well as the type of degree awarded, guide the applicant's choice of programs. Faculty are acutely attuned to the explicit curriculum as they discuss and alter various aspects in yearly or biyearly curriculum planning sessions. Clinical instructors receive explicit curricular information on student preparedness for their clinical affiliations (e.g., description of coursework completed by the affiliating students). When program outcomes are assessed, alumni are often asked to state their level of satisfaction with specific courses they completed. One easily might consider the explicit curriculum to be the only curriculum. However, students, alumni, clinicians, and new faculty can often distinguish and discuss the presence and power of a second type of curriculum, the implicit curriculum.

Implicit Curriculum

The implicit curriculum includes the values, beliefs, and expectations that are transmitted to students by the knowledge, language, and everyday actions of the academic and clinical faculty. The faculty themselves may be less aware of these values, beliefs, and expectations than students and alumni of the program. As we wrote in our 1990 article, ". . . students regularly receive from faculty members implicit messages about the relative importance of certain types of knowledge, what types of patients are most interesting and challenging, and what personal and professional behaviors are acceptable and unacceptable"[17] (Table 1-9).

Table 1-9 Examples of Implicit Curriculum in Physical Therapist and Physical Therapist Assistant Programs

Curriculum component	Example
Courses considered most important versus those considered least important	Courses that receive scheduling priorities for class time, location, and optimal examination times
Modeling of effective stress management	Faculty members* demonstrate calm and resiliency in response to no-show patients or guest lecturers, broken audiovisual equipment, sudden scheduling changes
Critical thinking considered inherent in professional behavior	Faculty members critically analyze information, brainstorm ideas, and demonstrate tolerance for ambiguity
Modeling of effective, professional behaviors	Faculty members demonstrate and expect of students courtesy, initiative, respect for other viewpoints, and willingness to act as moral agents
Expectations for lifelong learning	Faculty members display a continual quest for the latest information, are visible in the library, and attend and make presentations in health care settings and at clinical conferences
Respect for and trust in one's colleagues	Faculty members demonstrate enthusiasm for team teaching and treating and express fascination with alternative viewpoints
	Faculty members demonstrate respect for other health care professionals
Openness to innovation	Faculty members encourage students to explore alternative health care philosophies and models of practice (e.g., acupuncture, Feldenkrais method, Alexander technique)
Respect for and sensitivity to patients	Faculty members refer to patients as individuals characterized by complex and unique physical, social, and behavioral characteristics rather than by diagnosis or body parts
Expectations for lifelong service to the profession	Faculty members participate in committees and task forces and on boards at district, state, and national levels of the American Physical Therapy Association and other organizations

*The term *faculty members* implies academic and clinical faculty members.
Source: Adapted from KF Shepard, GM Jensen. Physical therapist curricula for the 1990s: educating the reflective practitioner. Phys Ther 1990;70:566.

Clinical and academic faculty are often unaware that every time they appear before students they are demonstrating behaviors they consider appropriate and professional. These often unconscious behaviors, for better or for worse, are powerful socializing elements that mold the future professional behaviors of students. For example, how faculty members engage in their own lifelong learning, make off-hand comments about patients and families or other faculty or students, participate in the concerns of professional organizations, and demonstrate caring are all absorbed by students as templates on which to model their own professional values, attitudes, and behaviors.

The implicit curriculum is also the basis for many decisions made about the explicit curriculum. For example, as discussed earlier, the sequence of coursework in a program (e.g., biological sciences first and social sciences last) and the length of time devoted to certain topics (e.g., prevention and wellness versus acute and chronic pathologic conditions) can give students a strong implicit message about what information is considered more or most important to the practice of physical therapy and what is considered less or least important. In fact, every aspect of explicit coursework contains an implicit message. For example, do the objectives of a course in clinical procedures include an emphasis on professional behaviors as well as on specific manual techniques? Do instructors expect the same careful draping techniques when students are working with each other in labs as when they are working with patients? Do examinations include clinical problems that challenge the student to think about the individual person who is receiving treatment as well as about the specific impairment problems they are treating?

Null Curriculum

The null curriculum includes those elements of physical therapy practice that are missing from the curriculum. Some elements are missing because there is no voice to champion their inclusion. This becomes a blind spot and is especially true about areas of physical therapy practice in which fewer physical therapists are currently engaged. For example, how much information do students receive about the role of physical therapists in obstetrics-gynecology care, hospice care, pro bono work with the homeless, or contributions that could be made in hospital emergency rooms and during times of disaster?

The null curriculum has the same impact on the professional attitudes and behaviors of students as the explicit and implicit curriculum. If, for example, students are never exposed to centers for adults who are developmentally delayed or well-elderly centers during their clinical internships, who will elect to seek a position in such a setting as a first choice after graduation?

Some curricular elements are missing because there simply is no time to teach any more information. Every academic and clinical faculty member grapples with how best to spend the limited time available for teaching. "More is better" is not the answer. Cramming more and more material into an unexpandable time sequence encourages rote memorization and repetition of tasks, drives out analytical and creative thinking, and, worst of all, snuffs out a desire to learn by setting unattainable goals that leave the students awash in fatigue and frustration.

Faculty must carefully consider and consciously weigh what to include and what to exclude from each course. Time for reflective thought and integration of concepts and ideas, as well as time for being presented with new information, must be consciously and deliberately built into the curricular structure from the beginning. In the same manner, clinical instructors must weigh whether to expose the student to an extensive potpourri of diagnoses and potential physical therapy treatment techniques or to teach students in-depth assessment and treatment skills for the most common clinical problems the student will encounter in practice. Trying to do both in depth will only promote anxiety and end in frustration for the clinical instructor and the student.

Decisions concerning the null curriculum are not easy to make. Two guideposts faculty might use in deciding what not to include are the current skills demanded in clinical practice and what skills students can attain after they are practicing in the field. To use the first guidepost, academic faculty benefit enormously from visiting students at clinical sites and having clinicians from different settings participate in curriculum planning sessions. For example, how much time are physical therapists and physical therapist assistants spending on hands-on care in comparison with teaching the patient and family to manage their own health care needs? The related curriculum issues are how much curricular emphasis is placed on teaching students to teach patients and families compared with how much time is devoted to presenting students with an ever-increasing array of physical modalities. What skills are physical therapists and physical therapist assistants currently performing? Are they working as teams? The related curriculum questions are: (1) Does the physical therapy curriculum contain information on physical therapists' and physical therapist assistants' roles, supervision, and the basic elements of effective teamwork? and (2) Do clinical education experiences allow guided experiences in physical therapist–physical therapist assistant teamwork?

The second guidepost, an emphasis on lifelong learning, can relieve the time constraint frustrations experienced by academic and clinical faculty and students. If faculty believe that the degree-granting educational program is only the start of the student's career and that the program provides only the most basic building blocks of that career, then attention can be turned from *what* to learn to *how* to learn. Thus, if students are taught how to gather and analyze information, to incubate ideas, to constantly reflect on their decisions and clinical performance, and to identify their learning needs (and observe academic and clinical faculty doing this), then they will become lifelong learners, learning as much each year in practice as they did during their matriculation in an academic program. A program cannot teach everything, but it can teach to the needs of the current clinical climate and prepare students to learn for all the years of their lives.

An effective educational program for physical therapist and physical therapist assistants is one in which the explicit, implicit, and null curricula are known to the faculty and are complementary. Faculty can identify strategies that will allow them to garner periodic input about their implicit, as well as explicit and null, curricula from students, alumni, clinicians, and on-site accreditation teams. Being able to assess and understand the power, influence, and outcome of one's curricular efforts through input from multiple parties is an intellectually challenging, rewarding, and joyful endeavor.

Conflicts between Professional and Liberal Arts Education

In 1974, Lewis Mayhew and Patrick Ford first described the inevitable conflicts that arise between educational programs for professionals (e.g., medicine, education, engineering, and law) and the traditional longstanding liberal arts educational programs (e.g., biology, English, philosophy, and physics).[19] Since that time, Patrick Ford has spoken about these issues directly to physical therapy educators.[20,21] The issues are fascinating because they are so pervasive. Twenty-five years after they first were revealed, the issues are still unresolved, which is a testament to the long-standing conservatism and resistance to change that characterizes American higher education.

The conflicts stem from the different educational outcomes that liberal arts programs and professional programs seek to attain. The goal of traditional liberal arts colleges is to create a learned person who has a grasp of many aspects of the world and is prepared to function in multiple settings. The focus is on discourse, theory, and the need to reason, argue, create, and, as graduation speakers exhort, "to make a difference in the world." The goal of professional programs, in general, and physical therapy programs, in particular, is to graduate students who will be prepared to function as professionals in a specifically defined field of endeavor. The focus is on attainment of practical skills, behaviors, and attitudes that reflect the ethos and functions, as bestowed by society, of that profession.

From these basic differences, five conflicts arise between liberal arts programs and physical therapy programs located within the same institution.

1. The curricular content of most physical therapy education programs is contested by college and university academicians and physical therapy practitioners. Academic faculty from liberal arts departments who have a strong voice on college and university curriculum committees often argue that physical therapy curricula focus too much on practical application and not enough on the theoretical underpinnings of knowledge. Conversely, clinicians chide physical therapy faculty for spending too much time on theory and not being responsive to the "real world" of clinical practice. (An unfortunate refrain often echoed by students returning from clinical internships.)

If the physical therapy faculty member has recently come from the clinical setting, she or he is more likely to teach knowledge that has been transformed by experience. Thus, these novice educators present students with a rich potpourri of clinically relevant information, only some of which can be found in textbooks. In contrast, the longer faculty members have been in the academic setting, the more socialized they are to the traditions of academia, and the more theory and critical analysis will play a prominent role in their courses. Of course, both perspectives are important and relevant to physical therapy curricula. However, conflict arises because there simply is not time to teach both perspectives in depth. Thus, the collective faculty continually struggle with (and faculty meetings are often permeated with) arguments about these somewhat antagonistic perspectives.

2. The university has traditionally been perceived as an agent of change in society. It is a place in which new ideas, skills, materials, and methods are created and shared with the world. However, to produce practitioners who must work in today's demanding health care environments, faculty must first ensure that their graduates are ready to practice. That is, they must focus their attention on codifying and transmitting the conventional lore that is accepted by the profession and will be tested by national licensing examinations. Creating new knowledge clearly has a secondary place in professional programs. This fact has placed many professional graduate physical therapy programs at odds with graduate curricular and promotion and tenure committees.

3. All physical therapy programs rely on the liberal arts programs of colleges and universities to supply prerequisite coursework for their entering students. The breadth and level of many of these prerequisite courses in the biological, physical, and social sciences are an anathema to physical therapy educators. Professional programs, of course, have little say in the content of these prerequisite courses, and similarly titled courses at community colleges, small private colleges, and large public universities yield strikingly

dissimilar educational backgrounds among students in an entering physical therapy class. Teaching students who enter with different levels of prerequisite coursework is frustrating to faculty (and the students themselves) who must continually readjust the foundation science, clinical science, and trans-curricular content of their coursework to meet a low to middle level of student knowledge.

4. The clinical education portion of the curriculum that takes place outside the walls of the university is not well understood nor particularly well supported by most institutions of higher education. Although students do pay a fee for clinical education coursework to the college or university to cover costs (e.g., salary for the academic coordinator of clinical education, travel to site visits, legal fees for preparation of clinical contracts, and administrative costs for maintaining student records), the clinical education site receives little or no compensation for its participation in physical therapy student education. The cries of clinical educators and administrators within health care environments who must figure out how to absorb the cost of clinical education programs long have fallen on the deaf ears of university administrators. The result is a smoldering conflict between the clinic and the academy that is fanned by resentment and fueled by little hope of resolution. As a result of current health care economics, many health care facilities have downsized or eliminated their student education programs. In response to the loss of clinical sites, different models of clinical education are being created that are more cost effective to health care organizations than the time-honored, effective but expensive model of one instructor to one student teaching. See Chapter 6 for further discussion of this issue.

5. Tenure and stability for any faculty member (and the program in which the faculty member teaches) come as a result of proven performance in three traditional areas of academic engagement: scholarship, teaching, and service. Of these three, scholarship, or success in developing a research program that garners external grants and provides the grist for research papers (creation of knowledge) acceptable for publication in peer-reviewed professional journals, is the area that has traditionally counted most toward tenure in universities. Most university arts and sciences faculty begin their academic careers with a doctorate degree in hand and their own well-defined and productive area of research. For these faculty, it is difficult, but not impossible, to juggle these three areas of endeavor with a high level of competence.

Historically, it has been a very different person who enters the academic world of a physical therapy program. The overwhelming preponderance of physical therapy educators have come directly from clinical settings, hold master's degrees, and have no well-developed areas of research. Although the number of doctoral faculty has clearly risen, in 1999 less than half of the faculty in professional physical therapy programs held doctoral degrees.[22] As Patrick Ford states, "Because physical therapy educators have, by and large, been socialized and mentored into a profession different from the profession of college and university teaching, they bring to the academy an ethos and a set of values and expectations that are frequently quite at odds with the prevailing value structure within higher education."[21] That is, physical therapy faculty are generally more than ready to teach students about clinical practice and to maintain their own clinical competence. However, many are exceedingly ill prepared to embrace the traditions of scholarship that are expected and needed for full acceptance in the academic world.

Physical therapy faculty who teach in the clinical sciences must, of course, keep their clinical skills and knowledge updated. Many faculty work at least part time in clinical settings, thus squeezing a fourth area of engagement into their busy academic schedules. However, this activity, which is so important to competent teaching in clinical courses, does not count toward tenure in the traditional university setting. It is difficult enough to do three things well (teaching, research, and service), but it is nearly impossible to do four things well (teaching, research, service, and clinical practice), especially if one does not have a PhD and is juggling the daily demands of family life. Many excellent clinician-educators have found themselves outside the university walls after 6 years because they were unable to fulfill the three classic tenure requirements.

Of course, knowing that these inevitable conflicts exist in the university is the starting place for resolution. At the heart of this resolution is the development of physical therapy educational programs that attract scholars who fit the traditional liberal arts model of excellence in teaching and research, as well as experienced clinicians who provide students with excellence in teaching and exposure to excellence in clinical practice. Creative thinking about ways to keep these clinical educators within the university has prompted such solutions as the development of faculty-run clinical practices and consultation and service contracts with nearby health care agencies. Other creative solutions include the creation of clinician-educator faculty tracks not subject to the traditional tenure time-limit constraints and scholarly demands, faculty positions shared between the university and health care settings, and the use of skilled clinicians as laboratory instructors in clinical science courses.

Professional Accreditation for Physical Therapist and Physical Therapist Assistant Programs

Accreditation is an American invention—in fact, it is uniquely American. Because it is a peer-review process carried out by volunteers and, at least as originally conceived, voluntary and non-governmental, it is not only American by intervention but in principle as well. Like American democracy, it is not a perfect system, but also like American democracy, no one has found a better way to do what it does. To our knowledge, every other nation in the world has a federal ministry of education that governs who shall teach what, and often who shall study what and at what level. That we in the United States rely on a non-governmental, voluntary system of quality assurance is partly because our founding fathers rejected the notion of a federal education system. They respected choice and they recognized the importance in an ideal democratic society that the intelligentsia not be controlled by the government.[23]

The primary function of accreditation is to set and ensure performance standards within disciplines across colleges and universities. Review Table 1-10 to gain an understanding of the breadth of purposes that support this quality assurance function.

Academic programs are judged by performance standards which include quantitative criteria and qualitative analysis. Quantitative criteria might include, for example, state board licensure examination scores of program graduates and professional qualifications of the faculty. Qualitative analysis might include the type of learning experiences students are engaged in and

Table 1-10 General Purposes of Accreditation

1. To foster excellence in postsecondary education through the development of criteria and guidelines for assessing educational effectiveness.
2. To encourage improvement of institutions and programs through continuous self-study and planning.
3. To assure other organizations and agencies, the educational community, and the general public that an institution or a particular program (a) has clearly defined and appropriate objectives, (b) maintains conditions under which its achievement can reasonably be expected, and (c) accomplishes its goals and continues to do so.
4. To provide counsel and assistance to established and developing programs and institutions.
5. To encourage the diversity of American postsecondary education and allow institutions to achieve their particular objectives and goals.
6. To endeavor to protect institutions against encroachments that might jeopardize their educational effectiveness or academic freedom.

Source: Reprinted with permission from KE Young, CM Chambers, HR Kells, et al. Understanding Accreditation. San Francisco: Jossey-Bass, 1983;23.

how these experiences impact the performance of the program graduates. These qualitative judgments can only be made by other people, and thus an on-site peer review visit is common practice. In this way, the public is assured that the institution meets or exceeds the general standards set for similar programs and institutions.

> Judging quality is not easy. It cannot be reduced to quantitative indices or formulas. Such judgments are made by gathering appropriate information about an institution or program and by having knowledgeable people appraise it. This is the essence of accreditation. (Council on Postsecondary Accreditation)[24]

Physical therapy educational programs can receive accreditation through a process established by the Commission on Accreditation in Physical Therapy Education (CAPTE).[24] This 26-member commission is comprised of physical therapy and physical therapist assistant academic and clinical educators, administrators from institutions of higher education, basic scientists, physicians, and public representatives. Since 1983, this commission has been the sole accrediting agency for physical therapy programs. CAPTE's authority currently is granted by the U.S. Department of Education and the Council on Higher Education Accreditation. As the sole accrediting agency, CAPTE makes autonomous decisions regarding the accreditation status of physical therapy and physical therapist assistant programs.

Although accreditation of physical therapy educational programs is considered a voluntary process because there are no federal laws requiring a program to be accredited, all viable physical therapy educational programs in the United States are accredited or in the process of becoming accredited. The reason, beyond assuring students and the public that the program conforms to general standards for the education of competent practitioners, is that all 50 states, the District of Columbia, and Puerto Rico require graduation from an accredited program as a prerequisite for acquiring a practice license.

The preaccreditation process for a new program is a lengthy one involving the APTA Accreditation Department staff and physical therapy educational consultants who work with an institution from the time it first inquires about developing a program. In this preaccreditation phase, the program submits substantive documentation 9 months before enrolling students. This documentation contains a comprehensive prospectus that includes an overview of the entire curriculum plan and identification of faculty, clinical sites, college or university resources (e.g., budget, space, and libraries) in place or needed to support the program, and a plan for evaluating performance of the graduates. This documentation is thoroughly reviewed and commented on by a reader-consultant who then makes a visit to the institution to further review the program's progress in development. The reader-consultant prepares a report that is discussed with the program director, faculty, and college administrators, and, along with updated materials, is forwarded to the commission for their decision regarding candidacy status. Candidacy status is required for a program to move forward in seeking accreditation status.

Self-Study Report

The accreditation process is somewhat parallel to the preaccreditation process in that a program prepares and submits a lengthy self-study report. The self-study process is a continual cycle fundamental to accreditation (Figure 1-5). During a self-study, the program's faculty is encouraged to use a system of ongoing review and evaluation for all program aspects.

With respect to the previous Council on Postsecondary Accreditation quotation, in physical therapy accreditation, "gathering appropriate information" would refer to the self-study report, and the "knowledgeable people" would be the members of the on-site team as well as members of CAPTE.

The program is guided in its ongoing program review and development of the self-study report by the Evaluative Criteria for Accreditation of Educational Programs for the Preparation of Physical Therapists or a comparable set of evaluative criteria for the physical therapist assistant program.[24] The

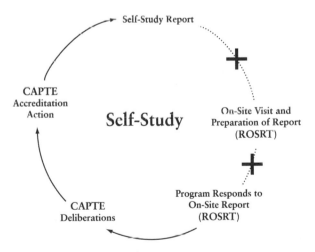

Figure 1-5 Ongoing self-study by the educational program is central to the accreditation process. (CAPTE = Commission on Accreditation in Physical Therapy Education; ROSRT= report of the on-site review team.)

evaluative criteria are periodically revised by CAPTE with input and feedback from many sources to reflect current standards of professional practice.

Reviewing these criteria will provide the reader with an excellent overview of the standards against which comparable physical therapy educational programs are assessed.[24,25] These criteria can be used on an ongoing basis by faculty for program evaluation. Reading these criteria also gives one an appreciation for the amount of extensive documentation regarding all phases of the program that is contained in a self-study report and reviewed and evaluated by the faculty as well as CAPTE.

The process of preparing a self-study report allows academic and clinical educators to review in depth all components of the curriculum to determine what is done and done well, what is done to an adequate or less than adequate degree, what is missing that should be included, and what can be omitted to update and strengthen the program. Thus, the process of compiling a self-study report is the first and most important aspect of ensuring and enhancing the quality of a physical therapy or physical therapist assistant educational program.

The self-study report contains extensive information in four major areas: organization, resources, curriculum, and program assessment (including performance of program graduates). The most important of these areas is the data that substantiate the outcome performance of the program graduates. All physical therapy and physical therapist assistant programs are urged to collect, compile, and review performance outcome data at frequent intervals. These data may include national physical therapy and physical therapist assistant licensing examination scores, surveys of graduates regarding their opinions about the strengths and weaknesses of the educational program, information that reflects the ongoing professional growth of graduates, input obtained from employers, and patient satisfaction surveys. Review Table 1-7 for a more complete list of examples of potential program evaluation data.

The self-study report is reviewed by a three-member on-site review team. The team consists of at least one physical therapy (or physical therapist assistant) educator and one physical therapist (or physical therapist assistant) clinician. The third team member may be a physician, basic scientist, or higher education administrator. The purpose of the on-site visit is to confirm the information presented in the self-study report, to describe the qualitative aspects of the program that cannot be determined by simply reading a paper document, and to provide summary information and consultation to the program.[26] The report of the on-site review team functions as a powerful "snapshot" of the program at the time of the site visit. The program's self-study report, along with the report of the on-site review team and any updated information the program wishes to present as a result of the report, is reviewed by members of CAPTE. Based on this review, the program is granted one of three general types of accreditation status: accreditation, probationary accreditation, or nonaccreditation. This intensive process is currently scheduled to occur 5 years after initial accreditation and then every 8 years, with smaller biennial accreditation reports containing updated program information due to CAPTE every other year.

Mary Jane Harris, MS, PT, Director of the APTA Department of Accreditation, states "CAPTE accreditation is all about fostering quality physical therapy education by encouraging program enhancement. In that way, CAPTE helps to assure that graduate physical therapists and physical therapist assistants are competent to enter the profession."

Faculty, clinicians, students, graduates, and administrators who have the opportunity to become involved with any aspect of the accreditation process are encouraged to do so with enthusiasm. In doing so, one witnesses an amazing process in which a community of professional peers works with unusual dedication to constantly strengthen and improve the educational foundations of physical therapy practice.

Summary

This chapter has given the reader an overview of the rational yet dynamic process of curricular design and has identified macro- and micro-level factors that influence curricular content. The three components of all curricula, implicit, explicit, and null, have been identified, as well as factors that have the potential to support or hinder implementation of a coherent, meaningful curriculum. Historic and pervasive conflicts between liberal arts and professional programs have been outlined and several strategies for resolution identified. Finally, this chapter presents a synthesized overview of accreditation, which is an engaging process that provides a stimulus and benchmark for quality physical therapy and physical therapist assistant education. The focus of all these efforts is to ensure excellence in clinical practice and provide learning experiences that will, as John Dewey states, "live fruitfully and creatively in subsequent experiences."[3]

References

1. Tyler RW. Basic Principles of Curriculum and Instruction. Chicago: University of Chicago Press, 1949.
2. Walker D. The process of curriculum development: a naturalistic model for curriculum development. School Review 1971;80:51.
3. Dewey J. Experience and Education. New York: Collier Books, 1938.

4. Eisner EW. The Educational Imagination: On the Design and Evaluation of School Programs (3rd ed). New York: Macmillan, 1994.
5. American Physical Therapy Association Education Division. A Normative Model of Physical Therapist Professional Education: Version 2000. Alexandria, VA: American Physical Therapy Association, 2000.
6. Siller C. Exploring the ethos of the physical therapy profession in the United States: Social, cultural and historical influences and their relationship to education. J Phys Ther Educ 2000;14:7–15.
7. O'Neil EH. Recreating Health Professions Practice for a New Century. San Francisco, CA: Pew Health Professions Commission, 1998.
8. Walker PH, Baldwin K, Fitzpatrick JJ, Ryan S. Building community: developing skills for interprofessional health professions education and relationship-centered care. J Allied Health 1998;27:173–178.
9. Rogers DE. The Education of Medical Students for Tomorrow. In Council on Graduate Medical Education, Reform in Medical Education and Medical Education in the Ambulatory Setting. Washington, DC: U.S. Department of Health and Human Services HRSA-P-DM-91-4;5, 1991.
10. Schön DA. Educating the Reflective Practitioner: Toward a New Design for Teaching and Learning in the Professions. San Francisco: Jossey-Bass, 1987.
11. Kern DE, Thomas PA, Howard DM, Bass EB. Curriculum Development for Medical Education: A Six-Step Approach. Baltimore: The Johns Hopkins University Press, 1998.
12. Miller SZ, Schmidt HJ. The habit of humanism: a framework for making humanistic care a reflexive clinical skill. Acad Med 1999;74:800–803.
13. Cruess RL, Cruess SR, Johnston SE. Renewing professionalism: an opportunity for medicine. Acad Med 1999;74:878–884.
14. Threlkeld AJ, Jensen GM, Royeen CB. The clinical doctorate: a framework for analysis in physical therapy education. Phys Ther 1999;79:567.
15. American Physical Therapy Association. A Guide to Physical Therapy Practice. Alexandria, VA: American Physical Therapy Association, 2001.
16. Mostrom E. Moral and ethical development in physical therapy practice and education: crossing the threshold. J Phys Ther Educ 2000;14:2.
17. American Physical Therapy Association Education Division. Curriculum Content in Physical Therapy Professional Education: Postbaccalaureate Level. A Resource from the IMPACT Conferences. Alexandria, VA: American Physical Therapy Association, 1993.
18. Shepard KF, Jensen GM. Physical therapist curricula for the 1990s: educating the reflective practitioner. Phys Ther 1990;70:566.
19. Mayhew LB, Ford PJ. Reform in Graduate and Professional Education. San Francisco: Jossey-Bass, 1974.

20. Ford PJ. The Nature of Professional Educations. In JS Barr (ed), Planning Curricula in Physical Therapy Education. Washington, DC: Section for Education, American Physical Therapy Association, 1982;22.
21. Ford PJ. The nature of graduate professional education: some implications for raising the entry level. J Phys Ther Educ 1990;4:3.
22. American Physical Therapy Association. 2000 Fact Sheet Physical Therapy Educational Programs. Alexandria, VA: American Physical Therapy Association, 2000.
23. Glidden R. The Contemporary Context of Accreditation: Challenges in a Changing Environment. Council for Higher Education Accreditation. Keynote address for 2nd CHEA "Usefulness" Conference, Washington, DC, June 25, 1998.
24. Commission on Accreditation in Physical Therapy Education 1997–1998 Accreditation Handbook. Alexandria, VA: American Physical Therapy Association, 1997.
25. Boucher B. Program assessment in physical therapy education: the transition to the new criteria. J Phys Ther Educ 1999;13:18–27.
26. Jensen GM. The work of accreditation on-site evaluators: enhancing the development of a profession. Phys Ther 1988;68:1517.

Annotated Bibliography

American Physical Therapy Association. Professional Education in Physical Therapy: Developing an Academic Program. Alexandria, VA: American Physical Therapy Association, 1993. Provides an overview of how to study the feasibility of establishing a physical therapy program and presents guidelines for planning and developing a professional education program. Especially useful for academic administrators who are considering developing a physical therapy program.

American Physical Therapy Association Education Division. A Normative Model of Physical Therapist Professional Education: Version 2000. Alexandria, VA: American Physical Therapy Association, 2000. This normative model originally was developed as a result of a series of national curricular conferences sponsored by the APTA Education Division. Using a framework of 19 practice expectations for entry into the field of physical therapy, this monograph contains examples of suggested curricular content in foundation and clinical sciences along with examples of terminal instructional objectives for classroom and clinical settings. Planned ongoing revisions of this model ensure responsiveness to changing practice, education, and health care environments. Physical therapy educators can glean many useful ideas for providing relevant classroom and clinical learning experiences from this monograph.

Commission on Accreditation in Physical Therapy Education. Accreditation Handbook. Alexandria, VA: American Physical Therapy Association, 1997. A "must" book for all physical therapy faculty. Contains the evaluative criteria for all physical therapy and physical therapist assistant programs. Interpretive comments and guidelines provided under the criteria are very useful in helping faculty to understand all relevant components of a physical therapy educational program and what is important to focus on to meet national standards.

Curry L, Wergin J. Educating Professionals: Responding to New Expectations for Competence and Accountability. San Francisco: Jossey-Bass, 1993. One of the few books in higher education written especially for those teaching in the professional fields. There are many excellent contributors, most of whom write from the perspective of the field of medicine. A central theme of the book is that a closer, more relevant, connection between education and practice is needed especially in light of the rapid economic, cultural, and technological changes looming in the twenty-first century.

Flinders DL, Thorton SJ (eds). The Curriculum Studies Reader. New York: Routledge, 1997. This edited reader contains chapters representing all of the classic works in curriculum: John Dewey, Franklin Bobbitt, Elliot Eisner, Philip Jackson, Joseph Schwab, Paulo Feire, James Popham, Herbert Kliebard, and others. For faculty who are interested in understanding curriculum theory and practice, this book provides a good historical and theoretical overview. Selected chapters would be excellent readings for graduate seminars.

Kern DE, Thomas PA, Howard DM, Bass EB. Curriculum Development for Medical Education: A Six-Step Approach. Baltimore: The Johns Hopkins University Press, 1998. The authors do an excellent job of explaining a simple six-step approach to curriculum development that includes: problem identification, needs assessment, goals and objectives, educational strategies, implementation and evaluation, and feedback. They provide several helpful tables and charts for mapping the relationship between goals and objectives, objectives and educational methods, and strengths and weaknesses of evaluation tools. This is an excellent resource for anyone who is involved in curriculum work with health professions faculty.

Tyler R. Basic Principles of Curriculum and Instruction. Chicago: The University of Chicago Press, 1949. This small (124 pages) classic book suggests ways to go about finding answers to the four questions Tyler posed as fundamental to curriculum development. The methods proposed to seek these answers have stood the test of time. An easy to read, enlightening, common sense approach to curriculum design.

Walker DF, Soltis JF. Curriculum and Aims (2nd ed). New York: Columbia University Teachers College Press, 1992. One of the Thinking About Education series of excellent paperback books produced by Teachers College Press. Summarizes and critiques major curriculum theorists. Argues that thinking and theorizing about curriculum help teachers to make their practice "intelligent, sensitive, responsible, and moral."

2

Preparation for Teaching Students in Academic Settings

Katherine F. Shepard and Gail M. Jensen

I went on a treasure hunt yesterday. It began in my kitchen. I found the flour, sugar, and butter but I couldn't find the recipe. I looked in every cookbook, on every shelf, in every cabinet. It was nowhere to be found. As I stood staring at the ingredients, my grandmother came to mind. "She would know what to do," I thought. I imagined adding a little of this, and a little of that, and finally created a small treasure, a cookie, just by feeling my way through the process. I closed my eyes, let my fingers do the baking . . . Voilà! Butter cookies galore.

As I turned from the kitchen into the living area of my apartment, I saw yet another treasure hunt unfold before me. There were piles of papers and books, empty book shelves, a long phone cord, and little Post-it notes strung all in a row. This "circle of knowledge" had no beginning and no end. Its main purpose was to design a 1-hour lecture for a group of students. Although I knew this purpose, questions of where I had begun and where I had learned all of this information ate at my very soul. How was I to compile all of this information into such a small package?

Looking down, I noted I had reread one of my favorite books, *Inspiration Sandwich*. In this book is my favorite phrase,

> "Creativity is all around you." Surveying the circle of papers, I knew there was no other way to accomplish the task. I organized the information with a little of this and a little of that. I added and subtracted, mixed it all together, and created my own little treasure—my first lecture. I found the experience to be just like baking: I identified, closed my eyes, and let my senses do the rest. Bon appétit! (Janice Franklin, first-year teacher)

Getting ready to teach a class or a course for the first time is almost always a perplexing situation. Where to start? Educators have suggested there are at least three kinds of knowledge essential to teaching effectively: (1) knowledge of the subject matter, (2) knowledge of the learners, and (3) knowledge of the general principles of teaching (i.e., knowledge of pedagogy).[1–4] This chapter presents an overview of the type of knowledge that physical therapy and physical therapist assistant educators are most often missing—knowledge of pedagogy.

Chapter Objectives

After completing this chapter, the reader will be able to

1. Identify and discuss the characteristics of five different philosophical orientations to curriculum design and give specific examples of how each applies to physical therapy or physical therapist assistant curricula.
2. Describe three learning theories that are based on three different views of how students can learn: (1) behaviorism, (2) gestalt–problem solving experience, and (3) Piaget/cognitive structure. Give specific examples of course materials that could best be taught by using each learning theory.
3. Discriminate among three major learning domains (i.e., cognitive, affective, and psychomotor) by citing elementary to complex levels within each that can be used to guide design of course content and assessment of student learning.
4. Identify the four learning styles described by Kolb[5] and give examples of student behavior that may be manifested by a high and low interest in each learning style.
5. Discuss construction of and specify the use of three different types of objectives that can be used to guide student learning: (1) behavioral, (2) problem solving, and (3) outcome.

6. Demonstrate how the delivery of course material and evaluation of students is linked to philosophical orientations, learning theories, learning domains, student learning styles, and course objectives.
7. List the items that could be included in a course syllabus.

Preactive and Interactive Teaching

Thirty-five years ago, a yellow paperback book titled *Handbook for Physical Therapy Teachers* was printed and distributed by the American Physical Therapy Association (APTA).[6] This small book was developed by a publication committee comprised of Ruth Dickinson at Columbia University, Hyman L. Dervitz at Temple University, and Helen Meida at Western Reserve University. This book was the only source of information regarding physical therapy education at the time and included information on how to develop, organize, and teach a physical therapy curriculum. The teaching focus of that pioneering book and this chapter is preactive teaching.

The terms *preactive* and *interactive* teaching were coined by psychologist Phillip Jackson.[7] *Preactive teaching* refers to those elements one considers when preparing to teach a course. Such activities include reading background information, preparing course syllabi, developing media, and even arranging the furniture in the classroom. These activities are highly rational—that is, the teacher reads, weighs evidence, reflects, organizes, relates the current class content to past and future classes the students are involved in, and creates an optimal environment for learning. Like the first-year teacher who was grappling with how to organize a 1-hour lecture, most of these activities occur when the teacher is alone and in an environment that allows for quiet, deliberative thought. Preactive preparation allows the teacher time to think through the breadth and depth of information that is to be presented (subject matter knowledge) to a particular group of students (knowledge of learners), as well as the most coherent and understandable way to present the information (pedagogical knowledge).

By contrast, *interactive teaching* refers to what happens when the teacher is face to face with students. Interactive teaching activities are more or less spontaneous—that is, when working with large groups of students, the teacher tends to do what he or she feels or knows is right. In the chaotic milieu of a classroom, laboratory, or clinic, little time is available to reflect on what are appropriate and useful teaching strategies. Obviously, experienced teachers are considerably more skilled in interactive teaching and "reflection-in-action" than novice teachers. This is similar to experienced clinicians who seem to know the right thing to do with patients with an ease and confidence that amazes novice clinicians.[8] However, thoughtful preactive teaching preparation

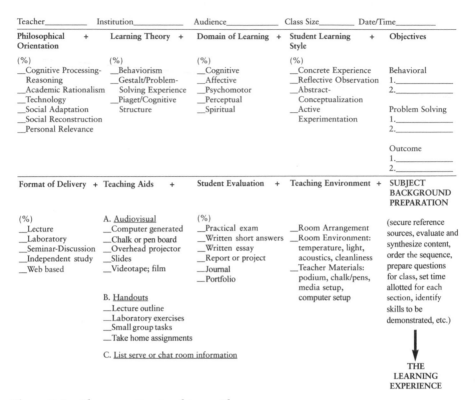

Figure 2-1 The preactive teaching grid.

can allow even the novice teacher the freedom to focus on student understanding and growth rather than lecture notes. Preactive teaching elements are covered in this chapter. Chapter 3 focuses on interactive teaching elements.

Preactive Teaching Grid

This handbook assumes that the teacher is extraordinarily competent regarding the subject matter to be taught (subject matter knowledge), and is a physical therapist (PT) or physical therapist assistant who has a good knowledge of the students to be taught and what information they need for competent clinical practice. However, to organize and present material in a manner that is responsive to the program mission and desired student outcomes, the teacher is urged to think through the components identified in the preactive teaching grid (Figure 2-1). This grid is useful whether designing a whole course or a single class. When all components of the grid have been identified and are related to each other in a coherent fashion, the delivery of the course content also tends to be coherent to student and teacher. Note that the grid encourages the teacher to think through how much percentage in time and effort each of the elements contributes to the presentation of a particular content area.

Philosophical Orientation

Eliot Eisner conceived of five philosophical orientations that can be used to guide curriculum design: development of cognitive processes, academic rationalism, technology, societal interests (social adaptation and social reconstruction), and personal relevance.[9] These orientations are based on what teachers think the aims of a curriculum, course, or class should be— that is, why they are teaching what they are teaching.

Cognitive Processing-Reasoning

The philosophical orientation of cognitive processing-reasoning focuses on teaching students to develop and refine their intellectual processes (e.g., how to gather and analyze data, how to pose and solve problems, how to infer, how to hypothesize, and how to make judgments based on limited information). The concern of the educator is on the *how* rather than the *what*. Little emphasis is placed on acquiring facts, as the development of cognitive processing-reasoning orientation proposes that by teaching students how to think, to reason, and to use resources, they will be able to identify, locate, evaluate, and apply whatever information they might need.

Problem-based curricula, such as that at MacMaster University in Canada described by Solomon, are entirely based on this philosophy.[10] In this orientation, faculty identify cognitive processes that are needed to practice as a PT. These problem-solving cognitive processes are then strengthened through a series of problem-based experiences that are similar to clinical situations that PTs encounter.

In a problem-based curriculum, the entire curriculum is comprised of clinical problems. For example, rather than a class of students sitting in traditional physical therapy courses, such as anatomy, pathology, therapeutic exercise, and health care policy, students in small groups guided by a mentor discuss patient problems. With any given patient problem, students learn to seek out, analyze, and act on the information they need. That is, students gather information from a variety of sources, including anatomy, pathology, therapeutic exercise, and health care economics, as these sources relate to the patient problem under consideration. For an excellent overview of the advantages and disadvantages of problem-based learning, read *The Challenge of Problem-Based Learning* by Boud and Feletti.[11]

Of course, in any class or any course in any curriculum one could be working toward the development of cognitive processes and reasoning. For example, you might ask students to use their "hunch" regarding the outcome of a patient care problem. Students could then identify and analyze what data their hunch was based on and what additional data they would need to confirm their hunch. By this process, the student is introduced to the cognitive processes of inductive and deductive thinking, and how both processes are used in health care decision making. As another example, students could be presented with a clinical problem that represents a moral dilemma. Analyzing such a problem involves the cognitive processes of identifying the student's own values, comparing and contrasting these values with the principles contained in a professional code of ethics, and working out a rational, empathetic decision. As time to evaluate and treat patients has declined in all health care settings, teaching students to think rationally, humanely, creatively, and quickly is time well spent in every course.

Academic Rationalism

The philosophical orientation of academic rationalism focuses on traditional areas of study that faculty think represent the most intellectually and artistically significant ideas within the field they are teaching. This approach relishes the history and the careful inquiry that have led to formulation of universal principles and philosophical, scientific, and artistic concepts useful in today's world. In this type of orientation, more time is spent on theory and less on practical application. The belief is that once students learn of the great ideas created by the most visionary people in their field (and related fields), they are able to perform as educated men and women. As Eisner states, "The central aim is to develop man's rational abilities by introducing his rationality to ideas and objects that represent reason's highest achievement."[9] Thus, college classes based on the works of great thinkers, such as Charles Darwin, Emily Dickinson, Albert Einstein, Mahatma Ghandi, Pablo Picasso, and Martin Luther King, Jr., would have as their focus academic rationalism.

Obviously, no health care curriculum could be based solely on academic rationalism because too much health care information and related patient care intervention strategies are outdated within a decade or less. However, physical therapy and physical therapist assistant educators struggle with how much academic rationalism to put into curriculum. For example, in one issue of *Neurology Report*, educators grappled with how much students should be taught about the historical perspectives of Margaret Rood, Maggie Knott, Berta and Karl Bobath, and Signe Brunnstrom, when compared with the time devoted to the current theories of motor control and motor behavior.[12]

Technology

The philosophical orientation of technology focuses on practical or technical behaviors that the student should attain to become proficient in her or his field. Using this orientation, a curriculum or a course would consist of a series of clearly delineated behavioral objectives the student is to master. The underlying approach is essentially a stimulus-response-reinforcement model. Computer-assisted instruction is an example of this orientation. The answers are predetermined to be clearly right or wrong, and students receive immediate corrective feedback. Using computer-assisted instruction, the student can repeat material until a certain proficiency level is attained.

In physical therapy and physical therapist assistant programs, there are many areas of content and skill knowledge that lend themselves to the technology orientation. For example, in anatomy there are clearly right and wrong answers, and the teacher's task is to determine how much anatomy, at what level, and what approach can be used that will help students memorize and apply the material accurately. Practical skills knowledge, such as the biomechanics of lifting or the steps involved in a wheelchair transfer, are often taught using this philosophical orientation.

Social Adaptation and Social Reconstruction

The philosophical orientation of social adaptation and social reconstruction focuses on societal interests. This is a two-pronged orientation, with one prong being social adaptation and the opposite prong being social reconstruction. Social adaptation curriculum orientation focuses on knowledge and skills students need to function in today's world—that is, on what society needs to maintain the status quo. Under this orientation, for example, physical therapy and physical therapist assistant students would be taught the information and technical skills that are needed to immediately fill those areas of practice with the greatest number of job vacancies.

In contrast, the philosophical orientation of social reconstruction focuses the curriculum on identifying the changing composition and projected needs of society and the skills that will be needed in the future to be responsive to these changes. Such skills might include working to change certain aspects of society, such as intolerance to ethnic and cultural differences, environmental pollution, or the rise of homelessness. For example, in a physical therapy or physical therapist assistant curriculum, students would be engaged in experiences designed to develop their tolerance for working with patients whose heritage and lifestyles differ considerably from their own, become involved in environmental health groups, or embrace participation in pro bono services for the homeless. Thus, although social adaptation and social reconstruction have different aims, they are tied by the common philosophical belief that societal needs should guide curriculum.

Personal Relevance

The philosophical orientation of personal relevance focuses on what is personally relevant to the student. In this orientation, the teacher and the student jointly plan educational experiences that are meaningful to the student. As Eisner states, "The task of the school is to provide a resource-rich environment so that the child will, without coercion, find what he or she needs in order to grow."[9] Probably the archetype of this orientation is portrayed in A. S. Neil's famous boarding school, Summerhill, founded in England in 1921 and designed to "make the school fit the child instead of making the child fit the school."[13]

This orientation probably has the least meaning to entry-level physical therapy and physical therapist assistant educators who have little enough time to teach groups of students the basic tenets and tasks of their profession without responding to the individual personal relevance requirements of each student. However, the personal relevance orientation is very much in evidence in continuing education programs as well as post-professional graduate degree programs. The most successful continuing education programs appear to be those that offer clinicians knowledge and advanced skills (e.g., in manual therapy), which can be immediately applied in an individual clinician's health care setting. The most successful post-professional graduate programs appear to be those that offer the student a great deal of latitude in what she or he chooses to pursue and where the faculty is dedicated to encouraging and supporting students in their individual pursuits.

Using the Five Curriculum Orientations to Guide Curriculum Design and Course Development

There are two useful ways to use these five curriculum orientations in developing a whole curriculum or a single course. In working with an entire curriculum design, the five philosophical orientations can be used to review the multiple courses that comprise the curriculum and to identify what philosophical orientation(s) the curriculum emphasis is built on. Faculty might realize that they are spending too much time on technology or academic rationalism and not enough time on developing cognitive processes and reasoning. You might find that the social reconstruction orientation is a nice thread throughout the curriculum or it may be left out altogether. This is an enjoyable and often revealing activity for individual faculty, as well as the collective faculty. It will clarify the faculty's own values and beliefs about the mission, structure, and outcomes of physical therapy or physical therapist assistant education as well as how any group of faculty envision the present and future practice of physical therapy.

In using the five philosophical orientations to develop a course, the teacher would first specify the goals of the course and then identify how much of each philosophical orientation will be used to help students reach those goals. For example, for a course in basic skills, the teacher probably wants a high percentage of class time devoted to technology (e.g., 60%). He or she might also want to teach students how to think about applying basic skills in a wide variety of clinical situations, so the teacher may plan to devote 20% of class time to stimulating cognitive processing-reasoning. Finally, the teacher might focus on some skills students will need to use immediately in clinical practice, such as taking a blood pressure or performing bed-to-wheelchair transfers. Thus, the remaining 20% of the time might be used for laboratory sessions organized around common clinical problems in which students can learn basic skills that are immediately applicable in their next internship. Going through the process of thinking about philosophical orientations related to the goals for each class can be an eye-opening experience, which can guide teachers in reapportioning classroom and laboratory time appropriately. Such a process can also ensure that all class time is not devoted inadvertently to a single philosophical orientation or an orientation that does not have a coherent fit with the overall curriculum design.

In Chapter 5, the Teaching Goals Inventory is presented and discussed. At that point, you will be able to see how the curriculum philosophy you are using is tied directly to your specific teaching goals.

Learning Theories

The next column in the upper part of the preactive teaching grid contains learning theories (see Figure 2-1). Phillips and Soltis, in their book *Perspectives on Learning*, provide an excellent synthesized overview of classical and current learning theories.[14] Theories about how people learn have been discussed at least since the time of the Greek philosopher Plato (428–347 BC). Plato postulated that knowledge was innate—that is, in place at the time of birth. The function of a teacher was to help the learner "recall" what one's soul had already experienced and learned. Nearly 2,000 years after Plato, the British philosopher John Locke (1632–1704) proposed an opposite view of the learner. Locke postulated that infants were born with the mind a blank slate, a tabula rasa. The teacher's role was to provide experiences that would fill this blank slate with knowledge.[14]

The current traditional learning theories fall somewhere within the pyramid model pictured in Figure 2-2. There are essentially three distinctly different theories about how people learn: (1) behaviorism, (2) gestalt–problem

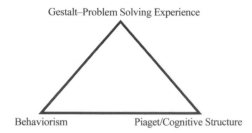

Figure 2-2   The pyramid of learning theories.

solving experience, and (3) Piaget/cognitive structure. Nearly all other learning theories are some combination of these three perspectives and, therefore, fall somewhere within the learning theory pyramid. Learning theories provide the teacher with ideas about how to present students with different types of knowledge and skill in a way that reinforces the underlying philosophical orientations the teacher is focusing on.

Behaviorism

The behaviorism theory was developed in the first half of the twentieth century as a result of numerous experiments, primarily on animals and birds, by the experimental psychologists E. L. Thorndike[15] and B. F. Skinner.[16] The basic theory of behaviorism rests on their observations that behaviors that were rewarded (positively reinforced) would reoccur. For behaviorists, the process of learning involves rewarding correct behavior until the behavioral change is consistently demonstrated.[14]

PTs and physical therapist assistants use behavioristic principles continually in patient care to teach psychomotor skills. For example, patients are reinforced with enthusiastic praise for attempting and subsequently achieving self-care activities, such as donning and doffing a prosthesis. In classrooms, acquiring accurate knowledge (i.e., knowing the right answer) is rewarded by receiving high grades and praise from faculty. Lack of responsiveness to acquiring the knowledge presented is quelled by poor grades and perhaps even failure to proceed in the program. Computer-assisted instruction is based almost exclusively on this learning theory. Students receive immediate feedback contingent on the accuracy of their responses. Clearly, many psychomotor skills and specific facts that need to be memorized are successfully taught using behavioristic principles. For a teacher whose main philosophical orientation to a course is technology, the predominant learning theory of choice would be behaviorism.

Gestalt–Problem Solving Experience

In the early to mid-1900s, gestalt psychologists presented a theory of human learning that was diametrically opposed to that of behaviorists. The word *gestalt* means organization. Gestalt psychologists believe people experience and organize the world in meaningful patterns or contexts. Therefore, information must make sense within some context or the learner will not be able to learn.[14] Gestalt psychologists believe that to identify and reinforce isolated behaviors (i.e., behaviorism) is a clear distortion of how humans actually learn.

This principle of learning within context clearly operates in clinical practice and academic settings. PTs, who in the past prepared patients for functional activities by working on strength and endurance of specific muscle groups, now ascribe to modern motor learning theories in which teaching movement within functional patterns hastens the acquisition of motor skills (see Chapter 11). In academic settings, it is known that students need a framework for information so that the knowledge "makes sense." For example, the tedious process of memorizing anatomical origins and insertions of muscle groups in an anatomy class has long been seen as an absolute necessity to the practice of physical therapy. However, students are quick to point out that learning this anatomical information is greatly enhanced by acquiring corresponding knowledge of the function of muscle groups in a kinesiology class and learning how to assist patients to improve the function of muscle groups in a therapeutic exercise class. In this manner, students learn and understand the origin and insertion of muscle groups in the context of muscle function and in the context of the use of this information in patient care. Thus, memorization of anatomical structures is easier because it has a useful context and therefore "makes sense."

John Dewey (1859–1952), who has been called America's greatest educational philosopher, expanded on the learning theory of gestalt or learning within a context.[17] For Dewey, the issue of activity (i.e., students being actively involved in an experience from which they could learn) was all important. Phillips and Soltis have clearly captured Dewey's beliefs about how learning occurs, and thus how teachers should teach using this gestalt–problem solving learning theory.

> Dewey described the process of human problem solving, reflective thinking, and learning in many slightly different ways because he knew that intelligent thinking and learning is not just following some standard recipe. He believed that intelligence is creative and flexible—we learn from engaging ourselves in a variety of experiences in the world. However, in all of his descriptions, the following elements always appeared in

some form: Thinking always gets started when a person genu-
inely feels a problem arise. Then the mind actively jumps back
and forth—struggling to find a clearer formulation of the problem, looking for suggestions for possible solutions, surveying
elements in the problematic situation that might be relevant,
drawing on prior knowledge in an attempt to better understand
the situation. Then the mind begins forming a plan of action, a
hypothesis about how best the problem might be solved. The
hypothesis is then tested; if the problem is solved, then according to Dewey something has been learned.[14]

Thus, in the classroom and in the clinic, when teachers present students
with clinical problems to solve, they are following the traditions of John
Dewey. Perhaps even more important, Dewey illuminates how we learn from
our experience in clinical practice. His postulation that learning occurs from
actively solving meaningful problems explains the accumulated wisdom of
experienced practitioners that is far beyond the knowledge contained in current textbooks. The concepts of *reflection in action* and *reflection on action*
described by Donald Schön and elaborated on in Chapter 3 of this book are the
present-day versions of this gestalt–problem solving learning theory that was
first articulated by Dewey.[8] For a teacher whose main philosophical orientation to a course is development of cognitive processing-reasoning, the predominant learning theory of choice would be the gestalt–problem solving
experience.

Piaget and Cognitive Structure

Jean Piaget (1896–1980) was a Swiss developmental psychologist
who looked at learning in terms of development of mental or cognitive abilities that make learning possible.[18] Much of his work is based on careful observation and description of the cognitive abilities of his three children from
their infancy to adolescence. From this work, he postulated that thinking and
learning were bound to the child's biological development. He suggested four
stages of biological development through which all children proceed:

1. Sensorimotor stage (birth–2 years): grasping, objects to mouth
2. Preoperational stage (2–7 years): concrete physical manipulation of
   objects
3. Concrete operations stage (7–11 years): beginning conceptualization
   (e.g., use of abstract numbers)
4. Formal operations stage (11–14 years): full conceptualization, solving
   problems in the abstract

Although there has been a good deal of criticism of the specific nature of Piaget's stages, he does present for us the useful concept that the mind develops through a series of stages that is limited as well as facilitated by biology and experience. Certainly, children at 2 years of age are not yet ready to understand abstract concepts that would help them deal more effectively with many issues with less emotional energy!

For students beyond Piaget's stages (the ages of physical therapy and physical therapist assistant students), the work of Robert Gagne proposes a hierarchy of learning that begins with the simple and concrete and moves to the complex and abstract.[19] The ideas contained within stages of a hierarchy suggest that higher-order cognitive abilities build on lower-order cognitive abilities. That is, students must master lower-order abilities before they can master higher-level ones. Gagne suggests the following hierarchy: (1) facts, (2) concepts, (3) principles, and (4) problem solving. Thus, for example, students should be able to identify the muscles, nerves, and connective tissues involved in the shoulder rotator cuff (facts) before they can understand conceptually how these structures fit together. After they understand how the structures are related, they can understand the biomechanical principles involved in the rotator cuff mechanism. After understanding these principles, they can solve problems related to rotator cuff injuries. If a student has missed any one of these steps it would be difficult to proceed to the next step. For example, if the student did not understand conceptually how the various tissue structures are related, then it would be difficult to understand the biomechanics of movement. Thus, cognitive structure learning theories that began with Piaget's observations are very useful in thinking about ways to organize and present information. For a teacher whose main philosophical orientation to a course is academic rationalism, the predominant learning theory of choice would be Piaget/cognitive structures.

Thinking Through the Relationship between Philosophical Orientations and Learning Theories

When the learning theory used is not compatible with the underlying philosophical orientation, course materials tend to be jumbled, leaving students and teachers frustrated with the teaching-learning process. For example, suppose a teacher believes strongly in the development of cognitive processing-reasoning (philosophical orientation) and regards that as the aim of teaching. In fact, the teacher sets up examinations in the format of patient cases about which he or she asks a series of open-ended questions. The questions are designed to require students to use cognitive reasoning skills. However, suppose the material was actually taught using the behaviorism learning theory. Behaviorism is the learning theory that has predominated in classroom life for most students since first grade, and they are well prepared for memorizing and parroting information. Does it seem that these students would be ready and able to take specific facts for which they know correct and incorrect responses and apply these facts without having had some learning that involved the patient care context—that is, gestalt–problem solving experiences? This "miss" between how the material has been taught and how the students are asked to apply it on a test is often apparent. The miss represents a discrepancy between the teacher's philosophical aim of the course and the learning theory that guides instruction.

Looking at the preactive teaching grid (see Figure 2-1), one can see that if a large percentage of the philosophical orientation to the material is technology (wanting students to learn specific facts and skills within a hierarchy of facts-to-principles involved), then the learning theories of behaviorism and cognitive structure could logically guide the presentation of the material. Likewise, if a teacher is interested in the social reconstruction philosophical orientation, then the gestalt–problem solving learning theory approach could be a useful way to present course materials. Remember that seldom are only one philosophical orientation and learning theory used in a class. However, just thinking through the emphasis to be placed on each orientation and learning theory and their resultant compatibility will help guide teaching and evaluation efforts in a way that will help students learn rather than be frustrated.

Domains of Learning

The third column in the upper part of the preactive teaching grid identifies the domains of learning (see Figure 2-1). In considering aspects of being human that are subject to growth and development and, thus, have implications for teaching and learning, at least five domains of learning can be identified.

- Cognitive (thinking)
- Affective (feeling, willing)
- Psychomotor (purposeful movement, doing)
- Perceptual (involving all the senses, including vision, olfactory, auditory, taste, and kinesthetic)
- Spiritual (faith)

The first three domains, the cognitive, affective, and psychomotor, are well known to physical therapy educators, as clinical practice obviously involves knowledge and skill in all three areas. These are the domains that have been most well defined and developed for educators.

In 1956, Benjamin Bloom and associates wrote the first book in this area entitled *Taxonomy of Educational Objectives, Handbook I: The Cognitive Domain.*[20] A companion book (*Handbook II: Affective Domain*) was produced

Knowledge	Comprehension	Application	Analysis	Synthesis	Evaluation
					appraise
					assess
				arrange	choose
				assemble	compare
			analyze	collect	criticize
		apply	appraise	compose	estimate
		calculate	calculate	construct	evaluate
compute	demonstrate	categorize	create	judge
describe	dramatize	compare	design	measure
cite	discuss	employ	contrast	formulate	rank
count	explain	examine	debate	integrate	rate
define	express	illustrate	diagram	manage	revise
draw	identify	interpret	differentiate	organize	score
list	locate	operate	examine	plan	select
name	report	practice	inventory	prescribe	
record	restate	schedule	question	propose	
relate	review	sketch	test		
repeat	tell	solve			
underline	translate	use			

Figure 2-3 Six levels of the cognitive domain. (Reprinted with permission from CW Ford [ed]. Clinical Education for the Allied Health Professions. St. Louis: Mosby, 1978.)

by Krathwohl, Bloom, and Masia in 1964.[21] In the 1970s, several books appeared on the psychomotor domain, one of the most useful being that by Simpson.[22] The primary reason these books have been so useful to teachers is that they clearly define lower-order and higher-order thinking, psychomotor, and affective abilities. Thus, similar to Piaget's and Gagne's contribution to cognitive structure learning theories, the domains of learning provide a guide to the order in which students can most easily acquire information, psychomotor skills, and values.

Cognitive Domain

The six levels of the cognitive domain are depicted in Figure 2-3.[19] The upward progression of steps illustrates that students must acquire some basic knowledge of the material before they can comprehend it, and they must comprehend the material before they can apply it. The three higher levels illustrate that it is easier for students to analyze information than to synthesize it, and only after achieving a sufficient understanding of analysis and synthesis can one learn to evaluate the material. The list of verbs under each level identifies the kind of behaviors students might exhibit when learning in that domain. For example, in learning how center of gravity is a key to moving one's body through space, the student might learn logically through the following steps in the cognitive domain.

1. *Knowledge*: Define the center of gravity.
2. *Comprehension*: Describe principles of the center of gravity involved in body movement.

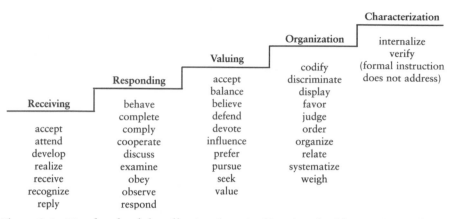

Figure 2-4   Five levels of the affective domain. (Reprinted with permission from CW Ford [ed]. Clinical Education for the Allied Health Professions. St. Louis: Mosby, 1978.)

3. *Application*: Demonstrate how center of gravity relates to balance.
4. *Analysis*: Compare how center of gravity differs in maintaining sitting, stooped, and standing postures.
5. *Synthesis*: Design a wheelchair-to-car transfer that uses the principles involved in the body's center of gravity.
6. *Evaluation*: Compare several different wheelchair-to-car transfers and determine which is the safest using the principles of the center of gravity.

Thus, knowing the various levels of the cognitive domain and deciding at which level(s) the student is ready to learn will help the teacher ensure that students have not missed any level of a knowledge component that would lead to full understanding. Similarly, the teacher can review examinations to determine if students are being asked to respond at the same domain levels that have been taught. This is similar to the need for coherency between philosophical orientation and learning theories in teaching and evaluation.

Affective Domain

The affective domain, which includes student interests, attitudes, appreciation, and values, is obviously more difficult to teach and evaluate.[21] Basically, behaviors in this domain are taught and measured by approach-avoidance tendencies, meaning positive attitudes are believed to exist if a student approaches and grapples with an issue rather than avoids it.

The levels of the affective domain are depicted in Figure 2-4. In this domain, the first step is to attend to an issue or "receive" it. After receiving an issue, one responds to that issue and subsequently may demonstrate that the issue is of value to her or him. The highest levels of organization and characterization include deciding the importance of that issue given other competing issues and acting consistently according to the value one places on the issue. The following is an example of how the affective domain could be used in physical therapy education regarding the issue of valuing diversity and embracing nondiscrimination.

1. *Receiving*: Realize that health care professionals may treat patients and families differently because of race, gender, or lifestyle.
2. *Responding*: Discuss how responding differently to patients because of race, gender, or lifestyle might affect treatment outcomes.
3. *Valuing*: Defend the right of each patient and family to receive the best health care possible regardless of their race, gender, or lifestyle.
4. *Organization*: Judge, or decide, when patients and families are being treated differently by health care professionals because of their race, gender, or lifestyle.
5. *Characterization*: Internalize the belief in individual patient and family rights regardless of race, gender, or lifestyle, and act consistently with those beliefs.

Krathwohl et al.[21] note that there is a good deal of hesitancy by teachers to evaluate students in the affective domain. Teachers, as well as students, often see it as inappropriate to grade on interest, attitudes, or character development, all of which are regarded as personal or private matters. Furthermore, education in the affective domain may be seen as indoctrination—that is, persuading or coercing students to adopt a particular viewpoint, act in a certain manner, or profess to a particular value or way of life.[21]

Certainly, the issue of professional socialization and ways that health care professionals are expected to behave is central to consideration of the affective domain. In physical therapy and physical therapist assistant curricula, clinical educators are regularly called on to evaluate students in affective areas, such as enthusiasm, dependability, judgment, and sensitivity in patient-family care. Clinical educators also evaluate how well students adjust to a department, how well they work with colleagues, how receptive they are to new ideas, and how they react to constructive criticism. In fact, it is unlikely that any clinical evaluation form exists that does not include these important affective professional attitudes and behaviors.

However, it is much less likely that academic educators deliberately teach and evaluate in the affective domain. Students see such evaluation as illegitimate. Take the example of the student who is perennially late to class, or students who leave the lab when their work is done regardless of

Table 2-1　Examples of Affective Behaviors Pertinent to Academic and Clinical Settings

	Satisfactory	Needs improvement	Unsatisfactory
Demonstrates ability to recognize and discuss own beliefs and values as different from others	_____	_____	_____
Seeks opportunities to augment learning and improve knowledge in theoretical and practical areas	_____	_____	_____
Works cooperatively with persons of varied ethnic, gender, lifestyle, and disability backgrounds	_____	_____	_____
Recognizes and handles personal and work-related frustrations in a non-disruptive and constructive manner	_____	_____	_____
Demonstrates ability to recognize, examine, and influence own strengths and limitations in academic and clinical settings	_____	_____	_____
Accepts role as a moral agent and moves to thoughtful deliberative action when moral dilemmas arise	_____	_____	_____

whether their colleagues have completed the scheduled group tasks. When students are reprimanded for these irresponsible professional behaviors, they often claim that they not only have good reasons for their behavior, but that they would not exhibit such behaviors in the clinic setting. Is this true?

For affective behaviors to be seen as legitimate in the academic setting, teachers must determine before the class begins what clinically related behaviors are acceptable and unacceptable and explicitly notify students that such behaviors will or will not be supported and will be evaluated. See Table 2-1 for examples of affective behaviors that can alert the student to expected clinical behaviors and guide the teaching and counseling efforts of educators in the academic setting.

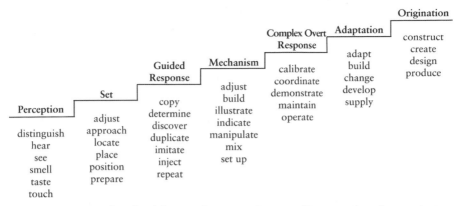

Figure 2-5   Seven levels of the psychomotor domain. (Reprinted with permission from CW Ford [ed]. Clinical Education for the Allied Health Professions. St. Louis: Mosby, 1978.)

Psychomotor Domain

The stages of the psychomotor domain are noted in Figure 2-5. The steps of these stages are self-evident, especially to the many physical therapy educators and students who have participated in sports. In fact, remembering how skill in a specific sport was acquired may be an excellent guide to teaching patients motor skills. (For more on the specific topic of learning motor skills, see Chapter 11.) The following examples of psychomotor domain stages could be applied to most sports as well as to patient tasks, such as gait training.

1. *Perception*: Distinguish among various maneuvers.
2. *Set*: Position oneself to engage in each maneuver.
3. *Guided response*: Duplicate the maneuver a skilled performer presents.
4. *Mechanism*: Adjust the maneuver to the needed response.
5. *Complex overt response*: Coordinate various maneuvers to accomplish successful play or task.
6. *Adaptation*: Adapt maneuvers to obtain the most successful response.
7. *Origination*: Create new maneuvers.

As with the other domains, thinking through the steps in the psychomotor domain before teaching, as well as before an evaluation such as a practical examination, helps the teacher determine at what levels he or she is presenting and requiring students to demonstrate motor skills.

Perceptual and Spiritual Domains

Neither the perceptual nor the spiritual domain has yet been fully described or classified in a series of learning steps, as has been done with the cognitive, affective, and psychomotor domains. However, neither of these domains should be neglected in physical therapy education. Clearly, the perceptual domain involving use of the senses plays a dominant role in how patients receive and use information regarding components of movement. For example, the psychomotor skill of balance is clearly enhanced with the use of kinesthetic proprioception and vision. Think about how the perceptual domain can be incorporated into classes with content in motor learning and motor control.

The spiritual domain appears to be very comfortable or very uncomfortable for health care professionals in their work with patients and families. The same is true of academic and clinical faculty in their work with students. The degree of comfort in presenting and discussing various beliefs related to spirituality with students appears to be directly related to one's own exploration and understanding of spirituality, as well as how colleagues support or dismiss attention to this domain. Certainly, this domain of learning plays a significant role in how patients and families perceive disease and manage illness within their lives and across their lifespan. Perhaps as we become more open to, comfortable with, and begin to introduce students to complementary and alternative health care practices, spirituality issues will enter the physical therapy curriculum naturally.[23]

Thinking Through the Relationship between Philosophical Orientations, Learning Theories, and Domains of Knowledge

Think about teaching a class in physiology of exercise. It is likely you will use some mix of philosophical orientations (e.g., technology [60%], cognitive processing-reasoning [30%], and academic rationalism [10%]). The predominant learning theories might be behaviorism (75%) and cognitive structure (25%). The learning domain might be the cognitive domain (100%). Contrast these choices with an approach to a class about sexuality of persons with spinal cord injury. For this class, you might choose to teach predominately from a social adaptation philosophy using the gestalt–problem solving experience learning theory and attending to the affective and psychomotor domains, as well as the cognitive domain. Is it clear how thinking through the preactive grid (knowledge of pedagogy) can lead to a course or class design that is as remarkably different as it is remarkably coherent?

Student Learning Styles

The fourth column in the upper part of the preactive teaching grid (see Figure 2-1) displays one example of how to think about student learning styles. Identifying your own learning style brings an understanding of how you prefer to learn. It is important for teachers to be aware that they are likely

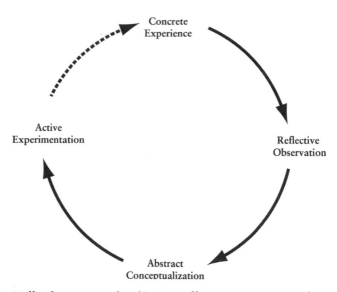

Figure 2-6 Kolb's learning styles. (From Kolb DA. Learning Styles Inventory. Boston: McBer and Co., 1985, with permission.)

to teach using the learning style they are most comfortable with. For example, if the teacher likes to learn by reading, an extensive assigned reading list will probably be in the course syllabi. Conversely, if the teacher likes to learn by doing, the course syllabi will be peppered with practical learning experiences for students. Thus, it is important for the teacher to be aware of her or his predominant learning styles, as well as the learning styles that she or he favors less. The less-favored learning styles may be ones that some students are most comfortable with and can learn the most from. Thus, one can become a more effective and appreciated teacher through devising activities that are responsive to a wide range of student learning styles.

Presented below is an example of one learning style inventory and how it can be used in academic and clinical teaching. (There are other learning style inventories, such as the Myers-Briggs Type Indicator[24] and the Canfield Learning Styles Inventory,[25] both of which are used by health professionals.)

Kolb postulated a model of normal learning processes that was eventually developed into the Learning Styles Inventory.[5] As seen in Figure 2-6, learning is depicted as a recurring cycle consisting of four stages, beginning with a concrete experience. Most concrete learning experiences involve other people in everyday situations. This type of learning relies on feeling and intuition rather than logic and reasoning. The second stage, reflective observation, involves learning by observing what happens to oneself as well as what happens to others during a concrete experience. In this stage, no action is taken, but through observation one learns to understand situations from different points of view. The third stage, abstract conceptualization, involves logic and reasoning. In this stage, theories or explanations are developed about what has been done and observed. Then actions may be taken and problems solved based on these theories. In the fourth and final stage, active experimentation, learning is through testing different approaches based on the theories generated. In this stage, the practical use of ideas, as well as theory, is evident.

PTs and physical therapist assistants use this cycle constantly in clinical practice when treating a patient (concrete experience), observing and reflecting on what happened to the patient as a result of that treatment (reflective observation), thinking about how a successful intervention with one patient may work on similar patients and theorizing why (abstract conceptualization), and then trying the intervention on other patients (active experimentation). By this learning process, clinicians create the ever-expanding knowledge base (tacit knowledge) they use in practice.

Kolb's Learning Styles Inventory consists of a series of choices the respondent ranks according to his or her learning preference. For example:

"When I learn,
___ I like to deal with my feelings. (Concrete experience)
___ I like to watch and listen. (Reflective observation)
___ I like to think about ideas. (Abstract conceptualization)
___ I like to be doing things." (Active experimentation)

Completing this inventory takes 5–10 minutes. You can then compute the scores and plot them on a grid comparing your individual scores with normative data using the self-scoring key. By looking at the grid, you can quickly see your most and least preferred learning styles.

In preparing for each class, think through the student learning styles that the presentation of material will most emphasize. That is, are students asked to observe, theorize, or engage in a practical activity? Whether one uses Kolb's Learning Styles Inventory or another learning inventory, the intent is to become aware of individual learning style preferences and how they influence teaching and student learning. The goal for academic and clinical educators is to expand their understanding and use of all possible learning styles so that individual students as well as collective groups of students can get the most out of each learning opportunity.

Objectives

The last column in the top of the preactive teaching grid contains objectives (see Figure 2-1). Objectives identify for student and teacher specifically what the student is to learn as a result of the class or course. There are three types of objectives: (1) behavioral, (2) problem solving, and (3) outcome.

Behavioral Objective

The most popular and most extensively used type of objective is the behavioral objective. The behavioral objective has three parts.

1. *Condition*: In what situation is the student to perform?
2. *Behavior*: In what action is the student to engage?
3. *Criterion*: What is considered acceptable and unacceptable performance?

An example of a behavioral objective is, "Given a patient immediate postop hip surgery (condition), the student will be able to identify and state the rationale (behavior) for three primary contraindications at a level of 90% accuracy or above (criterion)." The key to writing a behavioral objective is to specify an observable behavior, such as the behaviors identified under the cognitive, affective, and psychomotor domains in Figures 2-3, 2-4, and 2-5. Thus, the student is asked to engage in a behavior that can be seen and evaluated, such as describe (cognitive), demonstrate (psychomotor), or defend (affective). As more complex learning behaviors are required of students, action verbs in the higher levels of the three domains can be used to guide the teaching/learning content. By identifying specific behaviors rather than expecting students to "know" or "understand" material, the expected level of performance is much clearer to students and the teacher.

Even partial behavioral objectives, which identify at least the content area of knowledge to be acquired and the level of mastery (behavior) but not the grading criterion, are useful in identifying for the student what is to be achieved by her or his efforts. At the beginning of each chapter in this book, partial behavioral objectives are stated to identify for the reader what is to be gained from reading the chapter. Obviously, if the reader is able to perform the stated objectives there is no need to read the chapter!

The problem with focusing teaching only on a list of behavioral objectives is that education is and should be more than the sum of a list of behavioral objectives. Along with behaviors that can be seen and measured, teachers also hope to stimulate and accentuate in students such behaviors as insight, curiosity, creativity, and tolerance. Additionally, students will encounter an endless number of situations in the chaotic world of clinical practice for which they would be ill prepared if the curriculum focused solely on the competencies stated in behavioral objectives. Teaching students to learn constantly from the clinical practice environment (lifelong learning) requires setting up the type of objectives that alert students to the complex skills required of them in clinical practice.

Problem-Solving Objective

The problem-solving learning objective poses a "problem" for the student to solve. In solving a problem, the student will be asked to move beyond specific predictable behaviors, demonstrate analysis of a situation, and provide a reasonable solution. Often, many different solutions/behaviors will solve a single problem. For example, students might be given a series of short clinical cases. For each case, students individually or in small groups might be asked to determine additional evaluative information they will need to treat this patient and give a rationale for why they need that information. Each student or group of students might identify somewhat different evaluative information—and all may be "right."

The following is an example of a problem-solving objective and a brief clinical case. Problem-solving objective: Determine the additional evaluative information you need to provide treatment for the following clinical case(s) and provide a rationale for your evaluation choices.

> Mrs. Gonzales is a 76-year-old Hispanic female with a history of left hemiplegia of approximately 1 year. She fell 8 weeks ago and sustained a Colles' fracture of the right wrist. She was seen late last week by her orthopedist, Dr. Barbara Feigenbaum, who removed the cast and referred Mrs. Gonzales to physical therapy for evaluation and treatment.

Students at different levels of academic and clinical education will give different answers regarding evaluative information needed based on classroom materials and prior clinical encounters. Note that in stating a problem-solving objective, only general rather than specific student behaviors are identified. Thus, rather than focusing on a predetermined behavioral outcome, what is stressed is thinking through the materials or situations presented and "solving" the related problem(s).

Outcome Objective

Outcome objectives are comprehensive, broad-based objectives that specify practice expectations for students and teachers. The APTA's Normative Model of Physical Therapist Professional Education identifies 19 of these practice expectations, which can be used to guide course content and learning experiences for physical therapy students.[26] For example:

1. Demonstrate clinical decision-making skills, including clinical reasoning, clinical judgment, and reflective practice. (Practice expectation 4.2)
2. Educate others using a variety of teaching methods that are commensurate with the needs and unique characteristics of the learner. (Practice expectation 5.1)

3. Promote health by providing information on wellness, disease, impairment, functional limitation, disability, and health risks related to age, gender, culture, and lifestyle within the scope of physical therapy practice. (Practice expectation 15.2)

Under each of these outcome objectives (called Terminal Behavioral Objectives in the APTA document), specific behavioral objectives (called Instructional Objectives in the APTA document) are used to identify the knowledge and skills needed by the student to achieve the outcome objective. See the example in Table 1-2.

For any class, course, or curriculum any number of behavioral objectives and problem-solving objectives could be created to guide the coursework and student learning to prepare students for practice expectations (outcome objectives). Academic and clinical educators can use objectives to clarify and order learning experiences for different levels of physical therapy and physical therapist assistant students. In addition, writing objectives is the final step in stimulating student learning behaviors that are congruent with how the teacher has conceived the philosophical orientations, learning theories, domains of learning, and student learning styles that will receive focus for any class, course, or clinical experience.

Lower Half of the Preactive Teaching Grid

As can be seen in the lower half of the preactive teaching grid (see Figure 2-1), the next steps are to consider the types of delivery format and prepare relevant computer-based or audiovisual materials and handouts. The delivery format(s) selected should logically be related to the elements in the top half of the preactive teaching grid. Thus, for example, if the teacher was primarily interested in philosophical orientation of cognitive processing-reasoning, using the gestalt–problem solving learning theory, with a focus on the cognitive and affective domains of learning and emphasizing the abstract conceptualization student learning style, the format of delivery likely would be a seminar-discussion focused on case materials rather than a lecture. A thorough discussion of classroom delivery formats is presented in Chapters 3 and 4.

The teacher also must start thinking about how to evaluate students' knowledge well before the first day of class. Evaluations of students are events when students and faculty see how well they have engaged the teaching-learning process. Evaluations should be consistently related to the elements in the preactive teaching grid and specifically guided by the course objectives that have focused the course content and student learning. A basic educational truth is that the better students perform on all types of evaluations, the better the teacher has thoughtfully employed the pedagogical aspects of teaching to best engage students in their own learning. Thus, student evaluations demonstrate the level of success of teachers as well as students. Suggestions for different types of student evaluation are presented in Chapter 3.

Teaching Environment

Note that the last element in the preactive teaching grid before actually preparing the learning experience is attention given to the physical teaching environment. Preactive teaching includes content and format preparation well in advance as well as arriving at the classroom early to attend to the room arrangement and the room environment (including cleanliness and temperature) and being sure that all media and materials needed for teaching are available and working. Stand quietly in any empty classroom. Think of the impact on student learning of half-empty coffee cups and food wrappers from prior classes, dirty media equipment that is a rat's nest of electrical cords, bulletin boards that are empty or contain woefully outdated information, ceiling lights that have expired, and seating arrangements that make you invisible to students (and vice versa).

Make friends with the people from the housekeeping department, the media department, and administrative assistants in the dean's office. Work with them to create clean and inviting learning environments. Even if the classroom is used by many different faculty and student groups, assess and set up an effective learning climate for your students in your class. Your efforts, part of the implicit curriculum, will not go unnoticed or unappreciated by students or colleagues.

Preparing a Course Syllabus

Preparing a course syllabus is an excellent way of dealing with the often-paralyzing gap between what one would like to teach and the reality of the time available for teaching. From the students' perspective, a course syllabus provides a complete overview of the course content, course requirements, and timeline on the first day of class.[27] This overview allows students to organize their semester in a way that best promotes their learning and achievement. Table 2-2 contains a list of items that are often included in a course syllabus.

Note that in this course syllabus example, the course requirements are placed in Section A on the first page of the syllabus. Course requirements are the first thing students will want to see. Thus, placing these requirements on the first page of the syllabus (and detailing them later in Section D) will keep students from scrambling through the syllabus trying to find out how many

Table 2-2 Contents of a Course Syllabus

A. Name of university and department
Course title, course number and number of credits
Day(s) of week, time of day, and place course is held
Name and title of instructor
Phone number, FAX number, e-mail address
Office location and number
Office hours
Course requirements (e.g., type of exams, papers, small group projects, and so on, and the percentage each counts toward the final grade)
Classroom teaching philosophy
Attendance policy
Policy on incompletes and time extensions
B. List of course objectives
C. Required and recommended reading list
D. Detailed information regarding required papers, projects, and field experiences (e.g., content, length, resources needed, due date)
E. Course outline
Date
Topic to be covered
Required reading assignments to be accomplished

---

exams and projects will be included in the course and how much each will count while you are attempting to focus their attention on the course objectives (Section B).

Draw the student's attention to important items in your syllabus by bolding, bulleting, using graphics, color, etc. Early in the syllabus is also a good place to briefly share your classroom teaching philosophy and expectations for student presence and involvement in your class. The following example is from a course on the Psychology of Illness and Wellness Behaviors:

> **Philosophy and focus of this course related to your presence:**
> This class is about human beings—you and the people you interact with personally and professionally. The information presented and ideas exchanged during lectures or seminars and highlighted from required readings will be essential to the well-being of the patients and families you will treat and to your own health and effectiveness as a health care professional. As much active learning takes place during class time as during outside reflection and reading. A missed class means you miss stimulation for awareness of your personal attitudes, beliefs, and value judgments. You are urged to attend all lectures and

seminars. You may miss one class during the semester for your personal "low-ebb day," which may be taken for any reason.

Class participation: Each student is urged to participate freely and honestly in sharing the facts, impressions, and perceptions that constitute her or his reality. I believe that although students may hold some misinformation regarding their own and others' behaviors, there is very little right or wrong—only less effective and more effective ways to work with others. You will discover your own unique mode of effectiveness through active participation in class-related activities both in and out of the classroom setting.

Model good intellectual behaviors in your syllabus. Remember the implicit curriculum. What are you telling students by presenting incomplete information for reference sources, including last year's dates and misspelled words? Thus, give *complete* and *consistent citations* for required and recommended readings (e.g., author, title, journal [or publisher], year of publication, volume number, page numbers). Carefully review your syllabus for accuracy—dates, spelling, sentence structure, etc. Remember that preparing a good course syllabus takes time and that being only "one step ahead of the students" is reserved for first-year novice teachers.

Finally, give students a sense of fun and adventure about the learning they are to engage in. For example, ending your syllabus with a statement such as, "I am delighted to be your guide on this journey we are about to embark on together!" rather than a "law enforcement" message regarding poor performance sets the stage for a respectful and enjoyable mutual teaching-learning adventure.

Summary

This chapter has provided a broad overview of the elements a PT or physical therapy assistant educator should consider before, and in concert with, preparing the course content and conducting the academic teaching-learning experience. That is, it covers the preactive teaching elements or pedagogical principles, including philosophical orientations, learning theories, domains of learning, learning styles, and objectives that form the teaching-learning framework of a course. This chapter, along with Chapters 3 and 4, suggests a number of ways (pedagogical knowledge) to think about organizing, conducting, and evaluating classes and courses in a manner that supports learning and learning to love learning.

References

1. Brophy J. Teachers' Knowledge of Subject as it Relates to Their Teaching Practice. Greenwich, CT: JAI Press, 1991.
2. Grossman PL. The Making of a Teacher: Teacher Knowledge and Teacher Education. New York: Teachers College Press, 1990.
3. Reynolds A. What is competent beginning teaching? A review of the literature. Rev Educ Res 1992;62:1.
4. Irby D. What clinical teachers in medicine need to know. Acad Med 1994;69:333.
5. Kolb DA. Learning Styles Inventory. Boston: McBer and Co., 1985.
6. Dickinson R, Dervitz H, Meida H. Handbook for Physical Therapy Teachers. New York: American Physical Therapy Association, 1967.
7. Jackson P. The Practice of Teaching. New York: Teachers College Press, 1986;1–30.
8. Schön D. Educating the Reflective Practitioner. San Francisco: Jossey-Bass, 1987.
9. Eisner EW. The Educational Imagination. On the Design and Evaluation of School Programs. New York: Macmillan, 1979.
10. Solomon P. Problem-based learning: direction for physical therapy education? Physiother Theory Pract 1994;10:45.
11. Boud D, Feletti GE. The Challenge of Problem-Based Learning (2nd ed). London: Kogan Page, 1997.
12. Neurology Report. American Physical Therapy Association, 1996;20:1.
13. Neil AS. Summerhill: A Radical Approach to Child Rearing. New York: Hart, 1960.
14. Phillips DC, Soltis JF. Perspectives on Learning (2nd ed). New York: Teachers College Press, 1991.
15. Thorndike EL. Educational Psychology: The Psychology of Learning. New York: Teachers College Press, 1913.
16. Skinner BF. Science and Human Behavior. New York: Macmillan, 1966.
17. Archambault RD. John Dewey on Education: Selected Writings. Chicago: University of Chicago Press, 1974.
18. Piaget J. Psychology of Intelligence. Paterson, NJ: Littlefield Adams, 1969.
19. Gagne RM. The Conditions of Learning. New York: Holt, Rinehart & Winston, 1970.
20. Bloom B (ed). Taxonomy of Educational Objectives, Handbook I: The Cognitive Domain. New York: David McKay, 1956.
21. Krathwohl DR, Bloom BS, Masia BB. Taxonomy of Educational Objectives, Handbook II: Affective Domain. New York: David McKay, 1964.
22. Simpson EJ. The Classification of Educational Objectives in the Psychomotor Domain. Washington, DC: Gryphon House, 1972.

23. Sierpina VS. Progress Notes: University of Minnesota Center for Spirituality and Healing. Alternative Therapies 2001;7:85–86.

24. Harasym PH, Leong EJ, Juschka BB, et al. Myers-Briggs psychological type and achievement in anatomy and physiology. Am J Physiol 1995; 268:561.

25. Theis SL, Merritt SL. Learning style preferences of elderly coronary artery disease patients. Educ Gerontol 1992;18:677.

26. American Physical Therapy Association. A Normative Model of Physical Therapist Professional Education: Version 2000. Alexandria, VA: American Physical Therapy Association, 2000.

27. Davis BG. Tools for Teaching. San Francisco: Jossey-Bass, 1993.

Annotated Bibliography

Boud D, Feletti GE. The Challenge of Problem-Based Learning (2nd ed). London: Kogan Page, 1997. An excellent six-part book with 48 contributors that covers the use, strengths, and limitations of problem-based learning. The six parts include a description of what problem-based learning is and what it isn't, how to get started developing a problem-based curriculum, suggestions for design as well as how to implement problem-based learning (e.g., faculty training needed), examples of problem-based learning from different professions, such as engineering, social work, and nursing, how to assess student knowledge, as well as how to evaluate problem-based learning programs, and some unique models of problem-based learning. Strongly recommended for educators who are considering implementing a problem-based learning program.

Davis BJ. Tools for Teaching. San Francisco: Jossey-Bass, 1993. This book is filled with hundreds of good ideas that reinforce a nonpunitive approach to teaching and testing. Covers the gamut of teaching from producing a syllabus to teaching a diverse classroom of students to holding office hours. These tools can be used by novice, midlevel, and experienced educators to improve their teaching. There are especially good sections on evaluating students' written work and testing and grading that are guaranteed to stimulate your thinking regarding creative ideas for the use of testing to reinforce learning.

Gronlund NE. How to Write and Use Instructional Objectives (6th ed). Upper Saddle River, NJ: Merrill Education, Prentice-Hall, 2000. This is a classic paperback text for assisting teachers in writing instructional objectives. The book includes three major sections: (1) how to write instructional objectives, (2) writing objectives for various outcomes (across the cognitive, affective, and psychomotor domains), and (3) how to use objectives for teaching and assessment. The author provides extensive examples throughout the book, including a set of well-known appendices that give specific examples of objectives and "illustrative verbs" that can be used to identify student learning behaviors.

Phillips DC, Soltis JF. Perspectives on Learning (2nd ed). New York: Teachers College Press, 1991. Shortest, most interesting, and readable book available on learning theories.

Stage FK, Muller PA, Kinzie J, Simmons A. Creating Learning Centered Classrooms: What Does Learning Theory Have to Say? ASHE-ERIC Higher Education Report Volume 26, No. 4, Washington, DC: The George Washington University, Graduate School of Education and Human Development, 1998. This well-referenced monograph goes beyond traditional theories of learning to describe motivational and sociocultural theories relevant to higher education. Each theory (e.g., attribution theory) is presented along with examples, research, and implications for learning. Although the authors focus on undergraduate education, the theories and applications can be easily transferred into any learning environment.

3

Techniques for Teaching and Evaluating Students in Academic Settings

Gail M. Jensen and Katherine F. Shepard

As you walk into the physical therapy classroom—also used as the laboratory—you are hoping that you will be able to cover all of your material in the next 50 minutes. The students drag into the room having just finished a 3-hour anatomy dissection laboratory. They disperse themselves all over the classroom/laboratory and look like they could hardly stay awake for the next hour. You think to yourself, "Thank goodness, I don't want too many questions anyway and just need to get through this material so that we can get on with laboratory session tomorrow." In this coming hour, you are to give the overview lecture for the upcoming laboratory session on clinical measurement. You are very comfortable teaching the laboratory portion of goniometry and manual muscle testing, but a bit nervous about having to cover measurement concepts in this overview lecture; therefore, you have included several definitions of terms in your handout. You begin going through all of your overheads that complement the handout. You do try to ask a few questions of the class, but they appear to be dutifully taking notes and not very interested in interacting. So you

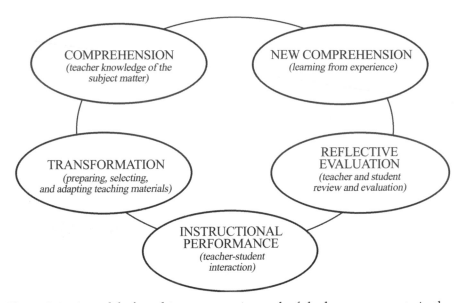

Figure 3-1   A model of teaching representing each of the key components in the teaching and learning process for teachers and students.

think to yourself, "Well that is all right, I will just get through the material and then we can have more interaction in the lab tomorrow where I am far more comfortable teaching the clinical skills."

If you were in the teaching situation described in the preceding anecdote, what could you do? How might you learn from this experience? What is going on? What are your options? Before focusing on specific techniques for teaching in academic settings, let's think about how teaching techniques or tools are part of a larger process of teaching and learning in academic settings. This chapter revisits the essential elements involved in any teaching situation: (1) content and knowledge that a teacher holds and must share with students, (2) transformation (transforming what is known into material that can be taught to others), (3) instruction (teaching performance), and (4) reflective evaluation (learning from one's teaching experience) (Figure 3-1).[1] The chapter then focuses on basic teaching and evaluation tools for large groups in the classroom from lectures to strategies for facilitating collaborative learning, teaching and evaluation tools for clinical laboratory performance, strategies for facilitating reflection and problem analysis, as well as a brief overview of teaching technologies.

Chapter Objectives

After completing this chapter, the reader will be able to

1. Describe how the four components of a "practical model for teaching" apply to experience in teaching and learning.
2. Discuss the design and implementation of effective lectures, including purposes, lecture planning, and lecture delivery. Describe techniques for facilitating interactive lectures.
3. Describe strategies for facilitating collaborative learning, including use of structured small group activities and peer teaching.
4. Justify the rationale that supports grading as a tool for learning. Describe and apply core principles that support this rationale.
5. Describe the pros and cons of various grading systems and written examination formats.
6. Apply the phases of learning psychomotor skills to teaching clinical laboratory skills.
7. Discuss how to enhance demonstrations of clinical skills and teach more complex psychomotor skills.
8. Outline the process for developing a clinical practical examination to assess psychomotor skills and reasoning/decision-making skills.
9. Identify and discuss techniques for facilitating reflection and problem analysis including case methods, concept mapping, and narratives.
10. Describe how to use portfolios and journals to facilitate and assess reflective thinking.
11. Identify the pros and cons of traditional educational technologies, including chalkboards, overhead transparencies, slides, and video and film.

A Practical Model for Teaching

Knowledge of the Subject Matter

Good teachers have a thorough knowledge of the subject matter that allows them to display more self-confidence and creativity in teaching. Investigations of teachers also demonstrate that teachers not only have information in the area but also understand how the key concepts or ideas are connected, as well as the ways in which new knowledge is created and validated.[1,2] Using the previous anecdote, remember that the instructor was nervous about having to cover measurement concepts and was unable to engage the students in any interaction during a lecture. The teacher ended up covering the material on the handout with little student interaction. Why did this happen? Perhaps the instructor, although very comfortable with teaching the clinical skills of measurement (i.e., goniometry and manual muscle testing), was much less certain of her or his knowledge of clinical measurement concepts; therefore, the instructor covered the content with little discussion. For example, in discussing the measurement concept of validity and manual muscle testing, a teacher with thorough knowledge of clinical measurement would move beyond the definition of validity to a discussion of the use of manual muscle testing for the assessment of muscle weakness. Use of muscle testing for assessing muscle strength raises a validity question.[3] Research on teachers supports this example; when teachers do not know the subject matter well, they tend to focus more on content, whereas teachers who know their subject well teach not only the content but also the practical application of key concepts and the current controversies of what is known and not known about the subject.[1,4,5]

Transformation

The transformation phase represents the teacher's ability to "transform" the material so students can understand. There are teachers who are quite expert in certain subjects, yet they are dismal teachers. A second component of teaching is the teacher's ability to do good "preactive teaching." As detailed in Chapter 2, there is specific knowledge and skill involved in taking what is known and *transforming* it in preparation for teaching. First, one must review any instructional materials in light of what is known about the subject: Are there any errors? Have things changed? Has the thinking changed in this subject? A second step in transformation is thinking about how to go about presenting the content. What learning theories will you use and what type of objectives will you focus on? Will you use a clinical case, a focused small class activity, or visual aids? A final step is deciding how to tailor your understanding of the content to students' understanding. Students are not likely to have the breadth and depth of knowledge that the instructor does. The critical issue is for the instructor to adapt what he or she knows and come up with examples or representations that fit the students' present understandings of the content.[6] In the anecdote of teaching clinical measurement, one may be discussing range of motion measures as they apply to physical impairment measures and challenge students that they will need to ultimately address any functional limitations the patient may have. In doing so, the teacher also assumes that the students remember the model of disablement that had been presented and discussed the previous week.[7] The instructor quickly discovers that the students do not understand; therefore, she or he must backtrack, using the overhead of the key model concepts and tying them in a simple and direct way to patient cases. The instructor should have students give examples of what functional limitations may result from physical impairments, and the instructor should write these on the blackboard (Figure 3-2).

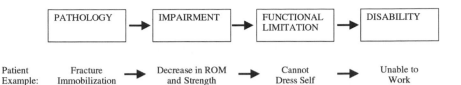

Figure 3-2 An example of a model that uses larger concepts to represent specific data from a patient case. (ROM = range of motion.) (Reprinted from A Jette. Physical disablement concepts for physical therapy research and practice. Phys Ther 1994;74:380, with permission of the American Physical Therapy Association.)

Instruction

Instruction is what is known as teaching, yet instruction is only the interactive phase or "performance" of teaching. It includes everything from pacing of the material, to classroom management, to asking and responding to questions. Many of the specific teaching tools discussed in this chapter are part of the instructional process. Active learning is frequently discussed as a key component of the instructional process.[8–10] Some general characteristics of and strategies for active learning have been suggested by Bonwell and Eison.[9] They are

1. Students do more than listen.
2. Less emphasis should be placed on transmitting information, and more emphasis should be placed on developing students' skills.
3. Students are involved in higher order thinking skills of the cognitive domain (e.g., analysis, synthesis, and evaluation).
4. Students are engaged in learning activities, such as writing, reading, or discussing.
5. Emphasis should be placed on students' exploration of their own attitudes and values.

Bonwell and Eison define *active learning* as learning that "involves students in doing things and thinking about the things they are doing."[9]

Reflective Evaluation and New Comprehension

The last two components of the model include processes of ongoing assessment and learning. This last component of the practical model for teaching is the ongoing process of learning from experience. This process of reviewing, reconstructing, and critically analyzing one's own performance and the class's performance is lifelong learning, a process that is central to teaching. For example, in the anecdote at the beginning of this chapter, the teacher found that after presenting a disablement model followed by the patient clinical measurement data the class looked perplexed and did not respond to questions. What could be done? The teacher could interrupt the class and admit that there appears to be some confusion. The teacher might then begin to go through the model again by asking students to provide their understanding of the concepts and the clinical application. The teacher could clarify each concept while going through the model with the class. This is an example of reflection. In the reflection process, a problem arises with some uncertainty, so one engages in a process of thinking critically about what is going on and alternative solution strategies. The first step involves seeing the problem. In this case, the instructor stops the class because he or she recognizes that students are confused. Then the group reviews the disablement model, which can then lead to a revised or new understanding with the instructor's guidance. The reflective process in this example is likely to lead to new understandings or comprehensions for students and teacher (see Figure 3-1). The last two sections of this chapter emphasize teaching techniques used to facilitate collaboration and reflection in the classroom.

Classroom Teaching with Large Groups

When thinking of a large class and limited time to cover a significant amount of material, the teaching tools that come to mind are lecture and discussion. If there is a great deal of content, there may be little discussion and a lot of lecture. This section addresses the formal, traditional lecture for large groups, including purposes, effective lecture design and delivery, and advantages and disadvantages of traditional lectures. This section is followed by active learning strategies for large groups, including discussion and questioning.

Lectures

A professor's response to why lecture: "It is tradition. It was part of my training, and seems like what I should be doing. I feel somehow guilty when I am not lecturing."[11]

The lecture method of teaching was a prominent method for disseminating information before the invention of mass print in the 1600s. In these lectures, the instructor would talk, while the students wrote everything down—in effect, creating their own "texts." Why is it that the lecture remains such a significant part of our teaching repertoire in the midst of ready access to information through many sources?[12,13]

What Purposes Do Lectures Serve?

Lectures are often used to transmit a lot of information efficiently to large groups of students. McKeachie summarizes the skills of a good lecturer, saying "[e]ffective lecturers combine the talents of scholar, writer, producer, comedian, showman, and teacher in ways that contribute to student learning."[12] Research comparing the lecture to other forms of teaching demonstrates that the lecture is as effective as other methods for teaching knowledge. In addition to the cognitive component, lectures can also motivate. A skilled lecturer can stimulate interest, challenge students to seek more information, and communicate passion and enthusiasm for the subject matter. Lectures can also be used as an efficient method to consolidate and integrate information from a number of different printed sources. Lecture material can be specifically adapted or tailored to the class, and difficult concepts can be clarified in lecture. Finally, lectures can set the stage for discussion or other learning activities.[12]

Perhaps the most important use of lecture is that it is a powerful tool for building the bridge between student knowledge and the structures of the subject matter. For example, imagine that a teacher is lecturing about kinesiology of the shoulder complex. The students have a strong anatomical understanding of the subject matter and some understanding of the basic biomechanical principles. It is important in this case for the teacher to use the lecture as an opportunity to facilitate mutual levels of application and understanding when presenting how concepts from anatomy and kinesiology apply to a clinical problem. The lecture also can be used to explore and analyze specific concepts or ideas, and the teacher can demonstrate her or his problem-solving process. As most teachers find out, lecture preparation involves seeking out a broad range of information and then analyzing, synthesizing, and integrating subject matter from various sources.

What Makes an Effective Lecture?

Planning

Teachers might plan a lecture as they approach writing a paper, by thinking about the overall organization, the introduction, body, and conclusion. Good overall questions to start with when planning a lecture, in contrast to "covering the subject matter," are (1) What do you really want students to remember from this lecture over time? (2) How should students process the information? (3) Are you trying to be a conclusion-oriented lecturer or is your aim to assist students to learn and think through a cognitive activity? (Review your preactive teaching grid [see Figure 2-1].)

One of the major concerns is keeping students' attention. One study reports that students recall 70% of the material covered in the first 10 minutes of class and only 20% of material covered in the last 10 minutes.[14] How does the instructor capture the students' attention? One effective strategy is to announce that the information presented will be tested; however, there are also many other ways to stimulate students' thinking and actively involve them in learning.

Introduction

An effective introduction focuses and engages the students and outlines the specific topics that will be covered and the order in which the topics will be discussed. The introduction should also identify the gap between the students' existing cognitive knowledge and the topic, or it should raise questions. Pre-questions can be used to focus students toward the intent of the lecture. For example, imagine that the topic is an introduction to the role of culture in professional-patient interactions. One may begin the lecture by standing in the back of the room (not the front) to talk to the class. The teacher may ask the class to share observations about the traditional role of the teacher and then proceed to ask questions about students' meanings of classroom behavior—that is, the culture of the classroom. Another useful technique is to begin with a story or a case that highlights the relevance and importance of the lecture subject matter.[12]

Body

The body of the lecture should fit with the students' ability to process information. Perhaps the most common error of the novice teacher is to try to put too much information into the lecture. This occurs when the teacher overestimates the students' ability to grasp the information and see the relationship between concepts and applications. Russell et al.[14] demonstrated that increasing the density of a lecture reduces the students' retention of basic information. Often, trying to present too much information is the result of inadequate preparation in which the teacher has not clearly identified the key concepts.

The lecture should not be written out verbatim, but an outline can be very effective in guiding the body of the lecture. The use of graphic representations, computer flow charts, or models can provide the class with a representation of the structure of the material presented. The instructor can also place cues in the lecture outline margins or notes that include learning strategies to be used along the way (e.g., the use of overheads, stimulating questions, different types of explanations, or brief dyad discussions among students).[12,15]

A single class usually represents a diverse group of learners. Some students may do better with a *deductive process*—that is, going from a sequence of generalizations to specific application—whereas other students may do better with a more *inductive process*—that is, moving from the specifics to the general concepts. The use of an outline and a visual structure provides cues for both groups.[16] An easy rule of thumb for a great lecture is a simple framework and lots of examples.[12] The following are additional tips for facilitating student comprehension[12]:

1. Use visual representations.
2. Develop the idea or concept, then give examples. Reiterate your initial point.
3. Pauses give students time to think—give periodic summaries in your lecture. You do not have to cover everything.
4. Check for understanding.

Conclusion

The conclusion is a time to summarize the important points of the lecture by going back over the outline or key graphics. The teacher may also use this as an opportunity to have students summarize the material orally or in writing. Other strategies include having the students do a 3-minute writing exercise summarizing the major points of the lecture or looking at student lecture notes to see what they are writing to determine if they grasped key concepts. These methods provide additional information about the students' understandings of the lecture.[12,15]

Lecture Delivery

Earlier in this chapter, we stated that instruction can be thought of as performance, and lecture delivery provides one of the most obvious chances to perform. Passion and enthusiasm for the subject matter are key aspects of any lecture. The teacher is a powerful role model in front of the class and represents a thoughtful scholar to the students. The following are five tips for improving lecture presentation[17]:

1. *Create movement.* Change your position in the room. Do not remain anchored at the podium.
2. *Use visuals.* Use various visual teaching tools (e.g., overheads, the blackboard, charts, graphs). These visuals are particularly good for highlighting key points. Videotapes can be powerful tools for illustrating examples from the real world in the clinic or community.
3. *Pay attention to the effect of the voice.* The voice can vary in terms of volume, rate, and tone. If your voice is not loud enough for the class to hear, a microphone may be necessary. Beware of avoiding a monotone delivery. Voice is one of the key ingredients for communicating enthusiasm to the

students. The use of audiotape or videotape can be a helpful feedback mechanism for assessing how you use your voice.

4. *Pay attention to body language.* In addition to the voice, teachers also communicate with students through nonverbal language. Be aware of nervous habits, such as playing with the pointer, jingling change, or any other persistent movement of the hands. Use body language to communicate points of emphasis and enthusiasm.

5. *Pace the delivery and clarify the material.* As stated earlier, two common elements of excellent lectures are a simple plan with a structure and the use of numerous examples.[12] The structure of the lecture provides the foundation for pacing the delivery of the material. Observe the audience to see if they are keeping up with note taking, are confused, or need more time for questions. A second consideration is how to go about clarifying difficult concepts. In the previous section on transformation, we advocated that teachers are responsible for transforming ideas to assist learning. Ideas can be represented through analogies or metaphors. For example, performing a grade-1 mobilization movement can be described as having "a fly doing deep knee bends" to over-illustrate how small the movement is. A metaphor can be useful for having students think expansively and creatively. For example, which metaphor best describes the work of a physical therapist or physical therapist assistant: teacher, gardener, business executive, or healer?

Perhaps the greatest advantage of the lecture is that it is economical, particularly when the teacher has lots of students and little time. The strongest disadvantages are the passive role of the students and the lack of student engagement in higher order cognitive objectives (e.g., analysis, evaluation). One quick classroom assessment technique for determining if sudents are attending to and grasping the lecture materials is called the *Punctuated Lecture*.[5] The Punctuated Lecture includes

- Listen: Students listen to the teacher's presentation
- Stop: Teacher stops the presentation
- Reflect: Students are asked to reflect on what they were doing while they were listening and how their behaviors enhanced or hindered their ability to listen and understand the material
- Write: Students then write down their reflections (anonymously)
- Feedback: Students provide feedback to the teacher

Many campuses have centers for instructional support that have additional resources and ideas for improving lecture presentations. One excellent resource, by Westberg and Jason, is listed in the annotated reference list at the end of this chapter.

The Interactive Lecture: Role of Discussion and Questioning in Large Group Settings

Initiating the Class Discussion

Questioning and discussion are two tools for moving to a more interactive lecture within a large group. The teacher can move from lecture, to discussion, to questioning, and then back to lecture. Class discussion, however, is not something to do when the lecture material runs out or as a way to extend the lecture. A good discussion, just as the lecture, is done with planning and purpose. A discussion usually starts with a question. This question could be focused on a common experience (e.g., a reaction to a visual, a videotape, or a story). Another good strategy is to begin with controversy or a debate. With this strategy, the class could be divided into two or more large groups and be given the task of developing a position. A third idea is to begin by having students brainstorm what they know about the topic; then the teacher can use these ideas to build a framework consistent with the students' understandings and discuss with the group any misconceptions.[9,10]

Another well-known technique is the use of Socratic dialogue or discussion. This approach has been used extensively in the education of lawyers. In this method, teachers focus on teaching from a known case to general principles, thus teaching students to think like a lawyer. The general questioning strategy is to use a known case to formulate general principles, and then these principles are applied to new cases.[12] For example, you might begin by discussing the following with students:

> Imagine that your patient asks you to not document in the medical record that he has been playing softball, even though he is still unable to return to work with his low back pain. Ask students to identify all the factors that might lead a patient to ask a therapist to do that. Then you might ask students what they would do if they were the therapist and why? Now ask the students to talk about the importance of the medical record and the professional's responsibility to be honest. As you discuss this case, you begin to introduce the general ethical principle of beneficence. Then you can move and talk about deception, and how the principle of beneficence would apply or not apply in this case. Then you propose a second case wherein the therapist does not exactly record the "truth" in the medical record. Now the therapist is involved in deception because he or she wants to make sure the patient gets the additional rehabilitation that is necessary to get the patient back to work.

These two cases can be discussed, looking for the differences and then applying the ethical principle of beneficence.

Common Discussion Problems

The two most common discussion problems are students who talk too much or too little. There are a number of reasons why students may be silent in the classroom (e.g., fear of looking stupid, prior bad experiences such as being mocked or berated, or even shyness). What can be done about students who do not talk during discussion? A supportive classroom environment is a key element. It involves more than encouraging students to participate. To have a supportive classroom environment, the teacher must create an emotional and intellectual climate supportive of risk taking. The following are suggestions for facilitating a supportive classroom environment[9,10]:

1. Learn the students' names.
2. Demonstrate a strong interest in students as individuals and be sensitive to subtle messages they give about the material or presentation.
3. Respond to students' feelings about class assignments and be willing to listen.
4. Encourage and invite students' questions and be interested in hearing their personal viewpoints. Consider having students write down their questions first then ask them to share with the class.
5. Demonstrate interest in the importance of students' understanding of the material.
6. Encourage students to be creative and independent in reacting to the material. Begin by asking students to share their perceptions or ideas about general questions that do not have a right or wrong answer.
7. Pay attention to the physical environment of the classroom. Even though you may be lecturing, you still want the physical environment to encourage active learning. For example in traditional classrooms and auditorium style classrooms where most lectures take place, think about having students sit so that they can easily do quick interactions in twos or threes as learning partners.[10]

What about the student who talks too much and responds to every question? McKeachie[12] suggests the following options for large groups:

1. Ask the class if they would like the participation more evenly distributed.
2. Audiotape a discussion and play it back for class analysis on how to improve the discussion.
3. Assign class observers who observe participation and report to the class.
4. Speak directly with the student outside of class.

Table 3-1 Teacher Behaviors That Inhibit Discussion

Insufficient waiting time for student response
Quick reinforcement of student responses, or "rapid rewards"
A programmed answer
Nonspecific feedback questions
Too much teacher talk
Low level of questions; questions with "yes" or "no" responses
Intrusive questions
Judgmental responses
Interrupting student responses
Hiding behind the role of the teacher

Source: Adapted from S Eaton, GL Davis, P Benner. Discussion stoppers in teaching. Nurs Outlook 1977;25:578.

Finally, what kinds of actions have the potential to stifle discussion? Frequently, a teacher can slow a discussion by talking more than engaging in actual discussion with students. Eaton et al.[16] identified several key teacher behaviors as inhibitory in student discussions (Table 3-1).

Questioning

Questioning is an important teaching strategy that can facilitate the process of active learning. In questioning, students are asked to link concepts, evaluate ideas, or apply knowledge. Skilled teachers use questions to guide the student's thought process. To be able to ask effective questions, one needs to understand more about levels or types of questions and when to apply them.

One simple model classifies questions under three types: (1) concrete, (2) abstract, and (3) creative.[12] Concrete questions generally focus on a recall of facts, literal meaning, and simple ideas. These are the "who, what, where, and when" questions. Abstract questions have students generalize, classify, or reason to a conclusion about the facts presented. These are the "how" and "why" questions. Creative questions ask students to reorganize concepts into a new pattern that may require abstract and concrete thinking. The teacher may ask, "What would happen if?" or "How else could you go about?"

A more frequently used classification system is based on the cognitive domain of Bloom's taxonomy, as discussed in Chapter 2. This domain has been used to classify educational objectives. Table 3-2 provides examples of each level of the cognitive domain along with key concepts and example words for initiating questions.

Table 3-2 Examples of Classifications of Questions in the Cognitive Domain

Category (cognitive domain)	Cognitive requirement	Concept	Examples of questions/words
Knowledge	Recall information	Memorization Description	What, when, who, which, list, name, describe
Comprehension	Understanding (questions can be answered by restating material in a literal manner)	Explanation Illustration	Compare, contrast, conclude, distinguish, explain, give an example of, illustrate
Application	Solving (questions involve problem solving in new situations)	Solution Application	Apply, build, consider, demonstrate (in a new situation) how would
Analysis	Exploration of reasoning (questions require the student to break the idea into its component parts)	Induction Deduction	Support your assumptions, what reasons, what evidence supports the conclusion, what behaviors
Synthesis	Creating (questions require students to combine ideas into a statement)	Productive thinking	Think of a way, create, propose a plan, suggest
Evaluation	Judging (questions require students to make a judgment about something by using judgment principles)	Judgment Selection	Choose, evaluate in terms of, judge, select on the basis of, which would you consider, defend, which policy

Source: Reprinted with permission from J Craig, G Page. The questioning skills of nursing instructors. J Nurs Educ 1981;20:20.

Questioning Techniques

In addition to being aware of the type of question being asked, a teacher should attend to technique or performance in the classroom. The following are recommendations for effective questioning techniques[9]:

1. Use open-ended, not closed-ended (i.e., questions that can be answered with "yes" or "no") questions.

2. Plan ahead to have key questions that will provide structure.
3. Avoid combining too many concepts or ideas and phrasing an ambiguous question.
4. Ask your questions logically and sequentially.
5. Use different levels of questions, going from simple to more complex, or higher order, questions.
6. Allow adequate thinking time for students—in other words, keep quiet. Research has shown that most teachers allow less than 1 second of silence before asking another question or reemphasizing, and that when teachers wait 3–5 seconds, the number and length of appropriate responses increase.[17]
7. Follow up with student responses by making a reflective statement or using deliberative silence.
8. Try to ask and use types of questions that are aimed at broad student participation. For example, after a response, ask for additions to the response.

Strategies for Facilitating Collaborative Learning

The best answer to the question, "What is the most effective method of teaching?" is that it depends on the goal, the student, the content, and the teacher. But the next best answer is, "Students teaching other students."[12]

This section covers several teaching strategies that provide opportunities for collaborative learning. These collaborative strategies include small group work for learning tasks, discussions, seminars, tutorials, peer teaching, and other strategies.

Small Groups Process: Why Group Work?

Group work is an effective teaching and learning strategy for achieving intellectual goals (e.g., conceptual learning, creative problem solving) and social goals (e.g., oral communication, decision making, conflict management). Working in groups is part of many professional workplace activities.[18,19] Two primary types of learning that lead to effective group work are collaboration and cooperative learning. Although not as much research on collaborative learning has been done in higher education, the findings from primary and secondary school research are relevant.[5,18,19] One of the most consistent findings is that students learn better through noncompetitive, collaborative group work than in classrooms that are highly individualized and competitive. A second element supporting group work is related to our understanding of knowledge. All knowledge, including scientific knowledge, has an element of "social construction" (i.e., knowledge includes the shared understandings within the group or discipline). Bruffee[19] argues that in higher education, teachers should work toward cultivating students' intellectual interdependence through collaborative learning. Students need to experience that knowledge is not transferred from one person's head to another, but that knowledge is a consensus among members of a community of knowledgeable peers; it is dynamic understandings among people.

The role of the lecture and discussions in large class settings was discussed earlier. Small group work is another teaching strategy to engage students in large classes in active learning. In any small-group process, there will always be issues of leadership, individual performance, and communication. Therefore, the use of small groups requires the same careful preparation and planning as a good lecture.

Preparation for Small Group Work

Students need to be prepared for successful group work. The following are two key concepts central to good small group work[18]:

1. *Learning to be responsive to the needs of the group.* Responsiveness to the needs of the group is a skill required for any cooperative task. Awareness of this skill can be facilitated through small-group game activities, such as "broken circles," in which the group must cooperate to solve the group problem[20] (see Appendix 3-A).

2. *Developing a norm of cooperation and working toward equal participation.* Having students learn about working toward equal participation is another important norm for small groups, whether the group's task is discussion, decision making, or creative problem solving. Only when students believe that everyone in the group should have a say can any future problems of dominance be handled. Students need to appreciate that group leadership is a function shared between group members.[18,19] A small-group exercise called Epstein's four-stage rocket[21] is a good preparatory exercise for facilitating small-group cooperative behaviors (see Appendix 3-B).

After students have gone through some initial group training, group work can be used as a teaching strategy. The following are basic ground rules for using small groups[18,19]:

1. A group size of five to seven is optimal. Larger groups may be used when the task is so large that it needs to be subdivided.

2. Groups should be diverse in terms of gender, academic achievement, and any other status characteristics that could influence group interaction. Allowing students to choose their own groups and work with their friends is usually not a good idea.
3. The teacher must delegate authority and let go. The teacher is the direct supervisor who defines the task and suggests how the group might go about accomplishing the task, but the teacher is not in charge.
4. If the overall goal is conceptual learning, then the learning task should require conceptual thinking rather than application of technique or information recall.
5. The group must have the necessary resources to complete the tasks or assignments.

Group Expert Technique

The group expert technique is an extremely powerful tool that builds confidence and collegiality among group members and can cover several example cases. The technique involves two divisions of the class into small groups (Figure 3-3). In the first division, each small group is given a different task (e.g., different patient cases to analyze). At this time, the teacher circulates around the class to make sure each group is on the right track. Each individual in the group must be an expert on solving the case, because the class is then divided again, mixing representatives from each of the patient case groups. In this second division, each group member is an expert on a particular patient case. The task for the second group division is to discuss each of the patient cases with the resident expert available to facilitate the discussion. This small-group strategy provides the class with a variety of patient problems to discuss in a short amount of time and gives each student equal status as a group expert for one case.[22]

Seminars

The seminar is another small-group teaching method usually associated with graduate study. The seminar also can be used in undergraduate and professional education after students master some content. The purpose of a seminar goes beyond discussion of an important topic and includes analysis, critique, and application of a topic. A seminar is not a class with small enrollment nor is it an undirected or unfocused discussion of a topic. A seminar is a guided discussion in which students take the intellectual initiative.[12,15] Using seminars as a teaching method requires prior planning,

Step 1: Initial Assignment:

Each student is given a handout with a number and letter assignment (e.g., 1A, 1B, 1C, 1D, 1E, 2A, 2B, 2C, 2D, 2E).

Step 2: First Group Division:

Class is divided according to numbers. Each group is given a patient case to analyze.

Step 3: Teacher Checks Out:

Teacher circulates around to all groups to make sure each group has analyzed case correctly.

Step 4: Second Division of Groups:

Class now divides a second time according to the letter assigned. This means each of the groups will have representation from each of the patient problems.

Step 5: Group Expert Discussion:

All groups discuss each of the patient problems. Every group will have a resident expert (a member from the original group) who can facilitate the discussion.

Figure 3-3   The steps involved in implementing the small-group expert technique. (Adapted from E Cohen. Designing Group Work. New York: Teachers College Press, 1986.)

explicit guidelines linked to objectives, and a clear structure for the students (see Table 3-2). The following are ideas for structuring a seminar:

1. Progress from teacher-led to student-led seminars.
2. Assign topics or allow students to select from a list of suggested topics.
3. Give responsibility for resources to students (e.g., a bibliography and readings).
4. Use guidelines for presentation format (e.g., use of audio-visuals, responsibility for facilitating discussion with entire seminar group).
5. Use peer evaluation.

Tutorials

A small-group tutorial is a specific application of group work. In recent years, several of the health professions have begun advocating the central importance of problem-based learning, using a small-group tutorial as the teaching strategy aimed at solving patient cases. Essentially, each small group of generally no more than 10 students and one facilitator is a learning group. A faculty tutor assists students in moving from teacher-centered to student-centered learning.[23] The tutor is responsible for guiding the process of learning at the metacognitive level—that is, the tutor helps students in thinking about their thinking as they work through the learning process.[5,23,24] This type of learning group can be a very effective means for students to practice skills they will need as professionals. Using learning groups may require changes in the faculty's teaching strategies as well as major or minor curriculum revisions. Refer to references in this section as well as Boud and Feletti (see the Annotated Bibliography in Chapter 2) for more information about the use of small group tutorials in problem-based learning.

Peer Teaching

Peer teaching is a critical tool for many of the collaborative learning experiences already discussed in this section. Peer teaching can be classified into five areas: (1) teaching or laboratory assistants, (2) peer tutors who work one-on-one with a student, (3) peer counseling involved in advising peers, (4) peer partnerships in which the partners alternate the roles of student and teacher, and (5) learning groups.[9] One particularly useful peer strategy is the "learning cell," a student dyad in which students alternate the role of teacher and student and ask one another questions. Use of learning cells in comparison to seminars, discussion, and independent study is a more effective teaching strategy regardless of class size, level, or the nature of the subject.[9]

Why does peer teaching and learning work? Remember that professionals read journals and attend conferences and seminars to stay up-to-date in their fields, yet most of the information is soon forgotten. If we run into a difficult case or problem, however, and have to read, consult colleagues or experts for advice, or research the literature for help, the information we gain is invariably far better retained.[24]

Peer teaching and learning provide the opportunity for elaboration of material so that students can put ideas in their own words. Successful peer interactions require that students question, explain, express opinions, admit when they are confused, listen, and correct misconceptions. Students are less threatened in peer settings, more likely to talk in small groups, and more likely to ask questions of their peers; thus, they are active participants in their learning process.[9,10,12]

Other Useful Collaborative Strategies

Brainstorming

Brainstorming is a useful initial classroom strategy for quickly facilitating creative thinking and group participation. The following is an example of guidelines for a brainstorming process applied to a physical therapist assistant laboratory session on teaching gait training activities to patients whose first language is not English[9,12]:

1. *All ideas are fair game and should be recorded even if they seem off the mark.* The class generates a list of ideas, such as demonstrate the task, draw pictures, get a translator, just take the patient through the motions (don't talk), and demonstrate the task on another person first.

2. *There is no judgment rendered of the initial list of ideas until all the ideas have been generated.* That is, no one in the class is allowed to judge any of the ideas until the class cannot come up with any more suggestions. This is the hardest part of brainstorming. Students have to be coached not to interrupt contributors with statements like "that won't work."

3. *The initial focus is on the quantity of ideas not the quality of ideas.* Again, keep the class focused on the number of ideas. Reward enthusiasm and creativity by cheering on the number of ideas that tumble forth.

4. *After the list is generated, combinations and transformation of ideas are encouraged.* After the list is complete, the class should discuss which of the ideas or combinations of ideas are the most practical and useful for the case. Then move the discussion to implementation.

Debate

Debate is a form of discussion that allows one to see the pros and cons of an issue. The following is an example of an issue and method for applying a framework that facilitates debate.[25] The issue is whether physical therapists or physical therapist assistants should support "cross training" of health care workers—that is, individuals trained to perform skills for more than one discipline. The following are suggested steps to debate this subject:

Step 1. Divide the class into three groups, one group that supports cross training, another group that does not support cross training, and a third group that serves as a panel of debate judges.

Step 2. The two debate groups meet to formulate a rationale in support of their position. Likewise, the panel of judges meets to discuss and formulate the criteria they will use to evaluate the debate. The criteria may include strength of the evidence, reasoning, rebuttal positions, flaws in the arguments, and so on.

Step 3. The initial affirmative and rebuttal arguments are given, using time limits.

Step 4. Debate teams meet briefly to formulate their strategy for the second round of the debate.

Step 5. Teams present timed presentations.

Step 6. Panel deliberates and presents findings.

Step 7. Entire class discusses process.

One criticism of debate is that it focuses on divergence and argument. Teachers may want students to assume positions that they are not committed to when making the initial group assignments. Remember that controversial issues work best for the debate format.

Role Play, Simulations, Games, and Expert Panels

Role playing is a form of drama in which the students spontaneously act out roles without detailed scripts. Role playing has been used in a variety of settings and most often deals with issues of human interaction. Role-playing exercises should maintain student interest and provide students with experiences that they can use to analyze their own feelings. Role playing can be used for the following purposes[12]:

1. Illustrate principles from course content and provide students practice in the skills they have learned. For example, in role playing a therapist working with a difficult patient, the principles of active listening can be applied, and both students will be practicing nonverbal and verbal skills in their interactions.

2. Develop insight into human relations problems that can be shared between students and can be used in class discussion. After students perform a brief role play, usually 3–5 minutes, they can each record their observations about the experience. These observations can be used for further analysis and discussion.

3. Develop increased awareness of one's own and others' feelings that can initially be expressed under the guise of make-believe. The role play exercise provides students with the opportunity to experience feelings in an engaging, yet controlled, setting.

Role-playing activities can be done with the entire class or with a few students as an example for the class. An essential aspect of role playing is analysis and discussion in a small or large group setting.

Games and simulations are advantageous in that students are active participants rather than passive observers. They are usually engaging, stimulating learning activities. Educational games usually involve students in some form of competition in relationship to a goal similar to an old fashioned spelling bee or television game such as Jeopardy. The use of games can be a refreshing change to traditional learning experiences, as long as the competition element does not facilitate negative behaviors among students. Whereas role playing involves a form of drama in which the learners act out roles, simulation exercises involve a controlled representation of a part of a real situation. The learner can then manipulate key elements to better understand the real situation.[17] Simulations can be fun and interesting and usually require students to use creative and divergent thinking.[12] Perhaps the most frequently used simulation in physical therapy is a disability field exercise, in which students assume the role of having a physical disability in the community. Another well-known simulation is the aging game,[26] in which students experience the changes that occur with aging.

Expert panels are another teaching strategy in which students are able to hear first-hand from experts about their experiences. These expert panels can be used to represent a broad array of expertise (e.g., physical therapists and physical therapist assistants talking about working partnerships, patients living with physical challenges, or parents coping with a child with special needs). Silberman's book, *Active Learning: 101 Strategies*, is an excellent resource for ideas on active learning strategies, many that engage students in collaborative learning.[10]

Grading in Classroom Teaching

For many teachers, making up tests, evaluating students, and assigning grades are difficult and, at times, unpleasant requirements of being a teacher. Physical therapy teachers want students to be motivated to study and learn not because of grades, but in pursuit of the knowledge and skills that will make them sound physical therapy or physical therapist assistant practitioners. Teachers also want students to be lifelong learners who are motivated by their own thirst for knowledge and are able to evaluate their own learning.[12]

Grading as a Tool for Learning

Appreciate the complexity of grading and use it as a tool for learning.[27(p10)]

No form of grading is absolutely objective; even multiple choice tests are not, as the selection and design of questions are *judgments* made by the teacher. When people say that grading systems are socially constructed and context dependent, what they mean is that there is no absolutely right system by external standards. Teachers construct grading systems to meet the needs and constraints of the teaching environment. So what can you do to facilitate using grading as a tool for learning? Here are some relevant principles of grading to consider[27]:

- Consider substituting the term "judgment" for objectivity. Your role is to establish the most thoughtful criteria and standards you can.
- Distribute your time effectively—that is, do not spend all of your time trying to render perfectly objective grades. There are other aspects of student learning that need your time.
- Be open to change. The social meaning of grading is changing all of the time. Grade inflation is a national problem and cannot be solved by an individual, but must be addressed across all institutions.
- Listen to and observe your students, as grades have different meanings to various kinds of students. Remember it is the meaning that students attach to grades that most affects their learning.
- Communicate and collaborate with your students. Grading does not have to bring on antagonism. Aim to facilitate a spirit of collaboration with students toward common goals.
- Make grading an integral part of your classroom as much as planning and teaching.
- Seize teachable moments around grading issues. Grades are powerful because they shape the interrelationships among students and teachers and carry high stakes. Informal feedback and discussion about grades can affect student attitudes and learning.
- Student learning is the primary goal, and learning should be the most important goal of grading versus reports to outsiders. There are three conditions of excellence for student learning: (1) student involvement (the amount of time and energy invested in learning), (2) high expectations, and (3) assessment and feedback.[28]

Remember your role as a teacher or guide first and a gatekeeper last. Ask yourself, How do I allocate time? You would like your emphasis to be less on grading and more on guiding (Figure 3-4). A traditional function of public school education in the United States has been the gatekeeper role in which grades are used to sort out those who are not "qualified" to advance. In professional education programs, teachers are gatekeepers at the end of the process, not the beginning. After we have demonstrated our belief in students, figure what they need and help them to learn, no matter what their backgrounds or academic history.

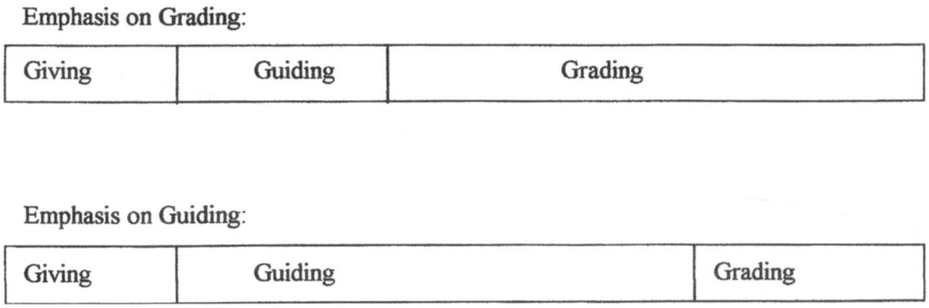

Emphasis on Grading:

Giving	Guiding	Grading

Emphasis on Guiding:

Giving	Guiding	Grading

Figure 3-4 Distribution of teaching time. (Adapted from B Walvoord, VJ Anderson. Effective Grading: A Tool for Learning and Assessment. San Francisco: Jossey-Bass, 1998.)

What do students, teachers, and employers want from grades? Students usually want to know how well they are doing and if they are succeeding in their pursuit of becoming a physical therapist or physical therapist assistant. For teachers, grading students is one of their required roles in academia. Grades provide information on how well the students are learning the material and provide a measure for assuring some minimal level of competence for preparing professionals. Employers may use grades as one factor in hiring decisions. How one feels about grades and grading is likely to depend on values and educational philosophy. Regardless of whether grades are seen as a motivator or a necessary evil, the following general guidelines should be considered[12]:

1. Avoid grading systems that put students in competition with classmates by limiting the number of high grades. This is called *grading on the curve* or the *norm-referenced model*.
2. Keep students apprised of their progress throughout the term.
3. Emphasize learning, not grades.
4. Consider allowing students some flexibility in selecting assignments for their grade (e.g., write a case report or create an educational module).
5. Deal directly with students who are upset about their grades. Listen to their complaints, think about their request, and resist pressure to change a grade because of a student's personal needs.
6. Keep accurate records of grades and use numerical grades for tests and assignments rather than letter grades whenever possible.

Grading Systems

Criterion-Referenced Grading

Criterion-referenced grading is a common system based on the student's level of achievement compared to a fixed standard, which is set by the instructor. So if all students obtained above 80 on the anatomy examination, they would all receive As or Bs. Institutions frequently set grading scales that schools and departments follow or have formulated their own numerical grading system.[12]

Norm-Referenced Grading

In norm-referenced grading, grades are assigned according to percentages of the class so that there is a normal distribution with few As, more Bs, quite a few Cs, some Ds, and a few Fs. The strict application of this system has received a fair amount of criticism and is often labeled as *educationally dysfunctional.*[12]

Competency-Based Grading

Competency-based grading is used frequently in the professions in which educational programs are responsible for preparing students for safe practice of a profession. Students are held to a standard and must demonstrate competency in performing skills or demonstrate knowledge according to specified objectives. Students who do not achieve certain objectives continue to be assessed until they demonstrate "competence." Often, an 80% cutoff is established as a definition of minimal competence.[12]

Contract Grading

In the contract-grading approach, the student must fulfill the designated aspects of the contract to receive a designated grade. The requirements for the level of contract (e.g., A or B) differ. This grading system allows the student some flexibility and opportunity to participate in the grading process. However, it is difficult to design a system in which the grade is determined not only by the fulfillment of the assigned activities but also by the quality of the work completed.[12]

Self-Grading and Peer Grading

Providing students opportunities to engage in self- and peer assessment should be an aspect of every professional educational program. Self- and peer-assessment activities will certainly be part of the student's future as an employed therapist. Self-assessment can be included as a component of a course grade for any kind of course. Portfolio development, discussed later in this chapter, is a method for facilitating self-assessment throughout the educational program. Peer assessment is frequently used for group projects and presentations. Students will provide better assessments if given explicit criteria for evaluation and if each student evaluates each of the group members.[12]

Tools for Student Evaluation

How do you motivate students to aim for high learning expectations? You must tightly integrate grading with learning and motivation. This takes us back to the central importance of carefully planned and delivered course goals. Evaluations of students are events when students and faculty see how well they have engaged the teaching-learning process. Evaluations should be consistently related to the elements in the preactive teaching grid discussed in Chapter 2. Remember the learning goals you have for your students are "operationalized" in your course objectives. These objectives focus on course content and student learning. Evaluations that closely follow the course objectives serve to reinforce this learning. A basic pedagogical truth is that the better students perform on tests, the better the teacher has organized the course materials and engaged students in their own learning. Thus, testing demonstrates the level of success of teachers as well as students.

As previously stated, the design and content of evaluation instruments should be thought through well before the first day of class. You might consider a number of different types of evaluation to give students a chance to shine in what they do best: Short answer tests, essays, projects, individual and small group work, portfolios, and class participation can all be factored into a final grade. Approach evaluation as a chance for all students to be involved in one more learning activity rather than as an event in which a number of students could fail.

The next section presents some commonly used methods of written evaluation, such as short answer tests, essays, and quick checks. Later in this chapter, a section on facilitating reflection and problem solving covers newer and perhaps even more powerful methods of evaluation that can promote students' learning and growth (e.g., the use of journals and portfolios).

Think broadly about activities that can be evaluated that could facilitate professional growth and emphasize student learning. For example, you might have the students do a book review that could be sent to a professional journal or magazine for consideration of publication. You could have students attend a research symposium and write a critique of presentation styles or attend an American Physical Therapy Association district or chapter business meeting and write a thought paper on one of the topics discussed. Evaluations should be filled with learning, fun, and professional growth whenever possible!

Examinations on Course Content

One of the best ways to identify questions to be used in written evaluations is to make notes of possible questions in color in the margins of the lecture and lab materials. Cross-check these questions with your course objective to be sure they cover important concepts and are not shallow or nitpicking. Then when it comes time to put together a test, you have already identified many good possible questions.

A word of caution: Be sure that the questions posed in any evaluation are culturally sensitive and do not reinforce stereotypes. For example, avoid "cutesy" or derogatory patient names (Mrs. Badhip), occupational and gender stereotypes (women are always housewives and men are always wage earners), and racial and socioeconomic biases (gunshot injuries are incurred only by Hispanic and African-American males). Students read examination questions with great intensity and are vulnerable to absorbing, somewhat unconsciously, these destructive stereotypes.

Short Answer Questions

Short answer questions typically require a student to identify, distinguish, state, or name something. Answers can be free format, such as simple questions or a fill-in-the-blank, or fixed format, such as true-false, multiple choice, or matching. Students can also be given a problem or case to read followed by a number of short answer questions.

Free Format Questions

The following are examples of free format questions:

- Describe bucket handle rib motion.
- Label the parts of the thoracic vertebrae in the diagram below.
- The type of justice concerned with every patient getting an appropriate share of the therapist's time is called _____ justice.
- Diagram the components of a muscle spindle.

The advantages of free format questions are that they minimize guessing, they give no clues as to correct response (tests recall not recognition), they are easy to write (alternative answers are not required as in multiple choice questions), and they can accommodate a figure, graph, or map. The disadvantages are they can be difficult to score because many different types of wording as well as content can arguably be correct, and they work best for very specific subject matter, such as anatomy and biomechanics. Fill-in-the-blank questions are more difficult to write because there must be a sufficient, but not overabundant, amount of clues that direct the student to a one- or two-word response.

Fixed Format Questions

TRUE OR FALSE QUESTIONS

The following are examples of true or false questions:

- T or F   The extensor digitorum, extensor indices, and extensor digiti minimi are the main muscles responsible for extending the interphalangeal joints of the fingers.

- T or F   The legal concept in which offensive touching is done without the consent of the person being touched is called battery.

The advantages of true or false questions are they are easy to write and can be answered quickly. The disadvantages and possible solutions are

- When guessing, a student has a 50% chance of being right. This can be remedied by asking the student to change a false item to read true, which decreases guessing.
- It is difficult to avoid ambiguity. This can be remedied by thinking about the key point you want to make and focusing on the accuracy of key names, actions, or concepts rather than on obscure points, such as whether a fact should be singular or plural.

MULTIPLE-CHOICE QUESTIONS

The following are examples of multiple-choice questions:

Which assistive device requires the least amount of coordination?
    a. Tripod cane
    b. Walker
    c. Forearm crutches
    d. Axillary crutches
Patients with genu vara tend to develop degenerative changes at the
    a. medial facet of the patellofemoral joint.
    b. medial aspect of the femorotibial joint.
    c. lateral aspect of the femorotibial joint.
    d. lateral facet of the femorotibial joint.

Advantages of multiple-choice questions are that well-constructed questions can measure knowledge and comprehension as well as application and analysis (i.e., higher levels of the cognitive domain), they are very easy to grade and can be scored by a computer, and a great deal of material can be covered quickly and in a single question.

The following are disadvantages of multiple-choice questions and possible solutions[12,15]:

- It is difficult to write plausible distractors. Try to think of at least three good distractors that are equal in length and parallel in structure to the correct answer. Do not overuse "all of the above" or "none of the above" for lack of inspiration in finding good distractors. Errors commonly made by students are a good source of distractors. Again, focus on major points related to your course objectives. Avoid triviality and irrelevance.
- Refrain from using words such as "always," "never," "all," or "none." Students know that few facts or concepts are always true.

- A certain degree of success can be obtained through guessing or figuring out in what order the instructor is likely to put the correct answer. Teachers are more systematic than they think. Given four choices in a multiple-choice question, the correct choice is most often in the middle (i.e., b or c). Use a table of random numbers to guide the placement of the correct response.
- Avoid trick questions, such as those using negatively worded stems along with negatively worded choices that test semantics and logic rather than knowledge of the subject matter.

Essay Tests

The following are examples of essay test questions:

- Read the research paper provided and give an assessment of the strengths and weaknesses of the method section.
- Discuss at least four strategies that would be effective in modifying public attitudes toward persons who have physical disabilities.
- Compare and contrast the major theories regarding therapeutic intervention in episodes of acute rheumatoid arthritis.
- Read the following community hospital case. As a consultant, outline the recommendations you would make to the hospital administration.

Advantages of essay questions are that they are especially good for measuring the upper three levels of the cognitive domain (analysis, synthesis, and evaluation); the student is free to decide how to approach the problem, what information to use, what aspects to emphasize, and how to organize the response; it is the easiest type of question to write quickly; and the teacher can determine the student's depth of knowledge and the quality of the student's critical thinking abilities.

The following are disadvantages of essay tests and possible solutions:

- Scoring is difficult and time consuming, especially as writing comments on each paper regarding the strengths and weakness of the essay are imperative for student understanding and learning. Fatigue during grading can lead to grading inconsistencies. If you use a series of short essay questions, grade the same question on all the papers (without looking at the student's name) before going to the next question to increase the consistency of your response.
- Writing ability influences the grade received. Suggest to students that they read over their answers quietly to themselves looking for incomplete or run-on sentences and spelling and punctuation errors. Reviewing common errors with the class highlights the importance and necessity of good writing skills for health care professionals.

Good in-depth information on all types of written tests is given by Davis (1993) and Linn and Gronlund (1995). (See Annotated Bibliography at the end of this chapter.)

Quick Checks

Quick checks are like pop quizzes with less anxiety and more learning imbedded in the process. Take the last few minutes of a class and ask students one short, focused question that will promote reflective thinking about the material that has just been presented, especially as it relates to the students' own thinking, feeling, or performing. The length of response should be no more than a few phrases or a couple of sentences. For example, you might ask students to give an example of one characteristic they exhibit that would promote effective physical therapist–physical therapist assistant interactions in the clinical setting and one characteristic they might consider working to change to avoid physical therapist–physical therapist assistant conflict. Quick checks also are one of many classroom assessment techniques that can be used for formative evaluation.[29]

Think about grading quick checks as "excellent," "good," or "try again." If the student receives a try again, he or she can do just that—that is, hand in another response within the week. When the second response is reviewed, the student's grade may be moved up to a good. This method of grading avoids the stress of a one-shot pop quiz and puts the focus on students grappling with ideas and transforming knowledge. Quick checks are easy to grade quickly and give the instructor information about how individual students are absorbing the information presented. (See Chapter 5 for a broad range of assessment techniques that can be used to facilitate the teaching-learning process.)

Clinical Laboratory Teaching: Development and Assessment of Clinical Practice Skills

You remember well entering your first laboratory class session with 30 eager students just dying to learn the "real thing" from a real clinician. Of course, just a few months ago you received a call from the director of the physical therapy program at your local university, and you were thrilled to be asked to coordinate this musculoskeletal assessment laboratory. After all, you have 15 years of clinical experience, have clinical specialty certification through the American Physical Therapy Association, and have served as a clinical instructor for several physical therapy students in the past. Now as you enter the laboratory for your first session, you realize this part-time teaching task may take much more of your time and energy than you imagined. You eagerly dive into the task, structuring your laboratory much like your own past experiences of learning clinical skills. You have picked up a few neat ideas along the way from your extensive continuing education background and wealth of clinical experience. Basically, you plan to demonstrate the skills to the class, have them perform the skills, and then circulate around the lab along with your other laboratory instructor providing pairs of students with feedback on their skill performance. As you go around the lab, you notice that there appears to be some diversity of effort among the students—some are wonderfully task-oriented, practicing diligently with their partners, while others do the activity once and are engaged in casual conversation. You also find students asking you to just tell them when to perform this or that technique. You think to yourself, "How do I know what to do in my clinical practice? And then, How should I structure this laboratory so that I am not only teaching these extremely important clinical skills but sharing my thinking and clinical knowledge with students as we go along? There must be a better way. . . ."

This anecdote describes the ultimate challenge of physical therapy faculty who teach in the clinical sciences. How do faculty in the professional education environment help students develop an effective system for learning that is responsive to practice needs and includes knowledge acquisition, problem solving, application of clinical judgment, and development of clinical skills? The profession of physical therapy is not alone here. The development of all aspects of professional competence, including clinical skills, knowledge, interpersonal attributes, problem-solving skills, clinical judgment, and technical skills/practice skills, is an ongoing challenge for faculty involved in all types of professional education.[4] It is certain that the field or clinical education portion of the programs is essential to the ultimate development of professional competence; however, teachers also have an obligation to begin developing all aspects of competence in the clinical laboratory. This section focuses on three critical concepts in laboratory teaching: (1) development of clinical practice skills, (2) development of clinical reasoning and judgment, and (3) assessment strategies.

Clinical Laboratory Teaching: Learning Psychomotor Skills

One of the major tasks in the clinical laboratory is to teach students new psychomotor skills, from the handling of their own bodies, to the handling of patients, to the sensing of changes of texture and mobility in soft tissue structures, to the ability to use touch as a way of communicating support and care. These tasks are an essential and fundamental aspect of professional competence. There is a growing body of literature in the area of motor learning that many therapists are applying to their work with patients.[30] Several of these concepts can also be applied to clinical laboratories. Chapter 11 covers the teaching of psychomotor skills in detail. This chapter highlights some key elements that can serve as a basic structure for planning the laboratory experience.

Phases of Skill Learning

Gentile[31] has a simple model for skill learning that includes two phases. The first phase is understanding the idea of the movement, which includes learning the skill that is specifically linked to the goal. After the skill is successfully performed, the learner can move to the second phase of refining the skill and committing the skill to memory. This phase is called the *stage of fixation and diversification*. In the learning process, the learner is exposed to many stimuli and needs to devote selective attention to the regulatory stimuli (i.e., those stimuli that affect accomplishment of the goal). These stimuli could be visual, verbal, written, tactile, auditory, and so on. Skills can also be categorized as *closed* or *open*. In a closed skill, environmental conditions and relevant stimuli remain stable throughout the performance. Consider the following example: You are teaching a lab in clinical measurement that starts with basic range-of-motion measurement with a goniometer. You would probably classify this skill as closed because the environment is the laboratory and the skill or measurement activity is being applied to a person with no limitation of movement. An open skill takes place in a changing environment, and the regulatory stimuli vary. Open skills are obviously more difficult for the learner because of the changing situation. After the learner can recognize and attend to the relevant stimuli, a plan for movement, or motor plan, that meets environmental demands can be formulated. When the skill or subset of skills is performed, the learner receives feedback on the skill execution. This feedback may be intrinsic (from the learner) or extrinsic (from the outside; a person or the environment).

Teaching a Skill

The following are suggestions for skill teaching:

1. *Establish a problem that leads to a goal and ensures adequate learner motivation.* Students will know that they (most likely) do not know how to go about measuring the range of motion. In this way, the problem (i.e., they don't know) and the goal (i.e., they need to know) are presented.

2. *Attend to regulatory stimuli that will help the learner perform the skill.* In doing this, the teacher must decide how to help the learner recognize the stimuli. This could be done in any of the following ways:

- Demonstrate the skill and give verbal instructions on the steps involved in performing the skill. (It is good to practice the skill ahead of time.)
- Use a visual, taped demonstration.
- Use the guided-discovery approach, in which the students use a text or manual and discover, through problem solving, the steps in the skill.

3. *Control the learning environment.* The teacher must decide how realistic the laboratory should be. There is some evidence that with nursing skills, when teaching open skills, the setting should be as realistic as possible. Teachers may provide students with different approaches they may try depending on a specific patient situation. Also, the laboratory can be structured to provide different stimuli (e.g., have students change partners, role play).

4. *Provide feedback.* Each learner needs intrinsic and extrinsic feedback. Intrinsic feedback should be given before extrinsic feedback. Intrinsic, or internal, feedback allows the learner to learn how to learn from his or her own feedback to self. Extrinsic, or external, feedback is feedback from the teacher. This feedback is most effective when there is no interfering activity between the skill performance and the feedback. The more detail a learner can be given about an error, the more readily it can be corrected.[32] With large lab groups, the instructor may use periodic time-outs or teachable moments when common mistakes are discovered and address the common mistake to the entire group.

5. *Have the students practice.* The final stage for the teacher is to move students to the fixation and diversification stage in which the general motor pattern is practiced and refined. If one is teaching simple closed skills, students may move quickly to this stage and thus lose motivation to continue practice. To improve skills, continued practice also requires ongoing feedback. Repetition without feedback is not likely to lead to improvement. Feedback could come in ways other than the extrinsic expert form. Students could provide ongoing feedback for one another. They could also review tapes of themselves or use other audiovisuals.

6. *Design effective timing and sequence of practice.* Is practice more effective if it is massed practice (no rest periods) or distributed practice (planned rest periods)? For motor skills, evidence supports that distributed practice is best. The rest periods must be short enough so that memory is not a problem, and reinforcement should follow after each practice session. After the learner reaches the fixation and diversification phase, then he or she is better able to attend to other stimuli in the environment.[17]

Suggestions for Clinical Skills Demonstrations

In the clinical laboratory setting, instructors are frequently involved in demonstrating to students how to perform skills. The following are suggestions for clinical skills demonstrations:

1. Plan and prepare ahead of time. Have the necessary equipment and practice the skill ahead of time. Determine how it will appear from the student's vantage point.

2. Perform the procedure step-by-step and explain as you go along. The entire skill will be demonstrated more than once. If the skill is complex, you may wish to demonstrate the entire skill first and then break it down into the step-by-step procedures.

3. It is best not to have students take notes so that they can concentrate on the demonstration. Have explanatory information in the text or a laboratory manual.

4. You may wish to videotape your demonstration or have someone take slides or digital images of key teaching points. These materials could then be made available to students for independent study and practice.

5. Ensure that the demonstration always adheres to fundamental principles of professional practice, such as proper body mechanics, patient positioning, and proper draping.

6. Demonstrate the skill from different angles or sides so that students can see what the skill looks like from different perspectives.

Suggestions for Teaching Open or More Complex Psychomotor Skills

Graduated Practice

Psychomotor skills that are difficult may need to be broken into subcomponents; this process is known as *graduated practice*. This gives the student the opportunity to concentrate on the component steps. For example, in teaching students how to perform proprioceptive neuromuscular facilitation patterns, one might begin by having the students learn the movements on themselves. The students can then proceed to doing simple, straight-arm patterns on a fellow classmate. Finally, the students should be ready to apply a pattern to a specific patient condition. Each of these subtasks takes students through guided practice—that is, practice with each of the components.[32]

Mental Practice

Mental practice, or imagery, is a technique that has been used by many athletes to help improve performance and reduce stress. For some clinical skills, students can learn by visualizing the sequence of steps involved in the mastery of the skill. The student would focus on mental rehearsal of a procedure (e.g., transferring a patient from a bed to a chair). With mental imagery, while students are waiting in the hallway for their practical examination, they can visualize themselves performing the steps and imagine the instructions they are giving the patient at each step.[32]

Clinical Laboratory Teaching: Learning How to Take Deliberate Action

When teaching in the clinical sciences, educators are not only interested in facilitating the development of students' psychomotor skills but also in developing the thinking skills (e.g., planning, analyzing, problem solving, evaluating, and decision making) that are essential to performing the deliberative processes of professional practice.[4,23,33] These deliberative processes are often referred to as being part of the clinical thinking, reasoning, and decision-making processes. They are "wise actions" that come from the professional's ongoing analysis, thinking, or reflection on practice. Such knowledge is frequently referred to as "knowing how"—that is, knowing how to apply or do what you know. A second category of professional knowledge is "knowing that"—that is, knowing about things. In professional education, students are exposed to increasing amounts of this kind of knowledge (knowing about things or facts), ranging from understanding how the body functions at cellular levels, to understanding system functions and human actions. Educators are more likely to focus on "knowing that," with emphasis on students' cognitive abilities, than on "knowing how," which occurs when students analyze and give a rationale for their practical skills and actions.[23,33]

In the clinical laboratory, teachers need to find ways to teach students the performance of skills. However, teachers also need to develop the inquiry processes that allow students to continue to learn through experience. Physical therapists are not just technical problem solvers but must be able to respond to the complex, uncertain situations routinely found in clinical practice. Schön[33] argues that students can be taught to reflect on or inquire about situations that are uncertain and that professional educators should design laboratory experiences that are more representative of real-life, clinical settings. He draws the analogy that educators should move from the more traditional "follow me" laboratory, in which technical skills are emphasized, to the "hall of mirrors" laboratory, in which students are challenged to not only perform the skill but also discuss and critique the performance among peers.

Providing structure or a conceptual framework for analysis can be one way of facilitating a student's thinking or reasoning process in a "hall of mirrors" laboratory. For example, in the area of musculoskeletal dysfunction,

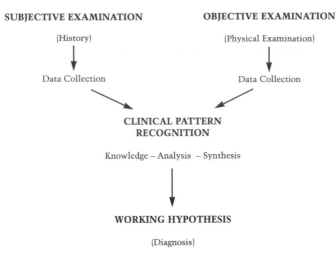

Figure 3-5   An example of how components of the musculoskeletal evaluation can be used to facilitate students' clinical thinking and reasoning processes. (Adapted from CJ Tichenor, J Davidson, G Jensen. Cases as shared inquiry: model for clinical reasoning. J Phys Ther Educ 1995;9:57.)

application of concepts from a clinical reasoning model can be used to assist students to think about integrating evaluative skills with their interpretive, ongoing thoughts about the data (Figure 3-5).[34]

A second example is the use of a conceptual model, like the disability model, that can assist students in seeing the larger issues involved in managing a patient (see Figure 3-2).[7] Even though much of laboratory teaching may be focused on skills development, these skills have to be understood as tools for gathering data, facilitating movement, and teaching patients and caregivers to ultimately have an effect on the patient's functional limitations and quality of life.

Clinical Laboratory Teaching: Assessment of Clinical Skills

It is your first experience with laboratory practical examinations. You remember how terrified you were as a student, but now you see the struggle from the other side, the tremendous number of hours that it may take to do a meaningful evaluation of students. How do you achieve consistency across evaluators? You remember again from your student days that sometimes these evaluation sessions can have a powerful effect on a student's self-confidence. How do you design an experience that provides the opportunity for a student's learning, demonstrates evidence of a student's competence and deficits, and can be done in less than 100 hours?

Practical Examinations: Design and Implementation

The basic ingredients for designing and implementing practical examinations include rationale (or aim of the evaluation), format, evaluation tools (including evaluators), and implementation.

1. *Rationale*. What is the overall purpose of the examination? Are you just checking competence of select clinical skills? Are you interested in how students think on their feet, their decision-making skills, how they synthesize information? Are you using the examination process to look at information across courses? Should the examination include any elements of self-assessment or only evaluator assessment?

2. *Format*. The format of the practical examinations will follow from the overall purpose of the examination. If you use the practicals as a formative assessment strategy to check out the basic level of skill performance, you may want to use a simple check-out strategy. With this strategy, you should identify a list of psychomotor behaviors and develop a checklist of the skills involved. Students perform the task(s) and are evaluated using the checklist. On the other hand, if the aim is to examine student performance of certain skills and the student's own analysis of the performance, you may choose to have the student create the "evaluation artifact" (e.g., videotape, audiotape, transcription, case description). For example, in looking at the patient interview process, you may want students to videotape their interview of another individual. They can do their own assessment of the tape, and, together, you and the students could do another assessment. Perhaps your faculty is interested in looking at student performance in a number of areas from the courses taught that semester. In this case, you may consider some form of examination stations in which each faculty member examines one area of performance, either by observing the student's performance or serving as the "standardized patient." If the faculty member serves as the patient, then she or he can experience the application of skills as well as assess the level of performance. This model is very similar to the objective structured clinical examination (OSCE) that has been used in medical education for assessing the clinical skills of medical students and residents.[35]

Laboratory situations can also be used to stimulate students' thinking and assess their attitudes and ability to reason and make decisions in ambiguous situations. For example, one area of importance and recent investigation in professional education clinical assessment is assessing behavioral skills such as patient-centered interviewing and student awareness and sensitivity to diverse health beliefs. A study by Oh et al.[36] found that residents trained in patient-centered interviewing were more effective in handling patients' emotions and more skillful in gathering patient data. The assessment was done through video recorded and scored interviews with standardized patients. The scoring tool, the Rhode Island Hospital Resident Interview Checklist, contained observable behaviors in core areas (opening of interview, exploration of problems, facilitation skills, and relationship skills).[37]

Another idea for working with students to assess their reasoning abilities and affective responses is use of a critical incident. Here are two examples of critical incidence techniques that can be used to look not at what an individual can do, but what an individual habitually does.[35]

- Impossible dilemma: Here you provide the student with a realistic and relevant task that poses mutually exclusive alternatives that represent different value positions that are more or less politically correct.

You are a member of the hospital's committee on health benefits. The committee must come up with recommendations for reducing the overall health plan by $3 million. Out of a list of provided services, you must now decide which of these services will no longer be part of the plan.

- Role play a situation in which a satisfactory resolution will be difficult to obtain:

You are a newly hired therapist in a large rehabilitation center. Steve, a patient well known to the department for his uncooperative behavior and substance abuse problems, is again being referred for physical therapy and is assigned to you. It is your task to establish a plan of care with Steve.

3. *Evaluation tools.* Unlike a multiple-choice test that can be scored by machine, practical examinations require human beings as part of the evaluation process. The evaluator will have to render some judgment about student performance. Because the evaluation of clinical skills is more subjective than evaluating cognitive performance, one should be absolutely clear about specific expectations in the course syllabus. To assist with the evaluation process, you will need to create an evaluation form that identifies the behaviors (cognitive, psychomotor, and affective) that you wish to assess. This also would be the first step in demonstrating consistency across evaluators.[38] A

drawback for the beginning teacher would be the lack of a data bank of experience regarding student performance. Even though your evaluation criteria are most likely criterion referenced on paper (i.e., identify the standardized expected behaviors of students to pass), there is likely to be an element of norm-referenced evaluation (i.e., student performance compared with other students who are taking the examination). When performing practical examinations, it is usually the case that you will judge not just the presence of a behavior but the quality of the behavior as well. In such situations, it is important to have a more experienced teacher and mentor to consult to learn what is average or excellent student performance. You may find that a videotape analysis of your own evaluation performance can be helpful.

4. *Implementation.* You may have wonderful ideas for your practical examinations, but are they realistic to implement? Time and personnel are perhaps the two biggest resources. Think creatively about how to stretch these resources. Perhaps there are clinical faculty who might love the idea of being involved in an assessment day or clinic. You may be able to recruit volunteers for patient role models (e.g., elders in the community, students from another year in the program, or students from other professions). If there are severe time constraints, you may want to provide students with the patient cases for the examination ahead of time. The students can then prepare and practice for all of the cases, even though they will only do selected elements in their examination time. However, because the students have prepared for all of the cases, your objective is accomplished. Also, think about ways to include peer assessment and self-assessment as part of the process.

Performance-Based Assessment: Use of Standardized Patients

Although performance-based assessment has been used in the health professions for many years, there has been increasing interest in the use of standardized patients.[35,39,40] Standardized patients are taught to portray patients in a standard and consistent manner. These patients are used in tests called *objective structured clinical examinations*. These tests are done by having students or examinees rotate through a circuit of stations where they perform a variety of clinical tasks, including patient history and physical examination. Standardized patients can be used to fill out check lists or rating forms regarding the students' interactions and performance. Although these kinds of examinations are more realistic simulations of clinical practice, they entail a great amount of time, coordination, cost, and effort for implementation.

In summary, it is recognized that performance-based assessment can identify skills that cannot be measured with traditional written examinations. It is also recognized that scores on performance-based assessments do not generalize well across situations (i.e., performance with one patient case does not necessarily predict performance in the clinic). Assessment experts in the health professions argue for continued use of a blend of assessment methods.[39]

Strategies for Facilitating Reflection and Problem Analysis

> None of us can ever teach students to think. We can, however, create experiences for students that will cause them to think and develop ideas. None of us can set thinking as our "terminal objective." Our obligation to the profession and to our students is to help them turn the wheel of their own minds with increasing power and ever clearer direction as they grow and learn.[24]

The greatest American philosopher of education, John Dewey, made many contributions to education. Perhaps one of his most important contributions was his writing about thinking—his "theory of inquiry."[8] Inquiry for Dewey was a combination of mental reasoning and action.[41] Schön[33] has furthered Dewey's theory in his writing on reflective practice. As discussed previously, reflection is the element that turns experience into learning. It is the process of purposeful thinking and inquiring about problems and how to solve them—that is, a process of deep and meaningful learning.[42] Physical therapist and physical therapist assistant students are faced with the challenge of many ill-structured problems in health care settings, for which the simple application of knowledge cannot produce a solution. How can teachers provide students with opportunities to "turn their own minds?"

Recall that in Bloom's taxonomy, knowledge and comprehension are the beginning levels of cognitive ability, and synthesis and evaluation are the upper levels.[43] Language can be one way in which a teacher can structure the students' thinking and discussion. For example, words like "argue," "explain," "hypothesize," "compare and contrast," and "provide evidence" all provide students with a more engaged and active image of how to think about their thinking.[44] A key term used in the thinking and learning process is *metacognition*. Cognition is the construction of meaning, whereas metacognition is the awareness and monitoring of one's own thinking and learning process.

The teacher's role is to facilitate this metacognition process through the instructional process. This section discusses two strategies for facilitating this process—the use of case method and concept mapping.[45–47]

Case Methods

> Educators have long been critical of academic programs dominated by the twin demons of lecture and textbook, each a method designed to predigest and deliver a body of key facts and principles through exposition to a rather passive audience of students.[45]

Case methods are widely used in business and law courses. The case method of teaching should be differentiated from a case report (usually a description of an intervention with a patient) or a case study (usually third-person accounts of detailed descriptions in which the focus varies from people to things). Cases are used in teaching to stimulate thought and discussion, often using Socratic questioning. In business, cases are used to train students to know and to act. Cases are used to help lawyers sharpen their analytical skills, and in case discussions students are challenged to defend their argument. Cases are frequently developed from problems in the field and are often constructed to represent a particular principle or problem.[12,45,46]

As discussed earlier in this chapter, cases have been used in problem-based learning in which small group tutorials work on the patient case. This requires that the group identify and gather the information necessary to analyze the case. In other words, the group must use processes of problem identification, problem solving, and analysis. The facilitator does not lead the group but questions and probes for student reasoning and analysis. Case formats can vary from a written paper case, to a videotape case, to a simulated or real patient.[12,45,46]

A critical dimension of case method is the formulation of the case as it relates to the broader issues of general principles and concepts. The case writer should ask, "What is this a case of?" Business education has perhaps the most detailed approach for assisting case writers. For the health professions, cases may go beyond the notion of the patient or client and include any number of real-world practice problems (e.g., management issues, staff problems, ethical dilemmas, reimbursement issues).

Writing cases that are grounded in real-life experience gives students and faculty the opportunity to address complexity of practice. Cases that are developed from practice or are adapted from situations in practice challenge faculty and students to move from a course orientation to integration and application of many courses.

Case 3-1: Example of a Patient Case Used by Students to Integrate Information across Courses in the Curriculum*

Betsy is a 27-year-old former fifth grade teacher referred to physical therapy for examination of bilateral lower extremity pain due to a peripheral neuropathy secondary to acquired immunodeficiency syndrome.

Social and Medical History
No one is aware of her diagnosis except health care workers involved with her treatment and immediate family members. Her husband is also human immunodeficiency virus (HIV) positive, and his work associates are unaware of the patient or the husband's diagnoses. The couple has a 2-year-old daughter who is HIV positive. They live in a one-story home with two bedrooms and a small bathroom. The patient has around-the-clock care and supervision when her husband is not home. Her husband and caregivers express concern over her declining function and their lack of knowledge of how to best help her. Previous medical history was negative before the diagnosis of HIV in 1997. Patient has had *Pneumocystis carinii* pneumonia twice, mycobacterium tuberculosis, and candidiasis. She was recently hospitalized for a deep vein thrombosis in her lower left extremity.

Current Medical Status
The patient is in the advanced stage of acquired immunodeficiency syndrome and requires 24-hour supervision. She requires assistance to transfer and is able to ambulate for very short distances with a walker and frequent verbal cueing to keep her knees and hips extended. She has periods of lethargy and confusion.

Medications
The patient takes Bactrim (antibiotic used to prevent recurrence of *Pneumocystis carinii* pneumonia), ciprofloxacin hydrochloride (Cipro, antibiotic), ethambutol hydrochloride (Myambutol, antitubercular agent), fluconazole (antifungal agent), sertraline (Zoloft, antidepressant), anticonvulsant (Neurotin, used for neuropathic pain), protease inhibitor (Crixivan), antiviral (Viramune), and antiviral (Epivir).

---

*From K Paschal, J Gale. Patient case materials. Creighton University Department of Physical Therapy, Omaha, NE, 2001.

Physical Therapy Examination Findings
Arrived in clinic in wheelchair assisted by her caregiver.
Chief complaint: Pain and weakness in legs
Range of motion: Grossly within functional limits
Strength:

Shoulder elevation 4/5	Hip flexors 3/5
Triceps 4/5	Hip extensors 2/5
Biceps 4/5	Knee extensors 3/5
Hands 5/5	Ankle dorsiflexors 4/5
Ankle planter flexors 2/5	

Transfers: Supine to sit with maximum assistance of 1; sit to stand with maximum assistance of 1.

Case 3-1 presents a patient case developed so that students would synthesize information learned in biological, physical, clinical, and behavioral science courses during the semester and integrate this information with prior knowledge. Student groups were given specific questions for each area (i.e., clinical medicine, physical therapy procedures, and psychosocial and cultural factors) to guide their case analysis (Table 3-3).

In designing a challenging case, one may want to gather and present data beyond the usual written patient cases. This might include information gathered from interviewing, documents, or the media or artifacts provided as part of the case (e.g., documentation and videotape). A critical element in the formulation of the case is consideration of the thinking dimensions stimulated by the case (e.g., knowledge, analytical thinking, and conceptual thinking).[45] A physical therapy community management case is used as an example in Case 3-1.

As stated earlier in the section on tutorials, cases engage the way in which practitioners think and continue to learn. As an instructional strategy, cases allow students to be actively involved in the information gathering, problem solving, and decision making that are applied to real practice problems.[46]

Concept Mapping

Concept mapping is a multipurpose, fun graphic technique that can be used to see how students "build what they know" (i.e., how they structure their prior knowledge). A concept map is an illustration of relationships between concepts and facts developed by moving from a general idea to specific instances. The technique can be used by teachers and students to identify the structure of prior knowledge, to organize or present

Table 3-3   Example Questions Used in the Case Analysis for Case 3-1

Clinical medicine (cognitive domain)	Physical therapy intervention	Psychosocial and cultural factors
How did the patient's medical diagnosis affect your evaluation and intervention?	What methods would your evaluation include? What is your justification for those methods?	What is your assessment of the patient's social support structure?
Could preventive measures, early intervention, or environmental adaptations minimize functional limitations?	Generate a problem list.	How would you go about establishing a therapeutic relationship with this patient?
What other health care professionals might this patient benefit from working with?	What is the working hypothesis(es)?	Identify any cultural variations that may have an effect on your interaction with the patient and caregivers.
Strategies	List your short- and long-term functional goals and your plan of care.	What specific verbal and nonverbal strategies would be most effective with this case?

Source: K Paschal, J Gale. Patient case materials. Creighton University Department of Physical Therapy, Omaha, NE, 2001.

new information, or to assess progress and change.[47,48] Figure 3-6 compares a student's concept map of evaluation to a clinical instructor's concept map.

Narrative: A Teaching Tool for Reflection

> The best physicians have always blended their understanding of psychology and culture with their biomedical knowledge, as they diagnosed health problems and treated patients. And they have called upon the resources of their faiths or philosophies, their senses of the meaning of the human experience, to give them the tensile strength to be healers and physicians rather than simply biomedical consultants.[49]

One of the assumptions of this book is that clinical practice in physical therapy demands expertise in all domains of learning: cognitive, affective,

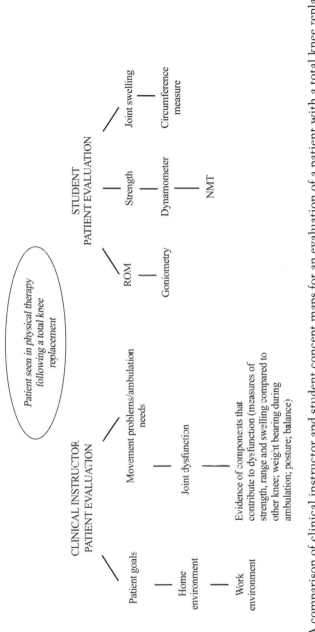

Figure 3-6 A comparison of clinical instructor and student concept maps for an evaluation of a patient with a total knee replacement. (NMT = neuromuscular tension; ROM = range of motion.)

psychomotor, perceptual, and spiritual. A student's identity as a physical therapist or physical therapist assistant depends not only on integrating the knowledge and skills of the discipline but also on developing self-knowledge through self-reflection. A very powerful teaching tool for facilitating this process of self-knowledge is the use of narrative, through one's own writing or the stories of others.[50] Experiences of therapists and patients provide insight in understanding the meaning of experiences, decisions, or events. For example, a student may be asked to write an account of a time in the clinic when he or she was confused. In this account, the student addresses questions such as: "What really happened here?" "Why did you do what you did?" "Would you do anything differently?" "What have you learned?" As another example: "You may have a patient with a terminal illness; how can you respond empathetically in the face of suffering and death?" "What inner resources can we develop to help us deal with our own limitations?" The student may also want to listen carefully to the patient's story and write a similar account.

Stories are useful not only as a vehicle for expressing one's thoughts, but they can also be read aloud in class. The reading aloud of narrative (stories or poems) brings yet another opportunity for students to hear and think about the meanings embedded in the narrative.

There are many learning exercises teachers can use to facilitate the role of narrative, such as journal writing, short free-writing or 5-minute writing exercises, reflection or reaction papers, and the sharing of short stories or poetry. All of these tools provide students the opportunity to seek meaning in the experiences of themselves and patients.[23,29]

Evaluation Methods That Promote Reflection

One of the central themes of this book is the role of educators in facilitating the development of "reflective practitioners." Dewey defined reflective thinking as a state of doubt or perplexity in which thinking originates and a process of inquiry begins that is aimed at finding ways to resolve the doubt or problem.[8] Schön, in studying several different professions, recognized reflection as an important vehicle for acquiring all types of professional knowledge.[33] More than a decade of research, dialogue, and writing has transpired since Schön's *Educating the Reflective Practitioner* struck the educational community. One recurring element is the use of structure to promote reflection, such as the use of portfolios and journals.[51,52] One suggestion for evaluating reflective work is the use of a Primary Trait Analysis, which clearly outlines differences between average and excellent reflective work (Figure 3-7).

Reflective Self-Assessment Paper Guidelines

Assignment: Perform a reflective self-assessment of expertise using the core dimensions from the expertise model (knowledge, clinical reasoning, movement, virtue, and philosophy of practice). The paper should be no longer than 8 to 10 pages (double-spaced, typed) and must include one figure or visual representation of your self-assessment. The excellent, good, and average categories represent A work, B work, and C work, respectively.

Papers will be reviewed according to the following criteria:

Clarity/ Organization	Excellent	Good	Average
	Clearly identified purpose; logical sequence and transitions throughout the paper	Adequately identified purpose; logical sequence and transitions	Poorly identified purpose; inconsistency in sequence and transitions
Supporting evidence	**Excellent**	**Good**	**Average**
	Multiple sources of evidence in support of assertions; fully developed quality links between assessment and evidence	Less thorough use of sources of evidence in support of assertions; visible links between assessment and evidence	Few sources of evidence; inconsistency in links between assessment and evidence
Reflection	**Excellent**	**Good**	**Average**
	Evidence of critical and deliberate reflection; quality connections are made among values, purpose, and action across all dimensions of expertise	Evidence of more technical and interpretive reflection less critical or deliberate; good connections among values, purpose, and action across all dimensions of expertise	Evidence of predominately technical reflection; inconsistent connections among values, purpose, and action across dimensions of expertise
Creativity	**Excellent**	**Good**	**Average**
	Strong evidence of original thought and risk taking	Good evidence of original thought and risk taking	Inconsistent evidence of original thought and risk taking

Figure 3-7 Examples of using Primary Trait Analysis as grading criteria for reflective work. (Adapted from R Lloyd-Jones. Primary Trait Analysis. In Cooper C, Odell L [eds]. Evaluating Writing: Describing, Measuring, Judging. Urbana, IL: National Council of Teachers of English, 1977.)

Student Portfolios

Student portfolios can be useful tools as formative and summative evaluation measures to assist students to invesigate their own learning experiences. It is important to provide some guidelines for students to follow in creating their portfolios. For example, you might ask students to include papers, reflective journal entries, and a self-assessment. The rule is variety; neither limit nor prescribe what the evidence must be in each of these categories.[53] Thus, the portfolio gives students permission to do creative self-assessment. One additional reflective strategy you might think about integrating into the portfolio process is VanManen's levels of reflection.[54] He describes three levels of reflection:

1. *Technical*: "How to" questions —thinking about application of technical skills and knowledge.
2. *Interpretive*: "What does this mean" questions—thinking about interpretation of words and actions.
3. *Critical*: "What ought to be" questions—thinking about the worth and nature of social conditions.

By encouraging students to question themselves and reflect on their classroom and clinic experiences at the three levels of reflection, the teacher can assist students to link their knowledge and skills with deliberate and moral actions.[55]

Student Journals

Writing is an essential tool in the reflective process.[51,52] Journal writing is a common learning activity used often in conjunction with clinical education experiences. Again, adding structure to the journal process is helpful in facilitating reflection.[56,57] For example, you may want to have students deliberately think about key aspects of a clinical environment—what they learn from patients, their views of the health care system, and how their clinical instructor teaches. The three levels of reflection (technical, interpretive, and critical) provide another structure students can use to facilitate reflective thinking and journal writing.

Educational Technology

Computer Technology

There is no question that computer-based technologies are rapidly transforming education. These technologies allow students and teachers to access and reconfigure information. Students can easily receive and interact with data of all kinds from all over the world. Some even argue that the electronic age is causing a paradigm shift in which the teacher is no longer the center of information but is the center of accumulated knowledge and experience.

One useful framework for approaching the use of computers in teaching is (1) learn about computers, (2) learn through computers, and (3) learn with computers.[58]

Learning through Computers

Learning through computers, with computer-assisted instruction, has been the emphasis in education. Hundreds of programs (e.g., on-line tutorials, simulations, and interactive learning programs) have been produced in medicine. There are a growing number of computer-based learning resources on the market (e.g., CD-ROM, multimedia databases, videodisc, and networked resources). Computer-based knowledge resources continue to expand.[58]

Learning with Computers

The most powerful approach to learning with computers is to require students to use computers on a day-to-day basis to support their classroom activities. Chapter 5 presents ways to use computer-based technologies as an integral part of a course and the teaching-learning process.

Traditional Instructional Technology

What about the use of more traditional instructional technology? The most commonly used instructional media include handouts, chalkboards, overhead transparencies, slides, and videotapes and films.

Chalkboards

Chalkboards (and the newer white felt-tip pen boards) have been in the front of classrooms for many generations of students. A writing surface in front of a class allows spontaneity of visual representation of words, phrases, or concepts. Some tips for the use of chalkboards include (1) write legibly and large enough for the class to see, (2) read aloud while writing on the board, (3) use the most visible parts of the board for critical points, (4) be selective in writing down only key principles, and (5) try to structure the board work with numbers or sections.[15]

Overhead Transparencies

Overhead transparencies can be used as a chalkboard for spontaneously writing down ideas or outlining content. Two positive features of using transparencies are (1) written materials can be made larger, and (2) the teacher can face the class while emphasizing key points. In addition, the classroom does not have to be dark as with slides, and the teacher can highlight words or phrases on the transparency while he or she is talking. Transparencies also are excellent tools for making copies of diagrams or drawings from texts. In general, use the same principles for writing on a chalkboard with transparencies. A few additional tips for using overhead transparencies include (1) prearrange the transparencies in the order in which they will be used; (2) when projecting a list, reveal only one item at a time; (3) after displaying an overhead, wait briefly before speaking; (4) make sure the transparency is not too busy and that the letters are legible; and (5) do not look at the screen—stand to the side of the projector.[15]

Slides

In teaching some topics, slides may be essential to helping students understand the necessary detail of the visual image. Slides are compact and easy to store, and the teacher can easily talk while presenting the slides. The biggest disadvantage of slides is that the room must be dark, which makes class interaction difficult.[15] The same disadvantage (dark room and little chance to interact with students) is present when a teacher uses computer technology to generate and display visual material. Slides can be generated quickly and multiplied rapidly with the advent of various software programs and the ability to run visual displays from a "smart" classroom. One caution: more slides, fancier slides, and multimedia slides, in and of themselves, will not result in more engaged student learning and better outcomes. The role of the media display should be linked carefully and thoughtfully to your learning goals for students.

Videotapes and Films

Videotapes and films can be used to bring a sense of reality into the classroom. Again, as with slides, one large disadvantage is that students are passive viewers of the media unless they have been prepared to be active viewers. This means that students need to know what the expectations are for viewing the video or film. The teacher, of course, is responsible for setting the stage for follow-up activities and discussion.[15]

Finally, visual teaching tools, such as flipcharts, chalkboards, overhead transparencies, and computers can be useful instruments for sharing small group tasks or results. For example, small group assignments can be posted on a course platform or Web site. You might even use laptops for small group work in the classroom.

Summary

There are many educators who say that teaching methods have not changed much in the last 100 years—that is, the students sit, and the teacher stands in front and uses a blackboard or another visual to dictate information to students. Most faculty find the traditional methods of teaching more comfortable because they provide the greatest control, and that is the way that they themselves were taught. Common barriers that inhibit change in the classroom include (1) the stable work setting, (2) the teacher's definition of self resists change, (3) the feedback cycle is stable, (4) innovative ideas cause feelings of discomfort and anxiety, and (5) faculty like to think aloud and lecture. However, the biggest barrier of all is risk.[9] Active learning for students and teachers requires learning new skills and taking risks.

In closing, diagnostic judgment and collaborative skills will continue to be essential capacities for students. Graham,[59] in a study investigating processes used by physical therapy students in developing conceptual knowledge, advocates that methods such as collaboration and group learning may enhance conceptual learning. Bruffee summarizes our challenge as educators quite well, saying,

> In any college or university today, mature, effective, interdependence—that is, social maturity integrated with intellectual maturity—may be the most important lesson students should be asked to learn. Students cannot learn this lesson if college and university teachers continue to teach the way most of them teach today. College and university teachers teach the way they do because they understand knowledge to be a certain kind of thing. Changing college and university teaching depends on changing teachers' understanding of what knowledge is. Most of us . . . assume a foundational (or cognitive) understanding of knowledge. Collaborative learning assumes instead that knowledge is a consensus among the members of a community of knowledgeable peers—something that people construct by talking together and reaching agreement.[19]

References

1. Shulman LS. Knowledge and teaching: foundations of the new reform. Harvard Educational Review 1987;57:1.
2. Hutchings P, Shulman LS. The scholarship of teaching. Change 1999;31 (5):11.
3. Rothstein JR, Ecternach J. Primer on Measurement: An Introductory Guide to Measurement Issues. Alexandria, VA: American Physical Therapy Association, 1993;59.

4. Eraut M. Developing Professional Knowledge and Competence. Washington, DC: Falmer Press, 1994;19.
5. Cross KP, Steadman MH. Classroom Research: Implementing the Scholarship of Teaching. San Francisco: Jossey-Bass, 1996:1.
6. Wiske M (ed). Teaching for Understanding: Linking Research with Practice. San Francisco: Jossey-Bass, 1998.
7. Jette A. Physical disablement concepts for physical therapy research and practice. Phys Ther 1994;74:380.
8. Dewey J. How We Think. Buffalo, NY: Prometheus Books, 1991;1.
9. Bonwell C, Eison J. Active Learning: Creating Excitement in the Classroom. Washington, DC: ASHE-ERIC Higher Education Report, George Washington University, 1991.
10. Silberman M. Active Learning: 101 Strategies to Teach Any Subject. Boston: Allyn & Bacon, 1996.
11. Creed T. Why we lecture. Symposium. St. John's Faculty Journal 1986;5:17.
12. McKeachie W. Teaching Tips (10th ed). Boston: Houghton Mifflin,1999; 66.
13. Bligh DE. What's the Use of Lectures? San Francisco: Jossey-Bass, 2000.
14. Russell I, Hendrieson W, Herbert R. Effects of information density on medical school achievement. J Med Educ 1984;59:881.
15. Davis BJ. Tools for Teaching. San Francisco: Jossey-Bass, 1993;63.
16. Eaton S, Davis GL, Benner P. Discussion stoppers in teaching. Nurs Outlook 1977;25:578.
17. DeYoung S. Teaching Nursing. Menlo Park, CA: Addison-Wesley, 1990;73.
18. Cohen E. Designing Group Work: Strategies for the Heterogeneous Classroom (2nd ed). New York: Teachers College Press, 1994.
19. Bruffee K. Collaborative Learning. Baltimore: Johns Hopkins University Press, 1993;1.
20. Bavelas A. The five squares problem—an instructional aid in group cooperation. Stud Personn Psychol 1973;5:29.
21. Epstein C. Affective Subjects in the Classroom: Exploring Race, Sex and Drugs. Scranton, PA: Intext Educational, 1972.
22. Gandy J, Jensen G. Group work and reflective practicums in physical therapy education: models for professional behavior development. J Phys Ther Educ 1992;6:6.
23. Higgs J, Edwards H (eds). Educating Beginning Practitioners: Challenges for Health Professional Education. Boston: Butterworth–Heinemann, 1999;1.
24. Bridges E, Hallinger P. Implementing Problem-Based Learning. Eugene, OR: Educational Resources Information Center, University of Oregon, 1995;3.

25. Fields E. Use of debate format to facilitate problem solving skills and critical thinking. J Phys Ther Educ 1992;6:3.
26. Dempsey-Lyle S, Hoffman T. Into Aging: Understanding Issues Affecting the Later Stage of Life (simulation game). Thorofare, NJ: Slack Publishing, 1990.
27. Walvoord B, Anderson V. Effective Grading: A Tool for Learning and Assessment. San Francisco: Jossey-Bass, 1998.
28. Astin AW. Involvement in learning revisited. Lessons we have learned. Coll Student Development 1996;37(2):123.
29. Angelo TA, Cross KP. Classroom Assessment Techniques: A Handbook for College Teachers (2nd ed). San Francisco: Jossey-Bass, 1993.
30. Winstein C, Knecht HG. Movement science and its relevance to physical therapy. Phys Ther 1990;70:759.
31. Gentile A. A working model for skill acquisition with application to teaching. Quest 1972;17:3.
32. Watts N. Handbook of Clinical Teaching. New York: Churchill Livingstone, 1990;139.
33. Schön D. Educating the Reflective Practitioner. San Francisco: Jossey-Bass, 1987;3.
34. Tichenor CJ, Davidson J, Jensen G. Cases as shared inquiry: model for clinical reasoning. J Phys Ther Educ 1995;9:57.
35. Tekian A, McGuire CH, McGaghie WC. Innovative Simulations for Assessing Professional Competence. Chicago: Department of Medical Education, 1999;73.
36. Oh J, Segal R, Gordon J, et al. Retention and use of patient-centered interviewing skills after intensive training. Acad Med 2001;76(6):647.
37. Novack DH, Dube C, Goldstein MG. Teaching medical interviewing. A basic course on interviewing and the physician-patient relationship. Arch Intern Med 1992;152:1814.
38. Riolo L. Reliability of assessing psychomotor tasks in physical therapy curricula. J Phys Ther Educ 1997;11(1):36.
39. Swanson D, Norman GR, Linn R. Performance-based assessment: lessons from the health professions. Educational Researcher 1995;24:5.
40. Robbins LS, White CB, Alexander GL, et al. Assessing medical students' awareness of and sensitivity to diverse health beliefs using a standardized patient station. Acad Med 2001;76(1):76.
41. Glassman M. Dewey and Vygotsky: Society, experience and inquiry in educational practice. Educational Researcher 2001;30(4):3.
42. Moon J. Reflection in Learning and Professional Development: Theory and Practice. London: Stylus,1999.
43. Bloom B. Taxonomy of Educational Objectives: The Classification of Educational Goals. New York: McKay, 1956.

44. Halpern D. Changing College Classrooms. San Francisco: Jossey-Bass, 1994;13.
45. Shulman J. Case Methods in Teacher Education. New York: Teachers College Press, 1992;1.
46. McGinty SM. Case-method teaching: an overview of the pedagogy and rationale for its use in physical therapy education. J Phys Ther Educ 2000;14(1):48.
47. Beissner K. Use of concept mapping to improve problem solving. J Phys Ther Educ 1992;6:22.
48. Daley BJ, Shaw CR, Balistrien T, et al. Concept maps: a strategy to teach and evaluate critical thinking. J Nurs Educ 1999;38:42.
49. Caelleigh AS, Dittrich LR. Preface. The humanities and medical education. Acad Med 1995;70:758.
50. Greenhalgh T, Hurwitz B. Narrative Based Medicine: Dialogue and Discourse in Medical Practice. London: BMJ Publishing Group, 1998; 3.
51. Loughran J. Developing Reflective Practice: Learning about Teaching and Learning through Modelling. Washington, DC: Falmer, 1996.
52. Russell T, Korthagen F. Teachers Who Teach Teachers. Washington, DC: Falmer, 1995.
53. Schön D. The theory of inquiry; Dewey's legacy to education. Curriculum Inquiry 1992;22:119.
54. VanManen M. Pedagogy, virtue, and narrative identity in teaching. Curriculum Inquiry 1994;24:135.
55. Jensen GM, Paschal KA. Habits of mind: student transition toward virtuous practice. J Phys Ther Educ 2000;14(3):42.
56. Jensen G, Denton B. Teaching physical therapy students to reflect: a suggestion for clinical education. J Phys Ther Educ 1991;5:33.
57. Hayward L. Becoming a self-reflective teacher: a meaningful research process. J Phys Ther Educ 2000;14(1):21.
58. Koschman T. Medical education and computer literacy: learning about, through and with computers. Acad Med 1995;70:818.
59. Graham C. Conceptual learning processes in physical therapy students. Phys Ther 1996;76:856.

Annotated Bibliography

Angelo T, Cross KP. Classroom Assessment Techniques: A Handbook for College Teachers (2nd ed). San Francisco: Jossey-Bass, 1993. This book is a must for every physical therapy education department. The book contains numerous examples of innovative classroom assessment strategies.

Bligh DE. **What's the Use of Lectures?** San Francisco: Jossey-Bass, 2000. A classic work that addresses the strengths and limitation of lectures. Well documented with clear expanations and examples.

Bonwell C, Eison J. **Active Learning: Creating Excitement in the Classroom.** Washington, DC: ASHE-ERIC Higher Education Report, George Washington University, 1991. A short book on practical teaching strategies for facilitating active learning in higher education classrooms. The authors argue that active learning is central to engaging students in higher order thinking tasks. The book provides several ideas for lectures, discussions, and creative learning strategies. An excellent resource for a quick introduction and idea source for changing your classroom.

Cohen E. **Designing Group Work: Strategies for the Heterogeneous Classroom (2nd ed).** New York: Teachers College Press, 1994. A very practical book for facilitating the small group process in the classroom. Cohen covers all aspects of group work, including research findings, goals, common problems, preparatory strategies, and planning group work tasks. Although much of the research on group work has been done in secondary education, the author does an excellent job of integrating the core theoretical concepts that apply to all levels of education.

Cross KP, Steadman MH. **Classroom Research: Implementing the Scholarship of Teaching.** San Francisco: Jossey-Bass, 1996;1. This book is designed to be a companion book to *Classroom Assessment Techniques: A Handbook for College Teachers* by Angelo and Cross. The book is designed to be used by faculty learning groups or in workshops. The authors use a case-based approach posing real questions about knowledge, critical thinking, and motivation for learning. Teachers can use this book to set up and carry out their own classroom research projects.

Davis BJ. **Tools for Teaching.** San Francisco: Jossey-Bass, 1993;63. This book is a wonderful resource for quick reference on specific teaching tools. The book covers everything from traditional teaching tools to educational technology. There is an excellent chapter on the use of instructional media.

Linn RL, Gronlund NE. **Measurement and Assessment in Teaching (7th ed).** Upper Saddle River, NJ: Prentice-Hall, 1995. Comprehensive treatment of instructional objectives and their role in planning tests. Helpful information on constructing objective and essay tests. Includes good information on how to tell if your tests are effective and fair. Very readable with clear examples. A classic in the field.

McKeachie W. **Teaching Tips (10th ed).** Boston: Houghton Mifflin, 1999;66. McKeachie's text is a classic, now out in a tenth edition. The text is a must for every teacher in higher education. The book provides quick answers and reference to any question you may have on course development and management. McKeachie does an excellent job of integrating the most recent research on teaching methods and evaluation. What the book lacks in depth, McKeachie compensates for with annotated references that direct the reader to key resources on the specific topic.

Moon J. Reflection in Learning and Professional Development: Theory and Practice. London: Stylus, 1999. Presents a powerful argument that reflection should be taught to students in all professions. Provides an interesting "concept map of learning" to demonstrate where reflection occurs. Provides a critique of the literature on reflections and learning and suggets a number of practical ways to encourage reflection by students.

Silberman M. Active Learning: 101 Strategies to Teach Any Subject. Boston: Allyn & Bacon, 1996. This book is a great quick reference for simple ways to implement active learning experiences in your classroom. The book is written as a quick reference guide and each technique includes step-by-step instructions.

Walvoord B, Anderson VJ. Effective Grading: A Tool for Learning and Assessment. San Francisco: Jossey-Bass, 1998. This book is another must for every physical therapy education department. Similar to the classroom assessment text, this book includes multiple examples of strategies and ideas that teachers can design and implement to enhance student learning through their grading process.

Westberg J, Jason H. Making Effective Presentations. A Center for Instructional Support (CIS) Guidebook for Health Professions Teachers. Boulder, CO: Johnson Printing, 1991. This is a video with accompanying teacher's guide that can be used in the classroom. The video contains several vignettes of common teacher presentation "pitfalls" with accompanying questions for the group to discuss. Other videos available from the Center for Instructional Support (CIS) include *Communicating with Patients, Clinical Teaching, Teaching Interpersonal Skills*, and *Using Video in Teaching*. Videos may be ordered from Johnson Printing, PO Box 1437, Boulder, CO, 80306-1437.

Appendix 3

Cooperative Group Training Exercise: Broken Circles

Instructions

Step 1. Divide the class into small groups (three to six persons per group). Give each person an envelope with different pieces of a circle.

Step 2. The goal is for each student to put together a complete circle. To do this, students must exchange some of the pieces.

Step 3. Rules of the game include

1. No talking. The game is done in complete silence.
2. A student may not point or signal any other player with his or her hands.
3. The focus of the game is giving. Students may give pieces one at a time. They may not place a piece in another person's circle. Students can hand a piece to a player or place it beside the other pieces in front of him or her.
4. Students must complete their own puzzle.

Step 4. This is a group task. Each group has 15–20 minutes.

After the time is up, the class should discuss the game using the following questions:

1. What do you think the game was about?
2. How did you feel as a group member?
3. What things helped your group be successful in solving the problem?
4. What things made it harder?
5. What could the group do differently?

Directions for Making Materials for Playing Advanced Broken Circles

1. Make a set from heavy cardboard. Cut the circles approximately 20 cm in diameter. Each set of six circles should be a different color with letters and

numbers marked on the back of each piece. Numbers indicate the group size and letters indicate the proper envelope. If a piece does not have a number on it, it remains in its lettered envelope regardless of group size.

2. Angles used include: 60, 90, 120, 150, 180, 210, 240, and 270 degrees. See the figure below.

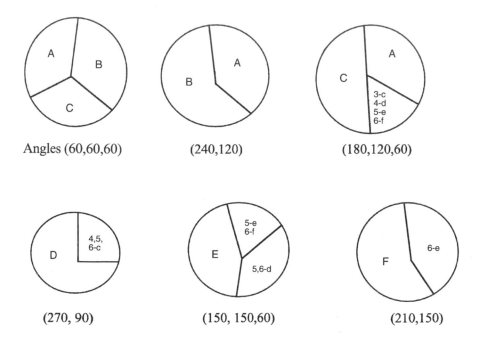

Angles (60,60,60)   (240,120)   (180,120,60)

(270, 90)   (150, 150,60)   (210,150)

3. Placement of the other four pieces varies with the size of the group. For example, if you have a six-person group, then 6-F (60-degree piece) goes into the F envelope, 6-E (150-degree piece) goes into the E envelope, 6-C (90-degree piece) goes into the C envelope, and 6-D (150-degree piece) goes into the D envelope. Repeat this pattern for each six-person group.

Sources: Broken squares game developed by A Bavelas. The five squares problem—an instructional aid in group cooperation. Stud Personn Psychol 1973;5:29. Broken circles game developed by T Graves, N Graves. (Game) Santa Cruz, CA: 1985. May be purchased by writing Graves, 136 Library St., Santa Cruz, CA 95060. Average class would need six to eight sets. Directions for preparation of game reprinted by permission of the publisher from EH Cohen. Designing Group work: Strategies for the Heterogeneous Classroom (2nd ed). New York: Teachers College Press, © 1994 by Teachers College, Columbia University. All rights reserved.

B

Cooperative Group Training Exercise: Epstein's Four-Stage Rocket

Group Activity

This training exercise involves having a small group discuss a topic that will generate interaction with different perspectives. The group is given a topic to discuss. As an example: For the next 20 minutes, you will discuss the role of research in physical therapy education. What should the role be? Consider you are a task force of students that is making recommendations to the faculty. Identify the driving and restraining forces and make a list of recommendations. Students can discuss what kind of research and scholarship they should do during their professional education (e.g., a literature review, a case report, a systematic literature review, a clinical research proposal, a full blown research project), the amount of content and experience in the curriculum, and whether students should generate independent projects or group projects.

Ground Rules

There will be four stages and 4 minutes of group discussion to practice these skills at each stage.

1. *Conciseness*. Select a timekeeper who will watch the clock and keep time for the group. The timekeeper must make sure that each person talks for only 15 seconds. Do this for 4 minutes.

2. *Listening*. Select a new timekeeper. Now the timekeeper must make sure that each person waits 3 seconds after each person has spoken before he or she talks. Do this for 4 minutes.

3. *Reflecting*. Select a new timekeeper. Now the timekeeper must make sure each person talks for only 15 seconds, followed by 3 seconds of silence.

The next person who speaks must begin by repeating to the group something that was said by the person who spoke before him or her. (The person who spoke before must nod his or her head to indicate if the repetition is correct.) Do this for 4 minutes.

4. *Everyone contributes*. Select a new timekeeper. All previous rules apply. In addition, no one may speak a second time until everyone in the group has spoken. Do this for 4 minutes.

Observers

The teacher can assign one or two observers to record examples of group members' skills for each of the four stages (conciseness, listening, reflecting, and contributions by all).

Debriefing Session

After the discussion, have the groups debrief using the following list of group behaviors as a structure for discussion.

Group Behavior and Process Skills

Work Behaviors: Skillful Members

- Have new ideas for the group
- Ask for or give information
- Help explain better
- Pull ideas together
- Find out if the group is ready to decide what to do

Helping Behaviors: Helpful Members

- Get people together
- Bring in other people
- Show interest and kindness
- Are willing to change own ideas if someone makes a good argument
- Tell others in a good way how they are behaving

Troublesome Behaviors: Troublesome Members

- Attack other people
- Refuse to go along with suggestions
- Talk too much

- Keep people from discussing because they do not like the argument
- Show that they do not care about what is happening
- Let someone boss the group
- Do not talk and contribute to ideas
- Tell stories and keep the group from getting their work done

Source: Adapted from C Epstein. Affective Subjects in the Classroom: Exploring Race, Sex and Drugs. Scranton, PA: Intext Educational, 1972.

4

Use of Computer Technology to Enhance Teaching and Learning

Tracy Chapman and
Gail M. Jensen

Not too many years ago, I was sitting in a classroom writing a "to-do" list in my notebook as my instructor struggled to get the data projector to work with his laptop computer. As he attempted several solutions, numerous thoughts ran through my mind: This is wasting my time! We have so much material to cover today, and now we will never get through it, let alone have time for questions. Why didn't he try this out before class to make sure it works? As the minutes ticked by, students began to visit, many voicing thoughts that mirrored mine. A few students offered suggestions to solve the technology snafu. After approximately 10 minutes, the instructor abandoned the technology endeavor, called the class back to order, and announced that he would present the material without the assistance of the audio and visual aids located on his computer.

Does this scenario serve to confirm that technology in education is just a passing phase and not worth the time, effort, and financial resources dedicated to it? Or does the scenario illustrate the need for better planning and education regarding effective and efficient use of technology? The purpose of this chapter is to provide information and guidance in the use of educational technology with an emphasis on computer technology. Specifically, we examine the role of educational technology in teaching and learning, including use in the classroom as well as in the distance education environment.

Chapter Objectives

After completing this chapter, the reader will be able to

1. Distinguish between what technology can do and what technology cannot do regarding learning.
2. Describe the four Cs essential in planning to use instructional technology.
3. State 10 criteria you would use to determine whether a Web site were credible.
4. Discuss how you would go about preparing materials, students, and yourself for using technology in traditional face-to-face classrooms.
5. Discuss how you would go about preparing materials, students, and yourself for teaching in a virtual classroom.
6. Describe how to create and facilitate a virtual learning community on the Web.
7. Describe the role of a learning community in transformative learning.

What Does Instructional Technology Include?

Technology tools have been part of teaching and learning for many years. Blackboards, chalk, and pencils are forms of early technology still used in classrooms. The International Society of Technology in Education has developed a set of standards for educational uses of technology.[1] There are six core areas that the standards address that are worth thinking about in terms of physical therapy education. The six areas include (1) technology operations and concepts; (2) planning and designing learning environments and experiences; (3) teaching, learning, and the curriculum; (4) assessment and evaluation; (5) productivity and professional practice; and (6) social, ethical, legal, and human issues. Although these standards are geared for K–12 teachers, they also may serve as a springboard for examining technology use in higher education. A list of these standards is found in Appendix 4-A.

The terms *instructional technology* and *educational technology* are often used interchangeably. Educational technology is defined by the Association for Educational Communications and Technology as "a complex, integrated process involving people, procedures, ideas, devices, and organizations, for analyzing problems and devising, implementing, evaluating, and managing solutions to those problems, involved in all aspects of human learning."[2(p164)] The Commission on Instructional Technology defines instructional technology as "a systematic way of designing, carrying out, and evaluating the total process of learning and communications, and employing a combination of human and nonhuman resources to bring about more effective instruction."[3(p19)] For the purposes of this chapter, we assume that the terms *instructional technology* and *educational technology* are synonymous.

Planning

As with most endeavors in education, planning leads to a greater chance for success. Using technology in the educational process is no different. Figure 4-1 represents an overview of this chapter as well as a working guide for an educational technology planning process. Often, technology exists on the periphery of a college's or university's instructional program. Technology is frequently implemented piecemeal, especially when year-end "extra monies" are available, with little or no long-range plan. Without a plan integrating the widespread use of technology in teaching, institutional support is likely to be meager. The planning process discussed in this chapter focuses on what you can do to plan for educational technology use in the classes you teach, as opposed to institution-wide planning.

The first step in the planning process is to accept some basic tenets or assumptions regarding the use of educational technology. These tenets include the following:

- Technology is not a panacea for many current problems plaguing education.
- Technology is not a substitute for good pedagogy.
- Technology is a *tool* for teaching and learning: objectives first, technology second.
- There is no single best use of technology.
- The potential benefit of technology is how it meets the needs of the learner.

Keeping these tenets in mind, you are ready to proceed with the process of planning for technology. We start with the four Cs of any planning process[4]: comprehensiveness, collaboration, commitment, and continuity.

Comprehensiveness

Your planning should cover all of the following elements:

- Equity issues—have you taken into account students with disabilities who may have difficulty interacting with the technology? Do all the students have easy access to the technology tools necessary to carry out your expectations?

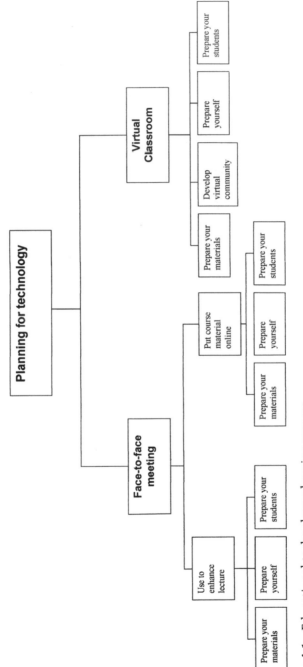

Figure 4-1 Educational technology planning process.

- Needs assessment—have you completed some type of formal or informal needs assessment to determine what areas of your teaching can best be enhanced by using technology and what types of technology will best meet your needs?
- What are your goals and objectives for incorporating technology into your instruction? If you cannot identify goals or objectives, you may want to think long and hard about why you are using technology. Remember, technology is only a tool for teaching and learning.
- What hardware and software do you need to accomplish your plan? Is it in place? Can it be purchased?
- What technology-related skills do the instructor and the students need?
- Development needs of the instructor and students—how and when will the instructor and students gain the skills necessary to successfully interact with the technology?
- Support—is the technology support you need available? (This topic is addressed further in Collaboration.)
- Financial—have you identified resources to finance the technology you are planning to use?
- Timeline—lay out a timeline for planning and implementation of the technology. Be sure to build in time for you and the students to learn the technology and additional time for installation (if necessary).
- Evaluation—how will you evaluate whether your goals and objectives related to use of the technology are accomplished?
- Do you have a backup plan in place in case the technology fails? (Remember the scenario from the beginning of the chapter?)

Collaboration

What human resources are available at your institution to assist in your technology use endeavor? Identify those resources, contact them, and determine how you will use them in the implementation of your plan. Collaboration resources may include

- Colleagues who are also attempting to incorporate technology into instruction, or those who have experience doing so effectively.
- An information technology department at your institution that may assist with hardware and software purchase suggestions, computing technology training opportunities, and help desk resources.
- Students—by bringing students in on the planning process, they may be more willing to endure any growing pains that may occur with the initial use of technology, and they may provide you with insights into the use of technology not previously considered.

- Professional organizations or technology partners outside of your institution—they may supply you with information relative to the attempts of others to incorporate technology.

Commitment

Ensure that those involved with your plan are committed to making it work. Are you sure those you are counting on for technical, financial, and moral support are actually behind you? Commitment stems from making your collaborative partners part of the planning process. Having partners participate in formulating the overall goals and objectives as well as developing specific implementation plans leads to commitment.[5]

Continuity

Your plan to implement technology will change as additional options are developed and made available. Typically, new technologies emerge as a result of the need to improve on older versions. Picciano[5] gives an excellent example. Once people migrated toward automobiles and away from horse and buggy for their primary mode of transportation, problems were noted (e.g., pollution and unreliability). Most did not go back to the horse and buggy but advocated for improvements in automobiles. Similarly, your planning process will need to continue, allowing you to incorporate future iterations of the technology. Once the planning process is complete, you are finally ready to actually try out all that you have planned for.

Implementation of Technology in the Traditional Face-to-Face Classroom

The face-to-face classroom is where you see the fruits of your labors. The first question to ask yourself is, "How will instruction in my classroom change as a result of incorporating technology?" The answer should start with a look at the goals and objectives for your course and how technology can help to move students toward accomplishing them. Generally, technology enhancements in the classroom fall into two categories: (1) lectures enhanced with visual aids or multimedia, and (2) making didactic content available to the students outside of class and spending class time in discussions and application exercises. Both scenarios require preparation of course materials, of students, and of yourself (the instructor). Let's take a look at both scenarios to see what groundwork is necessary.

Scenario 1: Face-to-Face Setting—Enhancing Your Lecture with Visual Aids or Multimedia

Preparing the Materials

Remember when preparing your materials for class meant organizing lecture notes and writing on transparencies for the overhead projector? Now, *preparation* often refers to PowerPoint presentations and video clips. Regardless of the media you use to enhance your lectures, keep in mind the basic tenet of using educational technology: It is a tool, useful only if it enhances the students' learning experience. Review your course objectives. Identify those concepts that can most benefit by multimedia illustration. Then identify and locate multimedia resources, evaluate the quality of those resources, and select those you will use. For example, showing a media clip of a patient on a ventilator and family decision making about life support is a powerful way to introduce a discussion on advanced directives.

As you identify possible multimedia resources, consider that "learners react favorably to situations involving the use of instructional technologies to present messages that are authentic, relevant, and technically stimulating."[6(p367)] Publishers are beginning to provide CD-ROMs with textbooks that include such features as slides of actual tissue samples, video clips of patient–physical therapist sessions, and animations of motion analysis. The World Wide Web has a plethora of resources, or you may produce your own such as reenactments of clinical practice filmed on digital video. If you decide to create your own multimedia resource, keep in mind that quality is important if students are to perceive the material as authentic and technically stimulating. You might want to identify professionals who can assist you in this endeavor. Creating multimedia can be very time consuming, with or without technical assistance, so allow yourself plenty of lead time.

When evaluating multimedia resources, the following checklist may be used:

- Can be seamlessly integrated into the instruction. Enhances the instruction; is not being used just because it is available.
- Classroom is equipped with equipment allowing students to easily see and hear source used.
- If animated, motion is smooth.
- If audio is used, quality is high; sounds can easily be heard and understood.

If you choose to use resources from the World Wide Web, it is important to evaluate them for credibility. The check list in Table 4-1 may be used to perform a general assessment of the credibility of a Web site. Additional evaluation check lists may be found at http://lme.mankato.msus.edu/class/629/Cred.HTML (Eval-

Table 4-1   Assessing the Credibility of a Web Site

Organization/group that maintains the site is evident
Mission, purpose of the site identified
Description of the content of the site provided
User is informed of controversial materials
Date of site creation identified
Author's name, professional institution affiliation, position title, e-mail, phone number are provided
A bibliography is present or references are cited
Links to resources used to develop the content are provided
A recognized style manual is followed to cite references
Bias of author is clearly stated when appropriate
No spelling or grammar errors
Links are clearly visible and understandable
Essential instructions appear before links and other interactive portions of the site
Users are informed when they are about to link off the site
Links are annotated
Links are relevant and appropriate to the content
Links are reliable

Adapted from http://www.waller.co.uk/eval.htm (Sixty Ticks for a Good Website); and Beer V. The Web Learning Field Book. San Francisco: Jossey-Bass, 1998:151–153.

uating Internet Based Information) and http://www.waller.co.uk/eval.htm (Sixty Ticks for a Good Website).

Once the possible resources have been identified and evaluated, select those you will use.

Preparing the Students

Generally, the technology used in the classroom illustrates and assists in the assimilation of concepts presented in lectures. In this situation, students need very little preparation. However, do not assume that students are familiar with technology used in the classroom. To illustrate this point, consider the following anecdote.

> I was assisting with a technology workshop for incoming students. The students were of traditional college age and, for the most part, from middle- to upper-income families—students who are generally thought to have basic computing technology skills. During the workshop, the students were participating in a tutorial about using particular features of Microsoft Word. At the conclusion of the Word tutorial, the students were told to click on the X in the upper right-hand corner of their screens to

close the program. I observed two students use their fingers to tap on the Xs, expecting the program to close.

Preparing Yourself

Although your students may need little or no preparation, you will require considerable preparation to ensure effective use of the technology. Identifying and locating high-quality material is only half the battle. You must be prepared to seamlessly integrate the material into your teaching, carefully ensuring that technology enhances, not overtakes, the instruction. To accomplish the seamless integration, you must be comfortable using the technology and practice before class time. A backup plan should also be in place in case the technology fails to function. No matter how much you prepare, some aspects of the technology are beyond your control (e.g., the classroom computer locks up, the data projector bulb burns out, your CD-ROM drive stops working).

You have prepared the materials you plan to use, prepared the students, and prepared yourself. Assuming your use of educational technology is for the purpose of enhancing your lecture with visual aids or multimedia, you are ready to go. But, what if you have a different scenario in mind for using educational technology?

Scenario 2: Face-to-Face Setting—Online Course Materials for a Campus-Based Course

The use of the Web for campus-based courses is frequently ignored or overlooked. Making didactic content available on the Web allows class time to be spent in discussions and application exercises. Beer[7] suggests the following uses for the Web in traditional classrooms:

- Source of updated content
- Repository for slides, lecture notes, and assignments
- Links to supplemental material on other sites
- Topical discussions moderated by the instructor
- Chat room for learners to discuss content and assignments
- "Teachers' lounge" where instructors can share ideas with each other
- Collaborative space for learners to publish or work on projects together electronically

Additionally, your Web site may allow virtual guest lecturers. Owing to scheduling and financing constraints, it may be difficult to include guest lecturers in your course. However, getting these lecturers to log into your course chat room or respond to discussion posting is often free and much easier to schedule.

Walvoord and Anderson[8] suggest that instructors examine the best use of time and space for students' first exposure to course material, for students' processing of the course material, and for instructors' responding to students' work. Typically, students' first exposure to course material is in the classroom, with the instructor and other students. Even given prior reading assignments, students are likely to come to class ready to "soak up" the material for that class session. In this instance, the opportunity for instructor-student interaction is diminished, because the instructor must cover a certain amount of material, which leaves very little time for interaction. Is this the best use of the instructor's time?

The most difficult part of the learning process often takes place when students are alone, away from the instructor. After the classroom lecture, students are given an assignment that requires them to apply the concepts presented in class, usually resulting in a product (paper, solving a set of problems, performance). Would it facilitate students' learning if the instructor were present during this part of the learning process?

The final part of the learning process usually involves the instructor's responding to the students' product. Often, the response is in the form of notes written on the product. Would it be more effective to have the instructor interact with the students face to face?

By restructuring *the time and place* for the first exposure to course materials, student processing, and instructor responses, the instructor's expertise can be used more effectively, and student–instructor interaction will increase.[8] For example, making your lecture available online allows students to gain the first exposure to course materials outside of class. Make the content as complete as possible, including all the anecdotes and examples you typically provide in class. Will students understand all the concepts presented in this way? Probably not. Will students read all the material you provide? Probably not. So . . . what do you do? Students generally need some incentive to read material before class. For example, require students to complete a 10-question multiple choice online quiz at least 24–36 hours before the start of class. This prompts them to read the material and lets you know what concepts they are having problems with, so you can design the next class session around these problematic areas. You could also have students e-mail you two or three specific questions they have about the materials, or give one or more suggestions for application of the material presented. During class time, your expertise is focused where it is most needed, addressing concepts students found difficult, helping students apply the concepts, and providing them with immediate feedback they can use for clear understanding and additional attempts at application. Thus, your limited face-to-face time with students is used to help students understand and apply concepts rather than relay ideas they can understand just by reading.

Preparing Teaching Materials for the Web

Preparing your material for students to access outside of the classroom can be achieved in several ways. You might provide students with printed copies of your didactic content, or provide a PowerPoint presentation to the students via the World Wide Web. The latter option allows students to access the material any time they are at a computer connected to the Internet. It also alleviates the "I lost my handout" problem. Moving your content to the Web allows you to

- Take advantage of the power of hyperlinking
- Make your content searchable
- Easily update your material
- Educate students about how to use the Internet and computing technology as tools for teaching and learning
- Decrease student note taking and increase their attention to content

So, where to start?

First, you need to find a "home" for your materials on a Web server. Most colleges and universities have servers and will assign you a space in which you may post your course materials. When you are assigned a server space, the server administrator will tell you the URL (uniform resource locator), or Web address, of your course site. Many institutions have purchased course management systems, such as WebCT (http://www.webct.com) or Blackboard (http://www.blackboard.com). These systems provide a structure into which you may put your course materials, as well as additional functionality, such as chat rooms, bulletin boards, and grade management. Course management systems are discussed further in the Virtual Classroom section of this chapter. If your institution is not able to provide you with server space, many independent companies have space available for free or for a modest monthly fee. Appendix 4-B lists some options for free and pay-by-the-month server space.

Once you have found a home for your course material, the next step is to find a piece of software that allows you to transfer your materials from a word processing format to HTML. (*HTML* stands for *hypertext markup language*, the language of the Web.) Assuming you have your course notes in electronic format (on your computer's hard drive, on a floppy disk, or on a zip disk), you should be able to copy and paste the material from the word processing format into HTML. The specifics of accomplishing this vary with the HTML software you select. Commonly used (and relatively easy to learn) HTML management and editing programs are Microsoft's FrontPage and Netscape Composer. If you are a novice at Web page creation, I recommend FrontPage, as the icons and basic functionality for creating text and including graphics are very similar to those for Microsoft Word. The software will instruct you on how to create hyperlinks, allowing your students to connect to other Web resources and move through the course material you put on a Web server. Transferring your materials into HTML essentially makes them a Web page. Once your materials are in HTML, your students are able to access them with a Web browser, such as Netscape or Internet Explorer. If you are interested in learning more about HTML, visit http://www.cwru.edu/help/introHTML/toc.html.

Wow! You are now the proud owner of a course Web site! Now, you need to educate your students about accessing and using the Web site and explain to them the changes in how class will be conducted.

Preparing Your Students

By the time students graduate from high school, they have experienced 12 years of classes in which the primary mode of teaching was lecture. You are now asking them to adapt to a new style of teaching. According to Rogers' diffusion theory,[9] we can expect any participants (in this case, your students) encountering a new innovation to progress through a series of stages that results in most participants adopting the innovation: knowledge, persuasion, decision, implementation, and confirmation.

Students predisposed to being innovators will adopt your new teaching mode faster than other students. To facilitate moving your students through these stages, provide them with detailed knowledge about why you are using this new approach to teaching, how to access your Web-based materials, and the changes in classroom procedures. Frequent feedback at the beginning of the course concerning expectations and student progress will also assist in adoption of this new teaching style. Allowing time at the beginning of the course for students to become familiar with your Web environment and ensuring that all students have convenient and reliable access to the material will increase students' comfort level and thereby increase the rate of adoption.

Your course materials have been adapted to incorporate educational technology. Your students have been prepared for this change in teaching style. Now, are you ready?

Preparing Yourself

We have already touched on several areas in which you will need to prepare yourself (e.g., learning to use HTML software and identifying how you will structure the time you spend in the classroom with the students). Attending a class or workshop, finding a colleague to serve as a tutor, or buying a how-to book can aid in learning to use the HTML software. You may find the Dummies series of books to be helpful, as they are very easy to use and understand. If you are putting course materials on the Web, you want them to be designed such that students can easily navigate and read them. The Virtual

Classroom section of this chapter provides an overview of Web design. The reference list and annotated bibliography at the end of the chapter contain some useful books and instructional design Web sites. Restructuring the time you spend in the classroom with the students will probably look something like

- Before coming to class, students are to read materials on the course Web site for Module 2.
- Before coming to class or at the beginning of class, students complete some type of assessment to demonstrate that they actually read the materials before class time.
- As class starts, you ask students for specific questions about Module 2 material they did not understand. You or other students answer these questions.
- Students break into discussion groups. Each group is given a case study to which it applies the knowledge it gained from Module 2.
- During the small group discussions, you move among groups, guide discussions when necessary, correct misinformation, and ensure that all students are participating.
- Groups report on their case studies.
- During group reporting time and class discussion, you facilitate the discussion, adding information and correcting erroneous information only when other students do not do so.
- Class discussion ensues on how each group addressed the case study issues.
- Students now individually apply their newly acquired knowledge to another case study or ongoing project.

Unfortunately, this model will not always work smoothly. What happens when students do not come to class prepared and do not participate in group discussions? This will probably happen quite often at the beginning of the semester; perhaps students will be at different stages of Rogers' adaptation to change (diffusion) theory[9] or testing you to see if you are serious about changing the way class is conducted. If your expectations remain consistent, students will eventually embrace the change, because they will come to realize that the only way they will successfully learn and be able to apply class material is by following your class structure.

Another aspect of preparing yourself is knowing the technology well enough so that you are comfortable with it and are able to assist students with basic technology-related questions. Thoroughly know your Web site, and be able to tell students exactly where particular information is located. If you are using a course management system (Blackboard, WebCT), know your way around the environment. Be prepared to assist students who want to print portions of the site. (Where can they print? How do they print just part of a page?)

Once you have put materials online for a traditional campus-based course, you may find yourself looking forward to or being assigned to teach an online course. Not to worry; you already have a good start!

Implementation of Technology in the Virtual Classroom

Up to now, we have been discussing the use of technology in a familiar environment: the traditional campus-based classroom. Using the technology may be a little scary, but you at least had the comfort of a familiar environment. If the technology failed, you could always wheel in the trusty overhead projector and pull out those transparencies. Well, hang on—we are about to explore a whole new environment: the virtual classroom. This is definitely part of the future of education. In *Forbes Best of the Web*, Danielle Svetcov makes the following statement about online education: "This is no fad. It is rather a stampede and nothing can stop it."[10] However, the recent shakeout of dotcom enterprises has shown the importance of combining an online presence with a physical presence. The dotcoms surviving the shakeout are, for the most part, those with accompanying brick and mortar enterprises.

Assumptions

Planning and implementing a virtual classroom can involve very sophisticated technology, including streaming audio and video, real-time sharing of resources, see-you-see-me virtual office hours, and more. Most institutions exploring or beginning to develop online distance education do not have the capability to offer these tools to their students; therefore, we focus on Web-based distance education that relies mainly on text, with basic synchronous and asynchronous interactivity.

A Course Site—Build It and They Will Come

A virtual classroom is more than just a repository of course content. It is a place where students can meet to collaborate on and participate in discussions related to the course and to issues on more personal levels. Ideally, you would like your course site to serve as a portal, providing students access to a variety of resources and services, all of which work together to develop a sense of community for the students. The first step in creating a virtual classroom is much the same as that for developing online materials for use in the face-to-face classroom: find a "home" for your Web site. As stated previously, many educational institutions have their own Web servers and will provide you with space to host your course Web site. Free or pay-by-the-month server space is also available from several companies. Next, identify communication options available, usually e-mail Listservs, discussion boards, and chat rooms.

Development of a home page is the next step. Your home page is the first page students access when logging into your course. It may take students to the following areas:

- Student and instructor biography page—a place where students can share information about themselves
- Virtual student center—a discussion or chat area where students can interact on a personal level, outside of course-related interactions
- Links and other resources—students can share interesting information they find relative to the course
- Links to the campus bookstore, library, institution's home page, or other resources the students might find useful
- Announcements—late-breaking information, usually relative to course content (e.g., a new module has been posted, you want to give reminders about approaching deadlines for assignment submissions or tests)
- Content area—entrance to course content
- Communication tools—usually discussion and chat to be used in conjunction with course content
- Assessment tools—online tests, quizzes
- Progress—a grade book

Your HTML editor may be used to create the home page, or, if you are using course management systems such as Blackboard or WebCT, home page creation is part of the course creation process. See Figure 4-2 for an example of a home page.

Plan Your Virtual Classroom

Before you actually create course materials for your virtual classroom, you need to develop a plan of what your classroom will look like. Web sites are generally organized using a flow chart type of configuration (Figure 4-3). You can then use sticky notes or index cards to represent the content of each Web page, laying them out on a flat surface and arranging them to reflect how students will move through your course.

Another strategy for organizing your course is to design a table of contents and use it as a course outline (Figure 4-4). Once you have determined the general organization of your site, you are ready to create Web pages and add content. The first few pages of your course Web site are generally an introductory page, syllabus, schedule, and contact information.

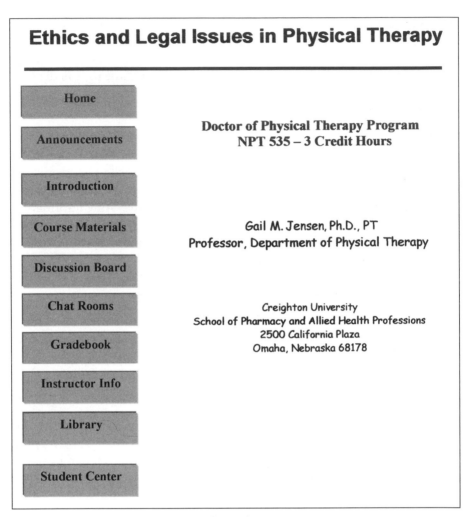

Ethics and Legal Issues in Physical Therapy

| Home |
| Announcements |
| Introduction |
| Course Materials |
| Discussion Board |
| Chat Rooms |
| Gradebook |
| Instructor Info |
| Library |
| Student Center |

**Doctor of Physical Therapy Program
NPT 535 – 3 Credit Hours**

Gail M. Jensen, Ph.D., PT
Professor, Department of Physical Therapy

Creighton University
School of Pharmacy and Allied Health Professions
2500 California Plaza
Omaha, Nebraska 68178

Figure 4-2   Example of a course Web site home page.

Preparing Your Materials

Introduction

Just as you would for the first day of a face-to-face class, begin your virtual course with an introduction. Include a little about yourself, an overview of how the class will run, an overview of the content to be covered in the course, and instructions guiding the students to read the schedule and syllabus. During the first few days of class, have students use each tool that will be used during the course. This assists students in learning the online environment and gives them a chance to work out any technical problems before the actual start of the course work.

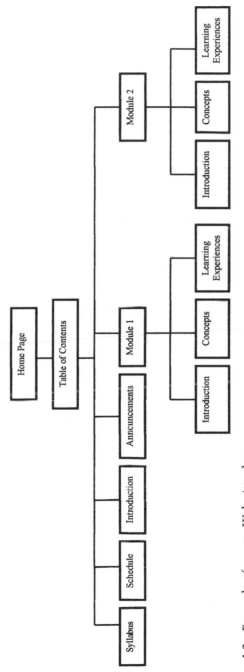

Figure 4-3 Example of course Web site plan.

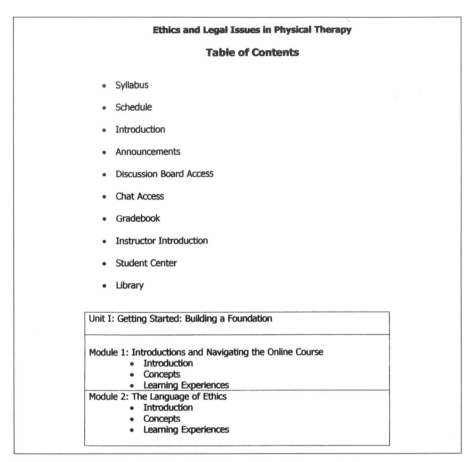

Figure 4-4   Example of a course Web site table of contents.

Syllabus

Items unique to the syllabus for your online class include virtual office hours, times when you can be reached by phone, response timelines for instructor response to e-mails and discussion postings, clear and detailed guidelines and expectations for class participation, and point of contact for technical problems (e.g., students are unable to log into the Web site, a hyperlink does not work). The syllabus should also clearly state your policy should students experience technical difficulties and be unable to access the course site for several days (e.g., a student's hard drive crashes, a monitor goes out, or a motherboard dies). All of these could take several days to resolve.

Schedule

Online learning is not synonymous with self-paced learning. Online students are just like your campus-based students in that they work to deadlines. Providing online students with a schedule increases the chance that they will move through the course and interact with each other on content in a timely and progressive manner. Consider building time into your schedule for students to get acquainted with the online environment.

Contact Information

This page provides names, phone numbers, e-mail addresses, and fax numbers for everyone the student may need to contact. This includes the instructor, technical support, and administrative support.

Creating Content Pages

Creating content pages for your online course is very similar to creating pages for your campus-based class. However, in online courses, instructional design becomes significantly more important because students rely heavily on the course Web pages to gain knowledge of concepts. The following is an example of a content page that presents new concepts to students.

Ethics and Legal Issues in Physical Therapy
Lesson 2: The Language of Ethics
Introduction

Done with Lesson 1 . . . moving right along to Lesson 2. Here, we start with an overview of terms and concepts used in ethics. You will find that having some familiarity with the terms will help with your reading.

Objectives

1. Define the basic ethical terms, including morality, moral character, context, virtue, ethics, consequences, duties, and rights.
2. Define, distinguish, and discuss application of theories, principles, and rules to ethical situations.
3. Define and apply the principles of beneficence, nonmaleficence, and autonomy.
4. Define and apply the principles of fidelity, veracity, and justice.
5. Describe how principles may be absolute, prima facie, or conditional.

Readings

Text: Chapter 1, pp. 5–19; Chapter 2, pp. 40–44; Physical Therapist Codes of Ethics (handout)
Web site: http://bioethics.georgetown.edu

Concepts

In Lesson 1, we discussed the difference between morality and ethics. *Ethics* is the "systematic reflection" on morality and therefore requires understanding and application of principles, concepts, and theories. Bioethics continues to emerge as an important element in health care. We have all experienced the changes in the health care system that often make health care and provision of rehabilitative services a scarce resource. Use of technology and genetic research offers choices often before any public discussion and societal consensus. So now, more than ever, ethics has come to the forefront. This course in ethics and legal issues will provide you with a sound foundation for integration of moral reasoning and ethical decision making in your practice setting. I tell our entry-level students that their 3–semester hour course in ethics should set them apart from their colleagues in their ability to integrate ethical principles and theories into their clinical decision making.

You will notice there are few pages for you to read in the book. Because the text integrates ethics and legal issues, it moves very quickly toward theory application. We are going to spend a bit more time reviewing terms so that we are all comfortable with the language.

Ethical Principles

Many of these concepts are taken from Ruth Purtilo's *Ethical Dimensions in the Health Professions*[11]; please refer to the text for more complete discussion of these concepts.

Nonmaleficence and Beneficence

Nonmaleficence (pronounced "non mal lif fi cence"): Do no harm. Refrain from doing harm to self or others. The Latin is *primum non nocere,* which you probably know is at the heart of traditional health care ethics and the Hippocratic Oath.

Beneficence (pronounced "be nef fi cence"): Promote good. In the position to bring about good. Sometimes these principles are thought of in terms of different levels:

Do no harm
Prevent harm
Remove harm when it is being inflicted
Bring about positive good

Autonomy: Self-determination or self-governance. Being in control of making one's own choices. Autonomy is a very powerful principle in our society. It is also a principle that has been the focus of criticism because of its focus on a person as an isolated unit standing alone over and against all other people. Carol Gilligan[12] and others argue for understanding ourselves as moral beings within the context of our relationships.

Justice: Fair distribution. In the position of distribution of benefits and burdens among individuals or groups in society who have legitimate claim on the benefits. In professional ethics, there are different types of justice to consider:

> *Distributive justice*: When there is more than one group competing for the same resources. Distributive justice requires equitable distribution of benefits and burdens.

> *Compensatory justice*: Compensations for wrongs that have been done.

> *Procedural justice*: "First come, first served." Impartiality is the key to this principle.

Fidelity: Promise keeping. Comes from Latin word meaning faithful. Purtilo's description of being faithful to patients entails meeting patients' reasonable expectations.

Veracity: Truth telling. Honesty.

Weighing the Principles—Are They All the SAME?

Absolute duties or rights are binding in all circumstances. They *never* give way to another compelling duty or right (e.g., prohibition of cruelty, torture, or murder).

Prima facie duties or rights allow you to make a choice among conflicting principles (e.g., do you stay late in the clinic and see a patient referred from the ER, or do you keep your promise to take your son to the basketball game?).

Conditional duties come only after certain conditions are met (e.g., the Americans with Disabilities Act outlines certain legal rights and responsibilities that apply only to people with disabilities).

Statement to Remember:

"Almost all ethical conflicts in health care arise from clashes among two or more duties, two or more competing rights, or duties competing with rights."[11] Just a note—most codes describe your "professional duties."

Learning Experiences

E-mail me your responses to the following questions:

1. Identify the ethical principles that are embedded in the American Physical Therapy Association Code of Ethics.
2. Review the first set of ethical principles for the American Physiotherapy Code of Ethics from 1935 through 1981 and record a few of your impressions. We will discuss further in the discussion group.
3. Would you call yourself more of a deontologist or a utilitarian in your thinking and decision making? Why?
4. Describe an example of an absolute duty in physical therapy practice. Describe an example of a prima facie duty in physical therapy practice.

Topics for the Discussion Page:

Topic 1: What is your interpretation of changes in the Code of Ethics over time? What does this tell you about physical therapy?

Topic 2: From what theoretical perspective are many of the health care decisions being made today?

See you on the discussion page . . .

Now that you have participated in the discussion and completed the learning experiences, here is a brief check of the core concepts in Lesson 2. Ask yourself the following questions:

1. What is autonomy? Give an example of its application in clinical practice.
2. What is the difference between nonmaleficence and beneficence?
3. How do the concepts of fidelity and veracity apply to clinical practice?
4. Would most situations in the clinic require absolute duties or prima facie duties?
5. What is the difference between deontology and teleology or utilitarianism?

Answers are on the next page.

How did you do? Are you ready to go on to Lesson 3? If so, click the Next button. If not, review the material from Lesson 2 or take a break and come back later.

Well-designed instructional material provides students with access to background knowledge they need to understand the new concepts being presented, opportunities to apply the concepts, feedback relative to their application attempts, and information to enhance retention and transfer of concepts. If the course is structured around a series of lessons or modules, create a template that could be used for each lesson. The following is an example of the content template for an online course:

> The following template is designed to be used for each lesson within the course.
> Introduction (first page of each lesson)
>
> - *Gain attention and stimulate recall of prior knowledge—a brief overview of the module.* Here you want to gain the learners' attention and stimulate any prior knowledge they should have that will help them understand the material included in the module.
> - *State objectives.* Specific to the lesson.
> - *Cite readings or other background material to be completed for the lesson.* Just because a course is online does not mean it all has to be online. This is where you refer students to offline content they need to read before or as they go through the module.
> - *Present concepts.* Depending on the course, the content you provide the students online may be very detailed and lengthy or just study notes to accompany offline reading assignments.
> - *Assess learning experiences.* This is where students are asked to produce some type of evidence that learning has occurred.
> - *Provide a self-assessment.* This is an opportunity for students to determine, without risking a grade, whether they understand the content for the module. Self-assessments are generally a series of questions that students answer and check themselves.
> - *Stimulate discussion or chat participation.* Students respond to instructor and student comments and questions relative to the course material. This is an opportunity for students to interact with each other.
> - *Give an assignment.* Students may be required to complete an assignment, a piece of an ongoing project, or a quiz or test.
> - *Provide a summary of the lesson.* This may include suggestions and information about how the content of the lesson may transfer to a variety of settings.

Using the HTML creation software of your choice (e.g. Microsoft's FrontPage), add content using your Web site plan and content templates as guides. When adding content, keep the following in mind:

- Putting your course materials on the Web for inclusion in a virtual classroom involves more than just copying and pasting course notes from a text document to a Web page created by an HTML editor. Instructional design issues must be considered. These are not difficult issues to address, but they can be time consuming. Grammatical and spelling errors should be eliminated.

- Writing style should be informal, conversational, written talk.
- Twelve- or 14-point plain fonts such as Arial are easiest to read online.
- Text should be broken into relatively small chunks, each chunk preceded by a heading. Headings should be of consistent color and size.
- Use of colored text can be very effective; just don't overdo it. Use no more than three to five colors per page, excluding graphics.
- Keep an eye on the load time for each page (the amount of time it takes for the page to appear in a browser); 30 seconds should be the maximum.
- Include the examples and anecdotes you use in your campus-based class. Your online students will benefit from these as much as or more than your face-to-face students.
- Online students do not have access to immediate answers to their questions as they would in a traditional class. Therefore, think about concepts that are typically problematic for students and include additional explanations and illustrations for these topics.

Navigation

Once you have created a set of content pages, students need a way to navigate through them. The structure should be intuitive and easy to read and follow. When developing a navigation structure, keep two things in mind: simplicity and consistency. The style and placement of the navigation structure should remain consistent on each page in your Web site. You want students to spend time with the content, not trying to figure out how to move through the Web site.

Site Map

The table of contents serves as the site map, providing students quick access to pages and a way to locate where they are in the site. The table of contents should list each and every page in the Web site in a type of hierarchical structure. Each page within a module also contains a navigational structure, links to all other pages in the module, and a link back to the table of contents.

Synchronous and Asynchronous Communication Tools

Adding access to synchronous (real time) and asynchronous (not occurring at the same time) communication tools to your course Web site must now be considered. These tools are used to provide opportunities for students to be actively engaged in the learning process. These learning experiences must include opportunities for students to learn with and from one another. Course management systems generally provide chat (synchronous communication) and discussion (asynchronous). It is imperative that students are provided with explicit instructions for using any communication tools included in your course. Instructions should include how to use the tools as well as expectations for frequency, timing, and length of contributions.

Network Etiquette: Netiquette

Awareness of acceptable etiquette in the online environment is important for online students. Because the online environment is new to most students, they are probably not familiar with commonly accepted rules for network etiquette, *netiquette*. To prevent or minimize misunderstandings among course participants, students should be aware of some basic, commonly accepted netiquette rules. Virginia Shea's book[13] *Netiquette* and its related Web site, Netiquette Home Page (http://www.albion.com/netiquette/index.html), are excellent sources of netiquette information. The core rules of netiquette as identified by Shea[13] are

- Rule 1: Remember the human being.
- Rule 2: Adhere to the same standard of behavior online that you follow in real life.
- Rule 3: Know where you are in cyberspace.
- Rule 4: Respect other people's time and bandwidth.
- Rule 5: Make yourself look good online.
- Rule 6: Share expert knowledge.
- Rule 7: Help keep flame wars under control.
- Rule 8: Respect other people's privacy.
- Rule 9: Don't abuse your power.
- Rule 10: Be forgiving of other people's mistakes.

In addition to learning about and getting comfortable with the online environment and gaining a working knowledge of netiquette, students also need to develop an awareness of the increased individual responsibility they are taking on by choosing to be online students. In the online environment, students have more freedom to choose what, how, where, and when they will study and interact with the course. They should be more proactive in seeking assistance and articulating their instructional and social needs. In a campus-based course, it is easier for students to seek and obtain assistance. It is also easier for the instructor to use nonverbal clues to identify students needing assistance, but not asking for it. Without the benefit of an instructor physically present, students should be able to identify when they need assistance and how to obtain it. Making this the topic of the first discussion postings is one way to ensure that students are aware of this responsibility.

Assignments

You need to decide how students will submit assignments. Will they send them to you as e-mail attachments? Will you accept assignments through the U.S. mail (snail mail)? Will they post assignments in your course discussion area? If you are using a course management system, does it include a digital drop box for turning in assignments? Regardless of which methods you use, your students need detailed instructions.

Assessments

Assessments for online courses may replicate those used in your traditional classroom-based courses; however, the issue of test security encompasses some additional considerations. Currently, there is no way to ensure that the online student is actually the one completing the assessments unless an instructor or proctor is present. Project-based assessments increase the likelihood that the assessment submitted was actually completed by the enrolled student. Owing to the time required to complete a project, it would be difficult for the student to find someone willing to complete a project for her or him. The chances of a student's finding someone willing to take a test or quiz for her or him is much greater. Therefore, you may want to consider using project-based assessments or proctored tests and quizzes. You might also want to assess students through their contributions in the course discussions and via submission of projects. Again, students should be provided with detailed information on how the assessments will occur in the course and how to access any online assessment tools you are using.

This section of the chapter has focused on steps to take in creating an online course site and preparing your material for online presentation. Another important element in online course creation, perhaps the most important, is the promotion of collaborative learning. The next section addresses which students are known to be particularly successful with online learning and how to create and facilitate learning communities for collaborative learning.

Attributes of Successful Online Students

Distance education has existed for more than a century, evolving through a number of stages: print-based correspondence courses, broadcast, teleconferencing, network, and multimedia. This long history of distance education has allowed researchers to identify variables correlated with being a successful distance education student. These variables apply to students in all genres of distance education, including those in Web-based courses. Categories and names given to particular variables differ among literature sources; however, most refer to basically the same characteristics. We look at categories and variables identified by Billings[14]:

Background variables. Higher standardized admission test (SAT) scores and college preparation lead to a greater chance for success.

Organizational variables. Grade point average (GPA), class level, experience with correspondence courses, and classmate support are all positively correlated with students' success.

Outcome-attitudinal variables. Perception of practical value, students' satisfaction with lessons within the course, timely and frequent feedback, and course's congruence with students' educational goals all lead to students' success. A feeling of isolation and difficulty with the course leads to dissatisfaction.

Environmental variables. Demands of employment and family responsibilities are negatively correlated to students' success. Employer support, family support, and proximity to instructor are identified as positively correlated to students' success.

Date of first lesson submission. The sooner a student submits or participates in a course, the more likely the student is to be successful in the course.

Intent to complete course. Students beginning a course with a definite goal to complete it are more likely to be successful than are students who are unsure about their ability to complete the course.

The ability or willingness of the student to accept responsibility for his or her own learning is also a variable in student success. The physical absence of an instructor makes it easier for students to procrastinate or put forth less effort. Students who take the initiative to learn the course material, seek assistance when needed, and complete assignments on time are more likely to be successful.

So, what do you, as an instructor, do with these variables? Obviously, you cannot influence all the variables, but you can have an impact on some. A good starting point is to provide prospective online students with some type of self-assessment, allowing them to decide if online learning is a good fit for their expectations and situation. Several sites provide self-assessment instruments: http://www.cod.edu/dept/CIL/CIL_Surv.htm (The Center for Independent Learning, Are Distance-Learning Courses for Me?) from the University of Illinois, http://illinois.online.uillinois.edu/model/ Studentprofile.htm (What Makes a Successful Online Student), and http:// illinois.online.uillinois.edu/IONresources/tips.html (Tips for Online Success) from the University of Illinois. You can also build interactivity features into your course to increase opportunities for peer support and to reduce feelings of isolation. (Interactivity is addressed in the following section, Development of a Virtual Community.) Providing frequent and timely feedback also lessens feelings of isolation and may also decrease difficulties students have with the course. Encouraging periodic feedback regarding student satisfaction with the course allows you to make changes and thereby increases the likelihood of students' success. Adjusting your course materials for optimal Web presentation increases students' satisfaction with the course and decreases difficulties, leading to increased probability for students' success.

Development of a Virtual Community

Developing a sense of a learning community among your online students where they can communicate and support one another is the most influential factor predicting student success. Hiltz states, "The greatest determinant of the extent to which students feel that the online mode of delivery is better or worse than traditional modes is the amount and quality of interaction between the instructor and students, and/or among the students."[15] To humanize the online environment, students should be provided with opportunities to form connections and build a sense of community. These opportunities must be planned and created. Palloff and Pratt[16] identify the following steps in the development of a virtual community:

- Clearly define the purpose of each group. The goals and objectives of the class somewhat define the purpose of some groups, but you may want to poll the students and develop additional shared purposes.
- Create a distinctive gathering place for each group—this will usually be discussion boards and chat rooms. Providing groups with their own space increases the chance that they will allow their personalities to emerge to group members. Encouraging students

to complete an online biography can facilitate the socialization process.

- Promote effective leadership from within—encourage students to assume leadership roles. In the online environment, the instructor steps back and becomes the "guide on the side."
- Define norms and a clear code of conduct—the netiquette rules previously identified may serve as a basis; allow students to come to a consensus on additional norms.
- Allow for and facilitate subgroups—project groups of four to five students work well online.
- Allow members to resolve their own disputes—provide suggestions if asked, but step in only if the disagreement escalates.

As the semester progresses, you may wonder if a virtual community has actually formed or if the class is still just a collection of students without the benefit of community. Palloff and Pratt[16] offer these indicators that an online community has formed:

- Active interaction among students involving course content and personal communication.
- Collaborative learning—comments are directed primarily student to student rather than student to instructor.
- Socially constructed meaning—agreement or questioning with the intent to achieve agreement.
- Sharing of resources among students.
- Expressions of support and encouragement exchanged between students.
- Willingness to critically evaluate each other's work.

Transformative Learning

The development of a virtual community is the part of online education that really makes transformative learning happen. Transformation of knowledge is discussed in Chapter 3. Similarly, *transformative learning* may be defined as learning that is based on reflection and on interpretation of the experiences, ideas, and assumptions gained through prior learning.[17] The power of a virtual community of learners is that the collaboration and interaction that occur facilitate reflection and the collective exploration of knowledge of practice. It is through thinking critically about real problems that learners are able to expose the "knowing how," which is the skill of practice (procedural knowledge). Our traditional classrooms are places in which we spend enormous amounts of time teaching students about the "knowing that"—that

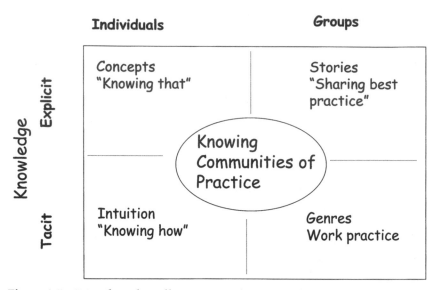

Figure 4-5 Distributed intelligence: insights into online learning. (Adapted from JS Brown. Growing up digital. Change 2000;32[2]:15.)

is, information, facts, and concepts (declarative knowledge). In the practice world, it is the procedural knowledge, or knowledge of practice and skills, that is essential. The computer becomes an important and engaging tool through which peer interaction around real-world problems can occur. So, when the instructor provides a structure for discussion of a patient case or students bring their own clinical cases to the discussion board, the community of learners can engage in a dialogue. For instance, they can ask questions of one another or pose suggestions for interventions, which contributes to the group discussion and participation in a community of practice. The computer, coupled with pedagogical structure, provides a stimulus for practitioners to share knowledge. Brown argues that this focus on the knowledge of practice facilitates a broader, more "distributed view of knowledge" versus the traditional view of knowledge as theoretical concepts and research-based evidence[18] (Figure 4-5).

This theory of transformative learning is perhaps best seen in an example. The course Ethics and Legal Issues in Physical Therapy Practice is designed for practitioners, so all students in this course are licensed physical therapists in either clinical practice or an academic setting. Each lesson in the course is designed to have students apply concepts and theory to their own real-life experiences. The students must then take that real-life application and do further analysis by responding to targeted questions. The following is an example of a threaded discussion in which students respond to discussion questions on one of the reading assignments:

Student A: The Thobaben article poses some interesting concepts about managed care. He states that utilitarianism will be insufficient for institutions that have as their purpose the prevention of impairments, quality treatment for improving function, and community reintegration. However, this might work out for institutions that are out to make the almighty dollar. A PTA I hired at the beginning of the year pointed out an example to me. He came from a facility in another state and was required to see a patient every 15 minutes, which meant the patient spent most of the time with the PT aide . . . He was treating (and billing) 30 patients per day . . . We must remember that this utilitarian style has difficulty protecting individual worth and rights as described in the Swisher text . . . I am interested to hear the thoughts of others on this topic.

Student B: Hi—I agree that this situation is horrible. I am writing my final paper on issues of overutilization of physical therapy aides. The case you discussed is similar. Why are patients being treated by aides? In our state, there are problems with Worker's Compensation Insurance not reimbursing for physical therapy treatments performed by a PTA. What is happening?

Instructor: Hi all—This discussion reminds me of a previous discussion we had on health care as a "commodity good" like selling cars or buying tires. Where is the focus of interest? On patient well-being or revenues? This discussion also relates to our American culture, with strong values such as self-determination and capitalism. How do we come to our own sense of "common good"? Do we have one?

Student C: I agree with Thobaben's concept of managed care and your analogy/case application to his construct. I continue to be amazed by persons who participate in a profession espousing compassion, beneficence, and justice but who seem to have no moral imagination when it comes to foregoing those attributes to make more money. The persons described by you can't go home at the end of the day and think they did a good job.

Student D: Hi all. This is what I am writing my final paper on for this class. There seems to be a conflict between utilitarianism and care for patients with chronic illness. I'm not sure what the answer is . . . but it seems that awareness of the importance of issues and ethical responsibility is a first step.

Instructor: Can you believe how far you have come? Look at your use of language and theory! Could you imagine using the term *utilitarianism* as part of your normal conversation? And look at the challenges that lie ahead for all of us. Keep up the great dialogue . . .

It is through the interactive, asynchronous discussion across learners that the group begins to form a learning community. The instructor provides key comments and corrects any misconceptions but essentially just gently guides the discussion. Often, those learners with more clinical and education experience and wisdom are able to assist others in the group with the analysis of their work.

Roles and Responsibilities of Online Instructors

Regardless of how outstanding a job you have done in preparing your course Web site, if you are not prepared to assume the role of an online instructor, students will be frustrated and less likely to be successful. As indicated in this chapter, instructors assume new roles in the online educational environment; they serve more as facilitators and guides than as purveyors of knowledge. Whitis[19] defines the characteristics of successful teachers in distance education as follows:

- Experienced, life-long learner
- Collaborative style of teaching
- Enjoys up-front conceptual work
- Skilled at group process
- Explicit expectations and evaluation schema
- Detailed, frequent, developmental feedback to students
- Takes risks and learns from experience
- Motivator, coach, and guide

This list of characteristics may explain why teachers who employ the traditional lecture style extensively may not be particularly successful when their lecture notes are simply transferred into an online learning format.

Hiltz[15] suggests the following guidelines for online instructors:

1. *Closely watch your use of language.* Students in your virtual classroom do not have the benefit of body language to assist them in interpreting your message. To compensate, they often read between the lines in e-mail messages, chat conversations, or discussion postings. See the netiquette guidelines.

2. *Keep Web lectures short.* If your course requires that extensive content be presented online, build in opportunities for students to participate early and often in each module.

3. *Constantly encourage learners to participate.* Refer to your students by name. Direct questions to individual students, and be generous with praise for students who participate with thoughtful contributions.

4. *Assign work that requires collaboration.* This humanizes the learning experience for online students and lessens their feelings of isolation. Design assignments that require students to form groups among classmates, contact experts, or collaborate with students in other online courses.

5. *Schedule and keep online office hours.* These may occur using a chat room or immediate-response e-mail. Online students also appreciate knowing when you are physically in your office, in case they wish to call. Be sensitive to the geographic locations of your students and schedule your hours so you are available at times convenient to all students.

6. *Provide a syllabus.* Include a schedule in your syllabus or as a separate page. If you plan to update materials on your site during the semester, let students know how you will notify them of changes.

7. *Provide frequent summaries and reviews.* Doing so is especially important in discussion postings. It provides students with a sense that you are engaged in the course and also allows you to keep students on track.

8. *Keep the class size between 10 and 20.* Enough students are needed to keep discussions robust and interesting, but too many students can be overwhelming. In fact, more than 15 is hard for faculty to handle in terms of discussion and online interaction. If it is necessary to have a large number of students in your online class, see about engaging some assistance to update content or facilitate some of the discussions, or both. Chat groups should be limited to five or six to allow all to participate and keep the thread of the conversation salient.

Online instructors must also take on a managerial role[20] that includes a wide range of responsibilities, such as

- Set and enforce objectives, rules, and, norms—intervene immediately to prevent and stop inappropriate online behavior (see Network Etiquette: Netiquette). Rules and norms for your class may also address the issue of plagiarism (which is more prolific online), model adherence to copyright, and fair use laws.
- Pace the course—be sensitive to students' technology-related problems.
- Make decisions relative to the course.
- Provide a list of all participants—doing so facilitates community building.
- Prompt students to maintain the pace of the course.
- Manage discussions (prompt students to keep the thread of the discussions, opening and closing discussions).
- Schedule and manage testing sessions.
- Keep records.

Record keeping in an online course can become very cumbersome and time consuming. A robust online course in which students are using online course tools to discuss materials, collaborate on projects, reflect on their experiences, and post projects may create large quantities of data that should be tracked and require responses. How do you keep track of all these data? A table or grid that lists all the students in the class down the left side and all required participation projects or communication across the top works well. As students complete a requirement, a check, plus, or minus is recorded. At a glance, the instructor can determine which students are participating and track their progress through the course requirements.

Online instructors must also help students overcome the temptation to procrastinate. The out of sight, out of mind thinking can lead to relatively large percentages of students not completing the class on time. Set a good example by responding to student communications and assignment submissions in a timely manner. Due dates should apply to papers, projects, and discussion postings. Students not meeting timelines should be contacted immediately to determine the reason for the timelines' not being met and to develop a solution if necessary. The online environment opens up a wide array of reasons why students may be late in submitting assignments. In addition to the traditional "the dog ate my homework," students may experience technical difficulties beyond their control. The following suggestions may help your students stay on track and submit assignments in a timely manner[21]:

- Save all assignments to the hard drive and to an additional media source (floppy disk, zip disk, CD-ROM).
- Have students complete all assignments offline, save, and copy or attach to the discussion posting or e-mail message; doing so decreases the chances that their work will become lost in cyberspace if they are kicked offline unexpectedly.
- Provide clear deadlines, discuss them during the first week of class, and stick to them.
- Develop multiple avenues to contact students. If the server housing your course goes down, you should be able to contact students quickly. Have fax and phone numbers in case the e-mail system becomes disabled.

Online instructors are often students' first line of defense when encountering technical problems. In this role, you should be prepared to assist students with basic technology difficulties and make students comfortable in the online environment. The goal is to make the technology transparent to the students, allowing them to focus on the course content. If you are comfortable and somewhat familiar with the technology used to deliver your online course, you are equipped to provide students with a basic level of assistance. This assistance usually involves helping them log into the class (ensure they are using the correct URL, user name, and password), helping them print course materials, and helping them use the course tools you have included in your class.

Now that your course materials are ready for students, you have plans in place to promote collaborative learning in your course, and you have prepared yourself for the role of online instructor, it is time to prepare your students for the online learning experience.

Preparing Your Students

Preparing your students for participation in a Web-based course encompasses many of the same issues addressed in preparing them for using online course components for traditional campus-based courses. For example, you first need to provide students with detailed knowledge about this new approach to teaching; then, provide them with frequent feedback concerning expectations and student progress at the beginning of the course.

Students are generally more anxious at the start of a Web-based course than a campus-based course, because the online learning environment is new to them. To make students feel comfortable in your class, allow them some time to explore the online environment. A scavenger hunt is a good way to accomplish this. The first day of class, send students an e-mail detailing a series of tasks they are to accomplish in the online course. Have them find and use each tool you plan to use in your course. You may have them find and print the syllabus, send an e-mail with an attachment to you and at least one classmate, post to the discussion, participate in a scheduled chat session, and complete their biography page. This exercise not only serves to increase students' comfort level in the environment, but also immediately engages them in the course and allows them time to work through technical issues before engaging in the content, all of which increase the likelihood they will complete the course successfully.

Summary

Technology is another tool in an instructor's arsenal to enhance the educational experience for students. Regardless of the educational setting or the type of technology used, technology should be used for the purpose of facilitating learning experiences that actively challenge and engage students. Teaching with technology may be accomplished in several scenarios: enhancing in-class lectures with multimedia, moving course materials to the Web and using class time for discussion and application exercises, or creating a virtual classroom. Regardless of the scenario used, planning and preparation are needed to maximize the effectiveness of the technology. As with a course low in technology, preparation of your teaching materials, yourself, and your students is crucial to a successful educational experience.

References

1. National Educational Technology Standards Project. International Society for Technology in Education, 2001, <http://cnets.iste.org>. Accessed: November 7, 2001.
2. Association for Educational Communications and Technology Task Force. Educational Technology: Definition and Glossary of Terms. Washington, DC: Association for Educational Communications and Technology, 1977.
3. Commission on Instructional Technology. To Improve Learning. A Report to the President and the Congress of the United States. Washington, DC: U.S. Government Printing Office, 1970.
4. Steathelm HH. Common Elements in the Planning Process. In RV Carlson, G Awkerman (eds), Education Planning: Concepts, Strategies and Practices. New York: Longman, 1991;267–278.
5. Picciano AG. Educational Leadership and Planning for Technology. Upper Saddle River, NJ: Prentice-Hall, 1998.
6. Simonson M. Instructional Technology and Attitude Change. In GJ Anglin, S Brown, S Haenel (eds), Instructional Technology: Past, Present and Future (2nd ed). Englewood, CO: Libraries Unlimited, 1995.
7. Beer V. The Web Learning Field Book. San Francisco: Jossey-Bass, 1998;43–63.
8. Walvoord B, Anderson V. Effective Grading: A Tool for Learning and Assessment. San Francisco: Jossey-Bass, 1998;43–63.
9. Rogers, EM. Diffusion of Innovations (4th ed). New York: The Free Press, 1995.
10. Svetcov, D. The virtual classroom vs. the real one. Forbes Best of the Web, 11 September 2000, <http://www.forbes.com/best/2000/0911/050.html>. Accessed: November 7, 2001.
11. Purtilo R. Ethical Dimensions in the Health Professions (3rd ed). Philadelphia: W.B. Saunders, 1999.
12. Gilligan C. In a Different Voice: Psychological Theory and Woman's Development. Cambridge, MA: Harvard University Press, 1982.
13. Shea V. Netiquette. San Francisco: Albion Books, 1994.

14. Billings DM. A Conceptual Model of Correspondence Course Completion. In MG Moore, GC Clark (eds), Readings in Distance Learning and Instruction. University Park, PA: American Center for the Study of Distance Education, 1989.

15. Hiltz SR. Teaching in a virtual classroom. Paper presented at the International Conference on Computer-Assisted Instruction, Hsinchu, Taiwan, March 1995.

16. Palloff R, Pratt K. Building Learning Communities in Cyberspace. San Francisco: Jossey-Bass, 1999.

17. Mezirow J and Associates. Fostering Critical Reflection in Adulthood: A Guide to Transformative and Emancipatory Learning. San Francisco: Jossey-Bass, 1990.

18. Brown JS. Growing up digital. Change 2000;32(2):11–20.

19. Whitis G. A Survey of Technology-Based Distance Education: Emerging Issues and Lessons Learned. Washington, DC: Association of Academic Health Centers, 2001.

20. Berge Z, Collins M. Computer-Mediated Communication and the Online Classroom, 3 vols. Cresskill, NJ: Hampton Press, 1995.

21. Schweizer H. Designing and Teaching an On-Line Course: Spinning Your Web Classroom. Boston: Allyn & Bacon, 1999.

Annotated Bibliography

Berge Z, Collins M. Computer Mediated Communication and the Online Classroom, 3 vols. Cresskill, NJ: Hampton Press, 1995. This collection provides a wealth of straightforward, concrete information relative to teaching and learning online. The practical, clear-cut suggestions for creating, teaching, managing, and assessing your course in the cyber classroom will make your and your students' experience more enjoyable and productive.

Brooks D. Web Teaching: A Guide to Designing Interactive Teaching for the World Wide Web. New York: Plenum Press, 1997. With the growth in the number of courses being offered on the Web across a variety of disciplines, instructors are often at a loss when attempting to identify the most appropriate Web-based tools available to assist in the achievement of desired student outcomes. This book provides a foundation of information on which instructors can draw in this endeavor. A wide array of topics is addressed, from pedagogy to managing the technology.

Palloff R, Pratt K. Lessons from the Cyberspace Classroom: The Realities of Online Teaching. San Francisco: Jossey-Bass, 2001. A must-read for anyone connected with moving teaching and learning to the online environment. This book is a comprehensive guide for preparing for online education. Palloff and Pratt begin by guiding you through the process of building a conceptual framework, then discuss the more pragmatic issues related to e-education, including numerous examples. The chapters include information and suggestions relative to the art of teaching, administrative issues and concerns, tools of online teaching, transforming courses for the online classroom, teaching courses developed by others, and working with the virtual student.

Palloff R, Pratt K. Building Learning Communities in Cyberspace. San Francisco: Jossey-Bass, 1999. Another must-read from Palloff and Pratt in which they lay out the process of creating a sense of community among online learners. As with *Lessons from the Cyberspace Classroom: The Realities of Online Teaching*, this book begins with the process of building a conceptual framework, then moves into practical advice for facilitating the creation of online learning communities.

Schweizer H. Designing and Teaching an On-Line Course: Spinning Your Web Classroom. Boston: Allyn & Bacon, 1999. Schweitzer provides step-by-step advice, including detailed examples, for developing and teaching an online course. The It's Your Turn section of each chapter gives you the opportunity to apply the practical, research-supported strategies presented. Comments from former online learners provide insight into what cyber students need and sometimes demand. Whether you are ready to develop an online course or are just contemplating the possibility, this book provides the steps necessary for course development, online teaching, and online assessment.

Whitis G. A Survey of Technology-Based Distance Education: Emerging Issues and Lessons Learned. Washington, DC: Association of Academic Health Centers, 2001. This publication, the result of a grant from the Robert Wood Johnson Foundation, focuses on key issues for distance educations in the health professions. The chapters are brief and to the point, highlighting the essential issues for faculty, students, and administrators in delivering distance education. This book is well referenced and has an extensive listing of resources and Web sites. This book is a must for any department launching a distance program in the health professions.

A

International Society for Technology in Education: National Educational Technology Standards and Performance Indicators

Educational Technology Foundations for All Teachers

I. Technology operations and concepts. Teachers demonstrate a sound understanding of technology operations and concepts. Teachers

  A. Demonstrate introductory knowledge, skills, and understanding of concepts related to technology (as described in the International Society for Technology in Education's *Technology Standards for Students*).

  B. Demonstrate continual growth in technology knowledge and skills to stay abreast of current and emerging technologies.

II. Planning and designing learning environments and experiences. Teachers plan and design effective learning environments and experiences supported by technology. Teachers

  A. Design developmentally appropriate learning opportunities that apply technology-enhanced instructional strategies to support the diverse needs of learners.

B. Apply current research on teaching and learning with technology when planning learning environments and experiences.

C. Identify and locate technology resources and evaluate them for accuracy and suitability. Plan for the management of technology resources within the context of learning activities.

D. Plan strategies to manage student learning in a technology-enhanced environment.

III. Teaching, learning, and the curriculum. Teachers implement curriculum plans that include methods and strategies for applying technology to maximize student learning. Teachers

A. Facilitate technology-enhanced experiences that address content standards and student technology standards.

B. Use technology to support learner-centered strategies that address the diverse needs of students.

C. Apply technology to develop students' higher-order skills and creativity.

D. Manage student learning activities in a technology-enhanced environment.

IV. Assessment and evaluation. Teachers apply technology to facilitate a variety of effective assessment and evaluation strategies. Teachers

A. Apply technology in assessing student learning of subject matter using a variety of assessment techniques.

B. Use technology resources to collect and analyze data, interpret results, and communicate findings to improve instructional practice and maximize student learning.

C. Apply multiple methods of evaluation to determine students' appropriate use of technology resources for learning, communication, and productivity.

V. Productivity and professional practice. Teachers use technology to enhance their productivity and professional practice. Teachers

A. Use technology resources to engage in ongoing professional development and lifelong learning.

B. Continually evaluate and reflect on professional practice to make informed decisions regarding the use of technology in support of student learning.

C. Apply technology to increase productivity.

D. Use technology to communicate and collaborate with peers, parents, and the larger community to nurture student learning.

VI. Social, ethical, legal, and human issues. Teachers understand the social, ethical, legal, and human issues surrounding the use of technology in preK–12 schools and apply those principles in practice. Teachers

A. Model and teach legal and ethical practice related to technology use.

B. Apply technology resources to enable and empower learners with diverse backgrounds, characteristics, and abilities.

C. Identify and use technology resources that affirm diversity.

D. Promote safe and healthy use of technology resources.

E. Facilitate equitable access to technology resources for all students.

For more information on the National Educational Technology Standards Project, contact

Lajeane Thomas, Project Director
Telephone: 318.257.3923
E-mail: lthomas@latech.edu
National Educational Technology Standards Web site: http://cnets.iste.org

B

Web Hosting Sites

http://www.homestead.com—Homestead's Web site provides you with tools to build your own Web site, share photos and images, and interact with others of similar interests.

http://www.yahoo.com—Yahoo! offers links to a wide variety of resources, including personal e-mail accounts, online shopping, current events, and Web site building and hosting.

http://www.blackboard.com—the Blackboard course management system provides server space to host your course materials, course discussions, and online testing.

5

Assessing and Improving the Teaching-Learning Process in Academic Settings

Gail M. Jensen and Katherine F. Shepard

Did you ever express or hear comments like these?

Well, you have to be careful about putting too much time into your teaching. Good teaching takes time away from the things you need to do to get tenure and promotion at this institution. What really matters is research, grant writing, and publications.

Isn't program assessment the function of the curriculum committee? Besides, I was hired as a neuroscientist, not an educator.

I know what the students need to know; that's why I need one more semester hour in my course to cover the material.

Whatever you do, don't volunteer for the self-study task force; leave those accreditation activities to the educators.

Sure, I evaluate my course. All students fill out an evaluation form the last day of class.

Now that the reader is well into using good pedagogy (see Chapters 1 and 2), which supports the use of carefully considered and effective techniques for teaching and evaluating students (see Chapters 3 and 4), we will turn our attention to the use of assessment techniques. Assessment techniques are used to assess one's teaching with the goal of improving student learning. Classroom educators focus on designing, evaluating, and revising the particular courses to which they are assigned. Intent on the subject matter they teach, educators often disconnect their teaching roles from the ongoing assessment and thoughtful scholarship of how their teaching actually influences student knowledge, understanding, attitudes, values, and behaviors. In this chapter, we explore practical mechanisms and tools that all educator-scholars can use for assessment and improvement of their teaching and resultant improvement in student learning.

Chapter Objectives

After completing this chapter, the reader will be able to

1. Define and give examples of the three main learning problems students have: amnesia, fantasia, and inertia.
2. Distinguish between assessment and evaluation, and describe the relationship between assessment and student learning across educational settings, including classroom, program, and institution.
3. Identify the four pillars of transformative assessment and describe how and why they undergird program assessment activities.
4. List six principles of good practice for assessing student learning suggested by the American Association for Higher Education (AAHE).
5. Take and score the Teaching Goals Inventory (TGI) to determine your primary course goals for each class that you teach (see Appendix 5-A). Determine whether these goals are synchronous with the preactive teaching grid (see Chapter 2) for each course.
6. Describe at least three classroom assessment techniques (CATs) that you could use to quickly assess the success of your teaching in any given class.
7. Apply the three levels of implementing an assessment program to the four areas of institutional assessment: institutional culture; shared responsibility among faculty, administration, and students; institutional support; and efficacy of assessment activities in your institution.
8. Distinguish the differences between scholarly teaching and the scholarship of teaching.
9. Describe key steps for implementing a process of peer assessment.
10. Discuss how the elements of design, enactment, and outcome apply to a course portfolio process.

Assessment

What is assessment? Is it that periodic bother that comes once every so many years when a program needs to go through a self-study and accreditation process? Is it the course evaluations that students fill out at the end of the semester? Is it a formal program review that institutions require of every department every few years or when a new president or provost is hired? Is it collecting data from graduate alumni? Assessment pertains to all of these major activities. But notice that all these activities are summative— that is, they occur *after* a teaching-learning experience has been completed. However, formative assessment activities, which occur *during* a teaching-learning experience, have equal or more importance in improving one's teaching skills and resultant student learning. It is these formative assessment techniques that are the focus of this chapter.

The terms *evaluation* and *assessment* are often used interchangeably. However, for the purposes of this chapter, we make the following distinction: *Evaluation* refers to an end point, determining whether an action is right or wrong (e.g., answers to questions on a classroom exam); *assessment* refers to looking closely at teaching events with a central emphasis on student learning and considerations of how to improve student outcomes.[1]

The assessment movement in education has been stimulated at the Federal level by both institutional and specialized (professional) accreditation agencies. This movement is having a powerful influence on higher education. The central focus is on accountability of the educational program related to student learning outcomes.[2] The American Association of Higher Education (AAHE) has been and continues to be a leader in the assessment movement in higher education. The AAHE's publications, *Change* magazine and the *AAHE Bulletin*, should be regular reading in physical therapy and physical therapist assistant programs for those interested in assessment. Why is ongoing educational assessment, which helps us determine ways to improve our teaching and resultant student outcomes, so important to physical therapy educators that we spend an entire chapter on it? The answer lies in the learning problems students bring with them when they enter physical therapy programs.

Student Learning Problems

Students come to our physical therapy programs with well-ingrained learning problems that hinder both the acquisition and the retention of information. Lee Shulman[3] identifies three of these common problems as amnesia, fantasia, and inertia. For those of us teaching the next generation of health care professionals, these problems with student learning are an anathema.

Amnesia refers to students' learning material for an exam but forgetting it immediately after the exam. This happens when our physical therapy programs are packed with courses with little time built in for students to reflect, integrate, and apply the information they are receiving. Students learn to survive such programs by focusing on whatever exam is next. Thus, for instance, cramming for an anatomy exam is followed by "dumping" the information to cram for a pathology examination. This practice might not have severe consequences in an undergraduate liberal arts program in which a biology course is not connected to an English course. However, amnesia obviously has serious consequences for students in health professional programs, in which inter-relating and building on information is a well-imbedded assumption of the faculty.

Fantasia refers to illusions students have about how things in the world work and how people behave. Cognitive psychologists have long argued that new learning grows out of prior learning; that is, learning will occur only when new information is linked to existing knowledge. Thus, Shulman points out that misconceptions that students hold hinder the appropriate reception of new information. For example, if a student believes from her or his past athletic experiences "no pain, no gain," how will that belief influence her or his understanding of pain management and ability to work with patients who have painful, chronic, debilitating conditions?

Inertia is the student's inability to apply what is known. This occurs when students are taught piecemeal facts that the student cannot organize or use in a problem-solving situation. For example, students who are asked to memorize origins and insertions of muscles without a functional movement context are very likely to forget this anatomical information by the time they are asked to assess gait deviations.

All academic faculty are familiar with these problems of learning. For physical therapy faculty, these problems must be dealt with for students to successfully attain the knowledge, skills, and values of a professional practitioner. Each new group of students enters our programs having done well in their prior academic endeavors in spite of exhibiting amnesia, fantasia, and inertia. Students may even believe they performed well because of amnesia, fantasia, and inertia! How do we deal with these three common learning problems, as well as the unique learning problems individual students bring with them (e.g., fear of asking questions in the classroom, competitiveness and the related unwillingness to share knowledge with peers, and the student-versus-the-teacher mentality)? A concerted, programmatic effort must be in place to diminish as much as possible these students' learning problems and give students the insights and skills they need to guide their own lifelong learning. Using the assessment ideas and tools presented in this

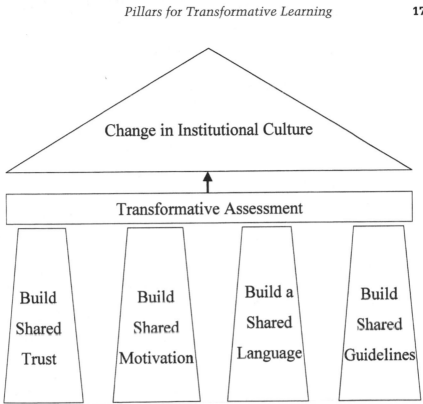

Figure 5-1 Angelo's four pillars of transformative assessment. (Adapted from TA Angelo. Doing assessment as if learning matters most. AAHE Bull 1999;51[9]:3–6.)

chapter is a powerful method to help teachers improve their teaching so that students learn and, equally important, find enjoyment in learning.

Pillars for Transformative Learning

Angelo states, "[D]o assessment as if learning matters most."[4] Assessment affects all levels of education, from individual classrooms and laboratories to programs and the institution in which the programs reside. Angelo argues that there are four essential components, or pillars, for transformative assessment (Figure 5-1). The term *transformative* is used with specific intent. It means that something actually will happen within an institution that leads to a change in the institutional culture. This change is facilitated through individuals who share common beliefs and values, work together to develop guidelines, and act on those guidelines.[5] An example of transformative change in higher education is the current emphasis on student learning, which is visible in many venues (e.g., highlighted in conference topics, discussed and debated in the research literature, and emphasized in accreditation documents).

The four pillars for transformative assessment include

1. *Build shared trust.* This is done through the faculty's building a productive learning community in which the faculty involved in assessment trust one another. All persons must feel respected, valued, and safe to share their experiences.

2. *Build shared motivation.* There have to be collective goals worth working toward and problems worth solving. This means a shift for some faculty, as faculty often focus on what they will teach rather than on what students will learn; students, in turn, often focus on getting through the program.

3. *Build a shared language.* Faculty need to develop a collective understanding of new concepts needed for transformative changes. Although *assessment* may mean only student course evaluations or standardized testing—and time wasted to some faculty members—a collaborative model would focus on assisting the entire faculty to see the broader conception of assessment that focuses on formative assessments and student learning.

4. *Build shared guidelines.* Faculty will benefit from a short list of research-based guidelines that can be used for assessment to promote student learning. An example of a research-based guideline in physical therapy or physical therapist assistant education might include gathering formative assessment data on the ability of students to demonstrate critical professional behaviors or ability-based outcomes. For example, do students demonstrate empathy across the curriculum? What evidence do students provide in support of their clinical decision-making skills?

Angelo's assessment vision includes the formation of learning communities that include groups of faculty and students working toward shared, significant learning goals. He proposes that assessment should be seen as less of a technical data collection process and more of a monitoring and problem-solving process. Moving from a focus on summative evaluation to formative assessment requires the faculty to think about and distinguish between these two concepts. Think about the last time your department went through an accreditation process. What type of approach did your department use in providing information?

The AAHE Assessment Forum provides nine principles of good practice for assessing student learning (Table 5-1) that are a good starting point for thinking about your current assessment activities. You might want to examine these nine principles and see which of them are included in the assessment activities in your classroom, program, or institution. For example, do

Table 5-1   Nine Principles of Good Practice for Assessing Student Learning

1. Assessment of student learning begins with educational values.
2. Assessment is most effective when it reflects an understanding of learning as multi-dimensional, integrated, and revealed in performance over time.
3. Assessment works best when the program has clearly, explicitly stated purposes.
4. Assessment requires equal attention to outcomes and to the experiences that lead to those outcomes.
5. Assessment works best when it is ongoing and not episodic.
6. Assessment fosters wider improvement when representatives from across the educational community are involved.
7. Assessment makes a difference when it begins with issues of use and illuminates questions that people really care about.
8. Assessment is most likely to lead to improvement when it is part of a larger set of conditions that promote change.
9. Through assessment, educators meet responsibilities to students and to the public.

Source: Adapted from AAHE Assessment Forum. Principles of Good Practice for Assessing Student Learning. Washington, DC: American Association for Higher Education, 1992.

your assessment activities attend equally to the teaching-learning experience and the learning outcomes?[6]

Classroom Assessment

> Learning can and often does take place without the benefit of teaching—and sometimes even in spite of it—but there is no such thing as effective teaching in the absence of learning. Teaching without learning is just talking.[7(p3)]

All of us in higher education, regardless of whether we are in a professional school or a graduate department, aim to produce graduates who achieve the highest possible quality of learning. As educators, our greatest reward is the success of our graduates. As we teach, we are constantly engaged in an "informal" process of classroom assessment—that is, what do students know, not know, need to know, and so on. To do this, we ask students questions, observe and react to body language that depicts confusion or boredom, and listen carefully to students' comments. In response to this input, we may speed up, slow down, review material, or change in other ways to react to student learning needs.

We rarely, however, do systematic and formal classroom assessment. As previously stated, classroom assessment techniques are well suited to formative assessment—that is, getting specific feedback from the entire class as we move through the course, thus gaining insight into student learning so that changes can be made to enhance the learning process *before* the end of the course.

Angelo and Cross's well-known book on classroom assessment techniques is an excellent resource for faculty.[7] This book is a practical guide for designing and implementing classroom assessment techniques for any faculty member, regardless of his or her background in education. One of their underlying assumptions is that the quality of student learning is directly related (not exclusively) to the quality of the teaching. One of the most promising ways to improve learning is to improve teaching. Their suggestions for improving teaching include the following:

- To improve effectiveness, teachers first must make their goals and objectives explicit and then obtain feedback to determine the extent to which these goals are being met. (See the preactive teaching grid in Chapter 2.)
- To improve learning, students need to receive appropriate and focused feedback early and often. They also need to learn how to assess their own learning.
- The type of assessment most likely to lead to improvement of teaching and learning is that conducted by faculty themselves, in which they formulate the questions specific to their own teaching concerns.
- The processes of systematic inquiry are an intellectual challenge and an important source of motivation for faculty. Classroom assessment provides this kind of challenge.
- Classroom assessment does *not* require specialized training. It can be carried out by any dedicated teacher within any discipline.
- Through collaborating with colleagues and actively involving students in classroom assessment efforts, faculty can enhance learning and personal satisfaction.

Teaching Goals Inventory

A useful way to initiate classroom assessment planning is for each faculty member to complete the TGI. The TGI is a questionnaire designed to assist faculty in identifying and ranking the relative importance of their teaching goals for any class. With one particular class in mind, the faculty member rates the importance of each of 52 teaching goals across six clustered areas: higher-order thinking skills, basic academic success skills, discipline-specific knowledge and skills, liberal arts and academic values, work and career preparation, and personal development. The complete TGI is available in Appendix 5-A. You will see that there are many parallels between the TGI and the philosophical orientations to curriculum discussed in Chapter 2.

The primary role of the TGI for classroom assessment is for teachers to identify what goals they view as important so that they may target their assessment efforts toward those teaching goals. Secondarily, the collective faculty can share its teaching goals across classes within a semester or across the entire curriculum to assess where its collective teaching and learning focus lies. As with sharing one's philosophical orientation and learning theory emphasis, sharing teaching goals is often an eye-opening experience.

Classroom Assessment Techniques

CATs, as proposed by Angelo and Cross, have the following characteristics[7]:

- The focus is on observing and improving learning rather than on observing and improving teaching.
- The individual teacher decides what and how to assess and how to respond to the information. Autonomy and professional judgment are respected, as the teacher is not obligated to share the results of her or his CATs with anyone else.
- Faculty improve their teaching by constantly asking themselves three questions: "What are the essential skills and knowledge I am trying to teach?, How can I find out whether students are learning these skills?, and How can I help students learn better?"[7(p5)]
- Student learning is reinforced just by doing CATs, as students are asked to reflect on what they are learning, give examples of how to use the information, and indicate points of confusion that can be clarified long before a midterm exam.
- As formative assessments with the purpose of improving the quality of student learning, CATs are usually anonymous as well as ungraded. Thus, students can focus on and provide honest feedback about what and how they are learning rather than searching for "the right answer." Students as well as teachers learn to enjoy CATs as both an intriguing and an intellectual process.
- Each class of students presents with a unique and diverse mix of student backgrounds, learning attitudes and skills, and learning problems, and, as such, each class develops a unique microculture. Thus, CATs need to be used sensitively and specifically with each different class being taught. A CAT that is successful for one teacher in one class with one group of students at one time of the year will not necessarily be similarly successful if any one of these variables changes.
- Classroom assessment is an ongoing process used throughout the semester.

What does a CAT look like? Here are simple examples of introductory assessment techniques for looking at student learning. Let's say you are teaching a unit in a neuromuscular course on motor learning. You are particularly interested in the students' ability to understand and apply core theoretical concepts. You know that the lecture and discussion materials you have for them in this area are complex and challenging, even for your strongest students. You want some quick way to assess students' ability to understand the theoretical concepts. Here are several very simple and quick ways to gather data from students:

- *Minute paper* (also known as the *one-minute paper* or *half-sheet response*). Stop your class a few minutes early and have students respond to two questions: (1) What was the most important concept you learned during this class?, and (2) What important question remains unanswered for you?
- *Muddiest point.* At the end of class, have students write down on a piece of paper a response to the question, "What was the muddiest point in this lecture today?"

By collecting and reviewing these CATs, you will gain immediate insight into students' learning experiences, which will help you direct your next class with them. Although CATs help teachers assess student learning problems, they also help enormously with actual student learning. That is, ongoing assessments of learning require that students stop and think about what they have learned and then synthesize and express in writing what they do and do not understand. Thus, CATs help to offset the global classroom problems of amnesia, fantasia, and inertia, as well as individual learning problems, such as reluctance to ask for help.

A CAT can also be used to determine whether students understand basic relationships among concepts. Be creative! For example, have students express concepts by drawing, moving their bodies through space, or using Tinker toys.

- *Modeling.* At any point in the class, have students draw a model that demonstrates the basic relationships among concepts. Have students discuss their models with each other and field their questions.

You can also use CATs to assess attitudes and perceptions. Metaphors are very helpful in identifying feeling states, often before the student is able to put feelings into words.

- *Metaphors.* Ask students to write a metaphor followed by a one- or two-sentence explanation. This is easily done as a fill-in-the-blank question. For example, the question is "Doing research is like _____." The answers—for example, "walking through molasses," "a puzzle," "going to the dentist," and "an adventure"—are very telling.

Table 5-2 Defining Features Matrix: Example from a Course on Health Behavior

Features	PRECEDE-PROCEED model	Readiness for change model	Self-efficacy model
Precontemplation		X	
Predisposing factors	X		
Social assessment	X		
Maintenance		X	
Outcome expectation			X
Reinforcing factors	X		
Confidence			X
Relapse		X	
Enabling factors	X		
Self-confidence			X
Behavior and lifestyle	X		
Importance			X
Action		X	
Educational assessment	X		
Contemplation		X	
Efficacy expectation			X

Source: Adapted from S Rollnick, P Mason, C Butler. Health Behavior Change: A Guide for Practitioners. New York: Churchill Livingstone, 1999.

You might be wondering how your teaching goals apply to your selection of CATs. The link between the TGI and your CATs is that you should do formative assessments on those targeted teaching goals that you value most. For example, many of us are interested in facilitating growth in students' critical thinking skills. How do we know that we are on the right track in our classroom experience with students? Here is one CAT that could be used to do a quick check on students' ability to distinguish core concepts:

- *Defining features matrix.* The purpose of this exercise is to assess students' skills at categorizing information using a given set of critical defining features. Faculty can then do a quick check of how well students can distinguish between similar concepts and make critical distinctions. This assessment technique is particularly good for helping learners make critical distinctions between apparently similar concepts. Table 5-2 provides an example from a course on health education and an assessment of health behaviors.

A quick scan of students' responses will help you identify points about which students are confused.

Here is another CAT that addresses students' problem-solving skills:

- *Documented problem solutions.* The aim of this assessment technique is to assess how students solve problems and how they understand and can express their problem-solving strategies. This technique is particularly good in helping students to explicate their thought processes and approaches to solving problems. For example, in a biomechanics course, you could divide the class into groups and give each group a problem. Have the groups solve the problem and document each step of the problem-solving process. Then have the groups do a show-and-tell on their problem solution approaches.

Similar to other CATs, this activity gives you good information about students' problem-solving skills, but it is equally useful in helping students identify how they solve problems, as well as in giving them ideas about other problem-solving approaches they might use.

For more examples of CATs, see Angelo and Cross's book, which has a compilation of more than 50 different classroom assessment techniques.[7]

Quality Circles

Quality circles have long been used by Japanese companies as a way to get input from employees on how to improve production. Although this practice has been adopted by many American companies, it has not been used in education, primarily because the issue of ongoing formative assessment has only recently been accepted.[7,8]

- *Quality circles.* On the first day of the course, ask for a small group of three or four volunteers who would be willing to meet with you every few weeks for 15 or 20 minutes to give you feedback about how the course is going. Ask for a diverse group—that is, those who are particularly interested in the subject matter to be taught, as well as those who are less interested. At the first meeting with students, ask them to be responsible for soliciting feedback from other students in the class and discuss with them how to give and receive feedback. That is, the quality circle will not be a "complaint session" but rather a discussion on what is going well in class and what might be improved in the course and how to improve it. The feedback is two way: Students give feedback to the instructor, and the instructor gives feedback to the students. The feedback is focused on anything that is happening in the classroom that facilitates or impedes student learning. Thus, discussions might include course assignments, classroom physical environment, use of cases and classroom exercises, communication between the instructor and the students, level of reading assignments, and evaluation and grading. The next time the whole class meets, members of the quality circle and the instructor make a brief report to the whole class on what can change and how, and what can't be changed and why.[7]

Students take their quality circle roles seriously, and the discussions are thoughtful joint problem-solving ventures during which the instructor is allowed to grow, and students gain insight as to their own responsibilities for learning. For example, the instructor can ask the quality circle to suggest ways to increase class participation or why an assignment was generally poorly done. The atmosphere is collegial, and change is supported and applauded.

Program Assessment

Another major area of assessment in educational programs is program assessment. One of the four major sections of the American Physical Therapy Association accreditation self study is devoted to program assessment: "Physical therapy education programs are accountable for an ongoing process of assessment of educational outcomes and for continuous improvement in all aspects of the program."[9] This ongoing process of assessment addresses all components of the program, including adjunct and support faculty; admissions criteria and prerequisites; clinical education facilities; clinical education faculty; core faculty; curriculum; institutional and program policies and procedures; program mission, philosophy, goals, and objectives; performance of recent graduates; and physical and human resources. Boucher surveyed physical therapy programs shortly after the revised accreditation criteria were implemented.[10] She found that the majority of programs addressed all of the components; however, some of the components (i.e., adjunct faculty, clinical education faculty, and admissions) were assessed on a more informal basis.

Remember that two of the "pillars of transformative assessment" include building a shared language and shared guidelines among program faculty. One powerful tool for doing this is to outline a formal, written assessment plan. It may be most helpful to look at an example from the Assessment Plan for the Doctor of Physical Therapy program at Creighton University. The Assessment Plan includes five core dimensions for assessment: student, faculty, curriculum, environment, and graduates. Each of these dimensions is broken into very specific subcategories. Then, each subcategory is mapped out according to what assessment method will be used, who will implement the task, and when the task will be done. In Table 5-3, you see an example from the student dimension—that is, admissions. Note that the specificity of the subcategories makes it easier to identify an assessment method as well as to determine the who and when.

Program assessment plans can identify and address the unique and innovative elements of the program and institution. These unique elements (e.g., producing graduates who will provide service to their community or an emphasis on rural health care) should be visible in mission and philosophy statements.

The crucial element in assessment is that a faculty "learning community" must be a real community that has shared motivation and trust. The assessment process is not the responsibility of one person, but that of the entire faculty. The departmental assessment plan needs to be monitored and updated annually, or more often if needed. This function can be done through the curriculum or assessment committee. If you are in a school or college with several health professions, you may find it worthwhile to have an assessment task force across health professions that can be used for sharing resources and designing instruments that target issues of the institutional mission.

One final suggestion to help make assessment a valued activity is to plan that assessment work to include a research component. Mentokowski and Loacker[11] have developed a model called the *triangulated validation model*. Figure 5-2 depicts an adaptation of this model applied to a physical therapy program. Here, the three core assessment dimensions include regular curricular activities, research and evaluation activities focused on tracking student and graduate progress, and review of external sources. The combination of these activities provides opportunities for triangulation of assessment findings as well as evolution and enhancement of the program.

Institutional Assessment

Most institutions now are required to submit annual updates of their assessment plans to their regional accreditation agency.[12] Health professions programs have much to offer other disciplines on campus, given the structure and accountability mechanisms in our specialized accreditation process. A useful tool for investigating how assessment is done on your campus or in your program is Assessment of Student Academic Achievement: Levels of Implementation, Chapter 4 in the North Central Association of Colleges and Schools' *Handbook of Accreditation*.[13] There are four areas of the institution that are targeted for assessment:

- Institutional culture: collective or shared values and mission
- Shared responsibility: faculty, administration, and students

Table 5-3   Example of the Student Component of Admissions for a Program Assessment Plan

Evaluation component/tasks	Method	Who	When
Students: Admissions			
1. Prerequisite courses/student preparation for doctor of physical therapy program	Review of prerequisite courses to determine fit between student preparation and curricular demands	Department Admissions Committee	Done annually before preparation of admissions material
2. Characteristics of students fit with admissions criteria	Database profile for enrolled students by class that includes academic background and performance upon entry	Department Admissions Committee	Data prepared annually at beginning of academic year with assistance from School Admissions Office
3. Student recruitment strategies	Comparison of database with School of Pharmacy and Allied Health Professions marketing plan (e.g., number of applicants, diversity of applicant pool)	School of Pharmacy and Allied Health Professions Admissions Office	Performed at the beginning of each academic year
4. Application process	Feedback gathered by Admissions Chair from faculty	Faculty/school admissions department	Immediately after admissions process each spring
	Applicant satisfaction surveys	Applicants	
5. Enrolled student review process by faculty for academic performance and professional behaviors	Academic performance: midterm and end-of-semester grade reports	Student faculty advisor	Ongoing—advisor follows up with students as needed
	Faculty group discussion of student professional behaviors from course interactions and other programmatic activities	Department Chair and faculty	Performed at the end of every semester/ongoing faculty meetings
	Clinical Competence Performance Exam	Faculty	Done at the end of every semester

Source: Adapted from Department of Physical Therapy, School of Pharmacy and Allied Health Professions, Creighton University, Omaha, NE.

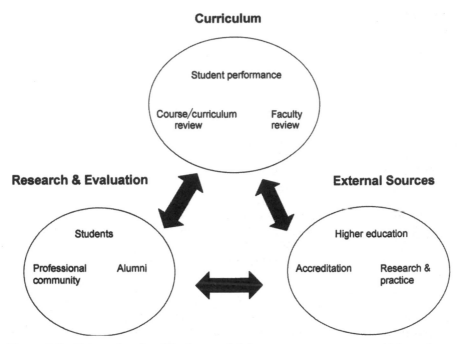

Figure 5-2   Triangulated validation model for program assessment. (Adapted from M Mentkowski, G Loacker. Assessing and Validating Outcomes of College. In PT Ewell [ed], Assessing Educational Outcomes. San Francisco: Jossey-Bass, 1985;47–64.)

- Institutional support: resources and structures
- Efficacy of assessment: evidence, outcomes data

Each of these four areas can be assessed according to three levels of increasing sophistication in examining and devising assessment strategies and collecting related evidence:

- Level 1: beginning implementation of assessment programs
- Level 2: making progress in implementing assessment programs
- Level 3: maturing stages of continuous improvement

Table 5-4 contains an example of the four areas of institutional assessment across the three levels of increasing sophistication in implementation. You may want to review the table to determine the status of your institution regarding level of implementation.

This chapter is about learning, assessment, and accountability. We began this chapter with a discussion of classroom assessment. We conclude the chapter by moving from a focus on classroom assessment to a discussion of classroom research, or the scholarship of teaching.

Table 5-4 Assessment of Student Academic Achievement: Examples of Patterns of Characteristics across Levels of Implementation

	Levels of Program Assessment		
	Level 1: beginning implementation of assessment program	*Level 2: making progress in implementing assessment program*	*Level 3: maturing stages of continuous improvement*
Institutional culture: shared values/mission	Shared understanding of assessment is just emerging. Institutional mission statement does not include wording about student learning. Some or all academic units do not show a relationship to the institutional mission.	Student learning and assessment are valued across institution, departments and programs. Institutional mission explicitly addresses student learning.	Assessment has become an institutional priority, a way of life. Assessment program materials developed at institutional level reflect emphasis on learning expectations, determining outcomes of student learning across academic programs, and using assessment to improve student learning.
Shared responsibility: faculty	Only a few academic departments have described measurable objectives for their educational goals. Faculty question the efficacy of the assessment program.	Most departments have developed measurable objectives for educational goals. Faculty members are taking responsibility for ensuring direct and indirect measures of student learning fit with educational goals.	Faculty speak publicly and informally with their peers in support of the assessment plan. Faculty are exploring uses of assessment in the context of research on learning theories and active learning strategies.

Table 5-4 *continued*

	Levels of Program Assessment		
	Level 1: beginning implementation of assessment program	*Level 2: making progress in implementing assessment program*	*Level 3: maturing stages of continuous improvement*
Institutional support: resources	Sufficient resources have yet to be allocated in the operating budget for a comprehensive assessment program. There are few provisions for collecting, interpreting, or using data about student learning.	There is an Office of Institutional Research and sufficient budget to support a viable assessment program. Resources are available for faculty serving on the Assessment Committee, faculty seeking to develop their skills in assessing student learning, and departments requesting funding to implement an assessment program.	Characteristics of Level Two are continued, sustained, and enhanced. A budget line has been established and sufficient resources are allocated to sustain a comprehensive program.
Efficacy of assessment: evidence and outcomes	Implementation of the assessment program is in initial stages and progressing at a slower-than-desired pace. Few, if any, programs are using assessment results.	Faculty members are increasingly engaged in interpreting assessment results, discussing implications, and recommending changes to improve student learning. Assessment findings about the state of student learning are beginning to be incorporated into reviews of academic programs.	Student learning has become central to the culture of the institution. A culture of evidence has emerged and is sustained by both faculty and administrative commitment to excellent teaching and effective learning.

Source: Adapted from North Central Association of Colleges and Schools Commission on Institutions of Higher Education. Handbook of Accreditation (2nd ed). Chicago: 1997.

Scholarship of Teaching

There continues to be interest in higher education about the meaning and scope of faculty scholarship and how the scholarly work of faculty is evaluated. Two books, Boyer's *Scholarship Reconsidered*[14] and Glassick, Huber, and Maeroff's *Scholarship Assessed*,[15] have had a profound effect on institutional discussions regarding standards for assessing faculty scholarship related to promotion and tenure. Boyer[14] advocates that *scholarship* is a broader term than *research*. In addition to basic research, which he calls *the scholarship of discovery*, he adds three additional forms of scholarship: the scholarships of integration, application, and teaching. The scholarship of integration is the need to make connections across the disciplines to a larger context, revealing the meaning of the data. The scholarship of application is asking how can this knowledge be "engaged" or applied to important real-world problems. The scholarship of teaching includes not only transmitting knowledge, but transforming and extending knowledge as well. Boyer's notion is that excellent teaching is visible through the same habits of mind that characterize scholarly work

A distinction can be made between excellent teaching and the scholarship of teaching (i.e., scholarly teaching versus the scholarship of teaching). Scholarly teaching is more in line with the original definition posed by Boyer. He sees scholarly teaching as being concerned not only with transmitting knowledge, but with transforming and extending knowledge as well; however, he makes no explicit reference to making this knowledge of teaching public or sharing in any way.

The scholarship of teaching includes a public account (community property) of some or all of the act of teaching that includes vision, design, enactment, outcome, and analysis that can be made available to critical review by peers. The scholarship of teaching also involves inquiry and investigation around issues of student learning.[16,17] Randy Bass,[18] a Carnegie Scholar, writes

> In scholarship and research, having a "problem" is at the heart of the investigative process. . . . But in one's teaching, a "problem" is something you don't want to have, and if you have one, you probably want to fix it. . . . Changing the status of the problem in teaching from terminal remediation to ongoing investigation is precisely what the movement for a scholarship of teaching is all about.

The scholarship of teaching is about bringing the process of inquiry to the classroom. It has also been described as "going meta"—that is, having faculty frame and systematically investigate questions related to student learning. What differentiates good teaching from scholarly teaching and scholarly teaching from the scholarship of teaching?

Case Example: Clinical Research Course—Reading the Literature

- Good teaching approach: The teacher gives a lecture on the core concepts for critical review of an article. Each step of the process is defined and discussed in class, with an exemplary article being used for application of each core concept. Students leave the class believing that they will be able to do an assigned article critique on their own.

Working definition for good teaching: often described in terms of presentational and interpersonal skill based on student evaluations. Are the lectures enjoyable? Does the instructor care about the students? Are needed resources available?

- Scholarly teaching approach: The teacher brings a manuscript that she has submitted; she has just received the review. After a brief review of concepts, she guides the students through the review process of her own manuscript. She then shares the actual review she received and discusses with the students how the paper will need to be revised to move the paper toward publication.

Working definition for scholarly teaching: The teacher brings the scholarship of discovery into class and works to connect current scholarship or knowledge development with the content of the course.

- Scholarship of teaching and learning: The teacher is interested in investigating what learning is taking place in small group work. Students are given a diagnostic quiz after an initial quick class review of core concepts in their assigned readings. In their assigned groups, they first exchange quizzes and correct the responses. Next, the group task is to critique an article that requires them to apply the concepts and supporting evidence for their judgment. Finally, they must go back to their initial quiz and do a self-assessment, answering these questions: (1) What were the most confusing concepts for you when you took the quiz?, (2) What did you learn from your group?, and (3) What did you contribute to the group?

Working definition for the scholarship of teaching: Teaching is examined from the perspective of the learner, examining student outcomes. What is the expected learning? The purpose is to improve the learning of students. Communication with one's peers is necessary in terms of making the work public for critical review and evaluation.

The issue of making the work public or community property is a critical issue for the scholarship of teaching. Here, we discuss the application of two different types of assessment that lend themselves well to the scholarship of teaching: peer assessment and course portfolios.

Peer Assessment

Teaching is a complex activity that is often done individually, within the confines of the classroom. Most faculty would agree that some combination of evidence from the person who is teaching, the students who are learning, and professional colleagues who observe is useful in evaluation of teaching. Although peer review and assessment could be used for either formative or summative evaluation, we focus here on its use as formative assessment. This means our aim is on improvement of teaching, not on administrative decision making. Remember, the central focus in assessment is on student learning.[19]

Peer review of teaching responds to two current concerns with teaching in higher education: (1) the needs to make teaching more public and promote the idea of teaching as "community property" through peer collaboration and discussion, and (2) the need to make teaching a topic for public examination, debate, and engagement (Figure 5-3).

An argument made about teaching is that it is difficult to assess; therefore, it is not valued. Research on teaching, however, has demonstrated a great deal of consensus on what is effective teaching. Here are 10 strategies and characteristics of good practice, supported by research, that effective teachers use[20]:

- Have students write about and discuss what they are learning.
- Encourage faculty-student contact, in and out of class.
- Get students working on substantive tasks, in and out of class.
- Give prompt and frequent feedback to students about their progress.
- Communicate high expectations.
- Make standards and grading explicit.
- Help students achieve those expectations and meet those criteria.
- Respect diverse talents and ways of learning.
- Use problems, questions, or issues, not merely content coverage, as points of entry into a subject and as sources of motivation for sustained inquiry.
- Make courses assignment-centered rather than text- or lecture-centered.

The use of these strategies and characteristics is what one would look for in a peer review process. We briefly outline an approach to peer assessment

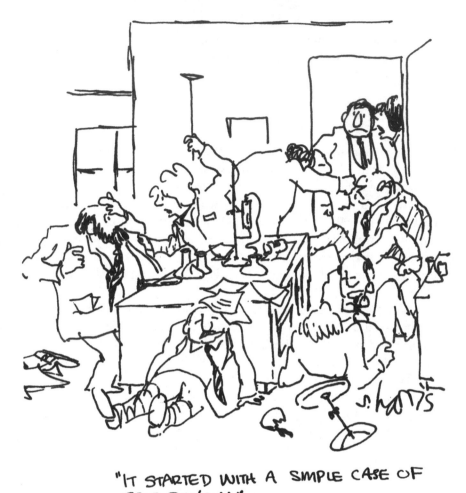

"IT STARTED WITH A SIMPLE CASE OF PEER-REVIEW."

Figure 5-3   Cartoon with permission from Harris S. Einstein Simplified: Cartoons on Science. New Brunswick, NJ: Rutgers University Press, 1992.

here that includes elements of constructive feedback, course review, and class observation. An excellent resource for peer review is Chism's sourcebook for peer review, *Peer Review of Teaching*.[19]

The peer reviewer assumes multiple roles, including developer, information gatherer, and evaluator. As our focus here is on formative assessment, we focus on the roles of developer and information gatherer. One of the most challenging tasks for a peer reviewer is to provide honest feedback that can be heard and understood by the teacher in a way that facilitates change. Here are some suggestions for providing feedback[19]:

Table 5-5 Examples of Course Materials for Peer Review

Course policy and practices
- Syllabus
- Ground rules for discussion
- Course guides
- Teaching evaluation instruments

Communication tools
- Course packets
- Texts
- Bibliographies
- Overhead transparencies
- Handouts
- Multimedia materials (e.g., computer simulations, videotapes)

Student performance instruments
- Tests, quizzes
- Project assignment directions, handouts
- Classroom exercises, worksheets

Instructor comments on student work
- Graded papers or tests
- Group projects
- Journals or posted messages from electronic communication

Source: Adapted from NV Chism. Peer Review of Teaching: A Sourcebook. Boston: Anker, 1999.

- Feedback should be authentic, in that it is based on a relationship of trust, honesty, and concern for your colleague.
- Descriptive information needs details and examples so the colleague can make decisions about change.
- Focus on teacher behavior, not personal attributes.
- Ground your feedback in the needs of your colleague from self-identified questions.
- Peer review activities require prompt feedback.
- Try to give feedback that looks forward, as well as feedback pertaining to the current classroom situation.
- Link your conclusions to evidence that you have gathered.

One core component of peer review is review of course materials. Course materials (preactive teaching) provide one component of the course, but they alone are not the course. Another core component of teaching is the enactment and interaction that occur in the classroom (interactive teaching). Materials that can be used for peer review include course policies and procedures, content, evidence of student performance, and teacher feedback (Table 5-5).

A second element of peer review is class observation. What do you look for while sitting in on a class? First, not everyone is a skilled observer, so some preparatory training is helpful. A pre-observation session may also provide the reviewer with a better sense of the context of the classroom. Second, research supports the idea that a single observation is not a reliable indicator of teaching quality.[21] A sufficient amount of time is important to allow the teacher and students to exhibit more typical behavior patterns. Finally, the observer should be as unobtrusive as possible.[19]

There are several different approaches one can use to help structure the classroom observation, from detailed checklists, to score sheets, to narrative prompt forms. We refer you to Chism's book for specific examples.[19] Here is a working outline of core elements that one might want to observe in a classroom:

- Instructor organization—for example, prepares self and students for classroom activities with creation of intriguing cases for discussion, interesting small group problem-solving tasks, and focused laboratory exercises
- Instructional strategies include variety and pace—for example, demonstrates effective balance between giving information and facilitating students' thinking
- Content knowledge—for example, presentation of current theories in relation to current practice implications
- Presentation skills—for example, actively engages student in learning; facilitates students' ability to transform knowledge into their own modes of thinking, conceptualization, and understanding
- Rapport with students—for example, creates a safe environment for the facilitation of student ideas, opinions, attitudes, values, and questions
- Clarity—for example, uses clinical examples, stories, metaphors, and the like to illustrate and clarify material

Another approach to classroom observation is through review and analysis of a videotape. The essential ingredient in all of peer assessment, again, is the central importance of student learning and how that can be improved through effective teaching.

Course Portfolios

A second technique for assessment of teaching is a course portfolio. Portfolios can take many forms and have various purposes, from looking at a faculty member's teaching across courses to a student's account of her or his learning and professional development, or a practitioner's account of professional development and achievement.[22] Here, we focus on the use of a course portfolio as a tool for continuous improvement of teaching and learning. The course portfolio is different from a teaching portfolio in that it is a wide-angle lens that focuses on teacher performance and learner performance.[23]

We begin by outlining our working assumptions for creating a course portfolio[22,24,25]:

- A portfolio is a tool for self-directed reflective learning, not just an exposé of good work.
- Portfolio development demands structure, yet allows for creativity, and provides a scaffold for reflective learning.
- A course portfolio should provide the teacher with a basis for improving teaching and student learning.
- Faculty will invest in this kind of assessment only to the extent that it connects goals, issues, and problems that really matter to them.
- Course portfolio assessment should be collaborative in that, just as a doctoral student works with a dissertation committee, following guidelines and seeking consultation, portfolio assessment includes coaching, deliberation, and collegial exchange.[25]

So how does one go about designing a course portfolio? Hutchings proposes three core components in a course portfolio: design, enactment, and outcome.[22]

1. *Design.* A useful way to start is to think about what purpose the course portfolio will serve. For example, are you trying to examine how to become more interactive with students and do less lecturing in your course? Cerbin[26] suggests that the course portfolio design begin with a teaching statement. This narrative will include a self-reflection on your beliefs and assumptions about teaching and learning, an explanation of your intended learning outcomes, the teaching practices you will use to reach those outcomes, and a rationale that connects the course goals to the teaching methods. It is this proposed relationship between your teaching methods and your learning outcomes that will serve as a framework for your analysis.

2. *Enactment.* Enactment is evidence or documentation of what happens in the class. This could take many forms, from the teacher's own self-reflections on the weekly progress of the course to the selection of class material samples that represent the connection between the course goals and the teaching strategies used to attain those goals. Following is a list of possibilities for documenting course enactment: videotapes, handouts, audiotapes of class interactions, hard copies of student-teacher online interactions, copies of lecture notes, examinations, readings, worksheets, and study guides. The important issue regarding evidence is not finding the evidence but selecting the evidence appropriate to your purpose.

3. *Results/outcome.* The defining feature of the course portfolio is the focus on student learning. How do you decide what student work to include? Samples of good and poor work? All work? Here are some suggestions: (1) Examples of student work should demonstrate a good fit between assessment and course goals. (2) Use existing assessment data whenever possible. You probably have evidence of student learning outcomes that comes from activities that are part of your course. (3) Include a variety of sources of evidence—for example, examinations, projects, worksheets, and minute papers. (4) Select your evidence of student learning with purpose. You might want to randomly select a small cohort of students to track their outcomes over the course so that you have longitudinal data. Focus on key assignments that represent links with your course goals. Hutchings states, "An ideal portfolio is both brief and complete."[22(p52)]

The final component of the course portfolio is your reflective analysis and conclusions about your teaching and your students' learning—that is, a focus on lessons learned. As an example of the scholarship of teaching, the course portfolio should make a connection between the activity and the results. Shulman describes the portfolio as a fruitful example of the scholarship of teaching: "The scholarship of teaching will entail a public account of some or all of the full act of teaching—vision, design, enactment, outcomes and analysis in a manner susceptible to critical review by teachers' professional peers."[22(p6)]

Summary

We have come full circle. We began the chapter by talking about student learning, classroom assessment, and the need to identify the teaching goals that we are working toward. We concluded the chapter by focusing on tools that teachers can use to examine their teaching in a way that will constantly advance their practice of teaching, improve student learning, and contribute to the scholarship of teaching.

References

1. Mentkowski M and Associates. Learning That Lasts: Integrating Learning, Development, and Performance in College and Beyond. San Francisco: Jossey-Bass, 2000;305, 359–405.
2. Wright BD. Assessing Student Learning. In D DeZure (ed), Learning from Change: Landmarks in Teaching and Learning in Higher

Education from Change Magazine, 1969–1999. Sterling, VA: Stylus, 2000;299–304.

3. Shulman L. Taking learning seriously. Change 1999;31(4):10–17.
4. Angelo TA. Doing assessment as if learning matters most. AAHE Bull 1999;51(9):3–6.
5. Eckel P, Green M, Hill B. Transformational Change: Defining a Journey. Washington, DC: American Council on Education, 1997.
6. AAHE Assessment Forum. Principles of Good Practice for Assessing Student Learning. American Association for Higher Education, Washington, DC: 1992. <http://www.aahe.org/assessment/principl.htm>. Accessed: November 8, 2001.
7. Angelo TA, Cross KP. Classroom Assessment Techniques: A Handbook for College Teachers (2nd ed). San Francisco: Jossey-Bass, 1993.
8. Kogut LS. Quality circles: a Japanese management technique for the classroom. Improving College and University Teaching 1984;32(2):123–127.
9. American Physical Therapy Association. CAPTE Accreditation Handbook, 2000.
10. Boucher B. Program assessment in physical therapy education: the transition to the new criteria. J Phys Ther Educ 1999;13:18–27.
11. Mentkowski M, Loacker G. Assessing and validating outcomes of college. In PT Ewell (ed), Assessing Educational Outcomes. San Francisco: Jossey-Bass, 1985;47–64.
12. Lazerson M, Wagener U, Shumanis N. Teaching and learning in higher education, 1980–2000. Change 2000;2(3):12–19.
13. North Central Association of Colleges and Schools Commission on Institutions of Higher Education. Handbook of Accreditation (2nd ed). Chicago: 1997.
14. Boyer EL. Scholarship Reconsidered: Priorities of the Professoriate. Princeton, NJ: Carnegie Foundation for the Advancement of Teaching, 1990.
15. Glassick CE, Huber MT, Maeroff GL. Scholarship Assessed: Evaluation of the Professoriate. San Francisco: Jossey-Bass, 1997.
16. Hutchings P, Shulman LS. The scholarship of teaching. Change 1999;31(5):11–15.
17. Hutchings P. Making Teaching Community Property. Washington, DC: American Association for Higher Education, 1996.
18. Bass R. The scholarship of teaching: what's the problem? Inventio [serial online]. February 1999;1(1). Available at: http://www.doiiit.gmu.edu/Archives/feb98/randybass.htm. Accessed: November 8, 2001.
19. Chism NV. Peer Review of Teaching: A Sourcebook. Boston: Anker, 1999.
20. Walvoord B, Anderson V. Effective Grading: A Tool for Learning and Assessment. San Francisco: Jossey-Bass, 1998.

21. Lewis K. Using an Objective System to Diagnose Teaching Problems. In K Lewis, J Lunde (eds), Face to Face. Stillwater, OK: New Forums, 1988; 137–157.

22. Hutchings P. The Course Portfolio. Washington, DC: American Association for Higher Education, 1998.

23. Bernstein D. Putting the Focus on Student Learning. In P Hutchings (ed), The Course Portfolio. Washington, DC: American Association for Higher Education, 1998;77–84.

24. Hutchings P. Opening Lines: Approaches to the Scholarship of Teaching and Learning. Menlo Park, CA: Carnegie Foundation for the Advancement of Teaching, 2000.

25. Shulman L. Teacher Portfolios: A Theoretical Act. In N Lyons (ed), With Portfolio in Hand. New York: Teachers College Press, 1998;23–38.

26. Cerbin W. The course portfolio as a tool for continuous improvement of teaching and learning. J Excel Coll Teach 1994;5(1):95–105.

Annotated Bibliography

Angelo TA, Cross KP. Classroom Assessment Techniques: A Handbook for College Teachers (2nd ed). San Francisco: Jossey-Bass, 1993. This is an outstanding resource for any academic department. The authors provide more than 50 examples of different CATs. The description of each technique includes an estimate of ease of use for the faculty, description of the technique, step-by-step procedures for adapting and administering the technique, practical advice, and pros and cons of the technique. The chapters focused on specific assessment techniques are grouped according to student learning goals (e.g., content knowledge, higher-order thinking skills, values, and attitudes).

Cross KP, Steadman MH. Classroom Research: Implementing the Scholarship of Teaching. San Francisco: Jossey-Bass, 1996. This is a good book for faculty learning groups interested in designing classroom research projects. The authors do an excellent job of integrating their first-hand experience with research and theory on student learning as well as providing concrete steps for your own classroom research project.

Glassick CE, Huber MT, Maeroff GL. Scholarship Assessed: Evaluation of the Professoriate. San Francisco: Jossey-Bass, 1997. This book is a sequel to the original Carnegie report published by Boyer. This book proposes new standards for assessing scholarship and evaluating faculty and is a good resource for an institutional debate on the role of scholarship in the academy. The book is based on the findings of Carnegie Foundation's National Survey on the Reexamination of Faculty Roles and Rewards.

Hutchings P. The Course Portfolio. Washington, DC: American Association for Higher Education, 1998. *The Course Portfolio* is one of the AAHE's teaching initiative projects. This book contains two excellent conceptual chapters by Lee Shulman and Pat Hutchings that set the stage for the nine case examples of course portfolios. The case examples cross a variety of disciplines, but the central focus of the cases remains the scholarship of teaching.

Palomba CA, Banta TW (eds). Assessing Student Competence in Accredited Disciplines. San Francisco: Jossey-Bass, 2001. The authors, who are well known experts in the area of assessment, have written the introductory core chapters of this book that focus on effective assessment of student competence. The remaining chapters are examples of assessments used in a number of applied fields, including pharmacy and nursing.

Palomba CA, Banta TW. Assessment Essentials: Planning, Implementing and Improving Assessment in Higher Education. San Francisco: Jossey-Bass, 1999. This book is the "bible" of assessment in higher education. The authors provide a step-by-step guide for developing assessment programs. Although the focus is on higher education, there are many core concepts that apply to professional education. The chapter on definitions, goals, and plans is fundamental to any good assessment plan.

Van Note Chism N, Stanley C. Peer Review of Teaching: A Sourcebook. Boston: Anker, 1999. Written as a sourcebook for administrators and faculty, this book is an outstanding resource for development of any peer review of the teaching process. The book is in two sections: The first provides a framework for designing and implementing peer review; the second provides guidelines, protocols, and forms for each task in the process.

A

Teaching Goals Inventory and Self-Scorable Worksheet

Teaching Goals Inventory and Self-Scorable Worksheet

Purpose: The Teaching Goals Inventory (TGI) is a self-assessment of instructional goals. Its purpose is threefold: (1) to help college teachers become more aware of what they want to accomplish in individual courses; (2) to help faculty locate Classroom Assessment Techniques they can adapt and use to assess how well they are achieving their teaching and learning goals; (3) to provide a starting point for discussions of teaching and learning goals among colleagues.

Directions: Please select ONE course you are currently teaching. Respond to each item on the Inventory in relation to that particular course. (Your responses might be quite different if you were asked about your overall teaching and learning goals, for example, or the appropriate instructional goals for your discipline.)

Please print the title of the specific course you are focusing on:

_____

Please rate the importance of each of the fifty-two goals listed below to the specific course you have selected. Assess each goal's importance to what you deliberately aim to have your students accomplish, rather than the goal's general worthiness or overall importance to your institution's mission. There are no "right" or "wrong" answers, only personally more or less accurate ones.

For each goal, circle only one response on the 1-to-5 rating scale. You may want to read quickly through all fifty-two goals before rating their relative importance.

In relation to the course you are focusing on, indicate whether each goal you rate is:

(5) Essential   a goal you always/nearly always try to achieve
(4) Very important a goal you often try to achieve
(3) Important   a goal you sometimes try to achieve
(2) Unimportant   a goal you rarely try to achieve
(1) Not applicable a goal you never try to achieve

Rate the importance of each goal to what you aim to have students accomplish in your course.	Essential	Very Important	Important	Unimportant	Not Applicable
1. Develop ability to apply principles and generalizations already learned to new problems and situations	5	4	3	2	1
2. Develop analytic skills	5	4	3	2	1
3. Develop problem-solving skills	5	4	3	2	1
4. Develop ability to draw reasonable inferences from observations	5	4	3	2	1
5. Develop ability to synthesize and integrate information and ideas	5	4	3	2	1
6. Develop ability to think holistically: to see the whole as well as the parts	5	4	3	2	1
7. Develop ability to think creatively	5	4	3	2	1
8. Develop ability to distinguish between fact and opinion	5	4	3	2	1
9. Improve skill at paying attention	5	4	3	2	1
10. Develop ability to concentrate	5	4	3	2	1
11. Improve memory skills	5	4	3	2	1
12. Improve listening skills	5	4	3	2	1
13. Improve speaking skills	5	4	3	2	1
14. Improve reading skills	5	4	3	2	1
15. Improve writing skills	5	4	3	2	1
16. Develop appropriate study skills, strategies, and habits	5	4	3	2	1
17. Improve mathematical skills	5	4	3	2	1
18. Learn terms and facts of this subject	5	4	3	2	1
19. Learn concepts and theories in this subject	5	4	3	2	1
20. Develop skill in using materials, tools, and/or technology central to this subject	5	4	3	2	1
21. Learn to understand perspectives and values of this subject	5	4	3	2	1
22. Prepare for transfer or graduate study	5	4	3	2	1
23. Learn techniques and methods used to gain new knowledge in this subject	5	4	3	2	1
24. Learn to evaluate methods and materials in this subject	5	4	3	2	1
25. Learn to appreciate important contributions to this subject	5	4	3	2	1

Rate the importance of each goal to what you aim to have students accomplish in your course.	*Essential*	*Very Important*	*Important*	*Unimportant*	*Not Applicable*
26. Develop an appreciation of the liberal arts and sciences	5	4	3	2	1
27. Develop an openness to new ideas	5	4	3	2	1
28. Develop an informed concern about contemporary social issues	5	4	3	2	1
29. Develop a commitment to exercise the rights and responsibilities of citizenship	5	4	3	2	1
30. Develop a lifelong love of learning	5	4	3	2	1
31. Develop aesthetic appreciations	5	4	3	2	1
32. Develop an informed historical perspective	5	4	3	2	1
33. Develop an informed understanding of the role of science and technology	5	4	3	2	1
34. Develop an informed appreciation of other cultures	5	4	3	2	1
35. Develop capacity to make informed ethical choices	5	4	3	2	1
36. Develop ability to work productively with others	5	4	3	2	1
37. Develop management skills	5	4	3	2	1
38. Develop leadership skills	5	4	3	2	1
39. Develop a commitment to accurate work	5	4	3	2	1
40. Improve ability to follow directions, instructions, and plans	5	4	3	2	1
41. Improve ability to organize and use time effectively	5	4	3	2	1
42. Develop a commitment to personal achievement	5	4	3	2	1
43. Develop ability to perform skillfully	5	4	3	2	1
44. Cultivate a sense of responsibility for one's own behavior	5	4	3	2	1
45. Improve self-esteem / self-confidence	5	4	3	2	1
46. Develop a commitment to one's own values	5	4	3	2	1
47. Develop respect for others	5	4	3	2	1
48. Cultivate emotional health and well-being	5	4	3	2	1
49. Cultivate physical health and well-being	5	4	3	2	1
50. Cultivate an active commitment to honesty	5	4	3	2	1
51. Develop capacity to think for oneself	5	4	3	2	1
52. Develop capacity to make wise decisions	5	4	3	2	1

53. In general, how do you see your primary role as a teacher?
(Although more than one statement may apply, please circle only one.)

1 Teaching students facts and principles of the subject matter

2 Providing a role model for students

3 Helping students develop higher-order thinking skills

4 Preparing students for jobs/careers

5 Fostering student development and personal growth

6 Helping students develop basic learning skills

Teaching Goals Inventory, Self-Scoring Worksheet

1. In all, how many of the fifty-two goals did you rate as "Essential"?

2. How many "Essential" goals did you have in each of the six clusters listed below?

Cluster Number and Name	Goals Included in Cluster	Total Number of "Essential" Goals in Each Cluster	Clusters Ranked— from 1st to 6th— by Number of "Essential" Goals
I Higher-Order Thinking Skills	1–8	_____	_____
II Basic Academic Success Skills	9–17	_____	_____
III Discipline-Specific Knowledge and Skills	18–25	_____	_____
IV Liberal Arts and Academic Values	26–35	_____	_____
V Work and Career Preparation	36–43	_____	_____
VI Personal Development	44–52	_____	_____

3. Compute your cluster scores (average item ratings by cluster) using the following worksheet.

A	B	C	D	E
		Sum of Ratings Given to Goals in That Cluster	*Divide C by This Number*	
Cluster Number and Name	*Goals Included*			*Your Cluster Scores*
I Higher-Order Thinking Skills	1–8	_____	8	_____
II Basic Academic Success Skills	9–17	_____	9	_____
III Discipline-Specific Knowledge and Skills	18–25	_____	8	_____
IV Liberal Arts and Academic Values	26–35	_____	10	_____
V Work and Career Preparation	36–43	_____	8	_____
VI Personal Development	44–52	_____	9	_____

Source: TA Angelo, KP Cross. Classroom Assessment Techniques: A Handbook for College Teachers (2nd ed). San Francisco: Jossey-Bass, 1993.

6

Preparation for Teaching Students in Clinical Settings

Jody S. Gandy

Teachers are those who use themselves as bridges, over which they invite their students to cross; then having facilitated their crossing, joyfully collapse, encouraging them to create bridges of their own.
—Nikos Kazantzakis in J. Canfield and M. V. Hansen's *A 3rd Serving of Chicken Soup for the Soul.*[1]

Case Situation 1

After earning a master's of physical therapy degree and 1 year of clinical practice, I was informed that I was now ready to serve as a clinical instructor (CI) for a student. I was finally comfortable with managing a full patient caseload and all related activities, including using the patient/client management approach to care, related documentation, case and family conferences, peer evaluations, implementation of a plan of care to achieve established functional goals within expected time duration, establishing and seeking positive relationships with other professionals, participating in journal club and weekly in-services, directing and supervising physical therapist assistants and other support personnel, and attending monthly professional meetings. Now, without more than a simple proclamation, I was to be assigned to a student for her first clinical education experience from a 3-year master's of physical therapy program. Just when I was feeling like I finally had a handle on performing as a competent practitioner and meeting departmental expectations, one more responsibility was "dumped" on me.

The center coordinator of clinical education (CCCE) hastily reviewed with me a copy of the academic program's curriculum and course objectives, dates of clinical experience, name of the academic coordinator of clinical education (ACCE), and evaluation tool to be used to assess the student's performance for this first clinical experience. In addition, there was a brief student profile that was written in the student's handwriting, albeit somewhat illegibly, that indicated her address, preferred learning style, and specific learning objectives. After this brief discussion, I was informed that the student would arrive at our clinical facility in 1 week and would need an orientation, "good" patients (whose care is reimbursable) with whom to practice her skills, and assurance that any patients selected would consent to care provided by a student under line-of-sight supervision. The center coordinator asked me if I had any questions. After a brief pause, I quietly replied, "No." Not only did I not know where to begin to ask the first question, but also I was absolutely overwhelmed by the responsibility. I assumed that everyone who was assigned a student after 1 year of clinical practice must be capable of serving as a CI, and I did not want to respond any differently than my peers.

Afterwards, I realized that in 1 week I would be responsible for this student's clinical learning experience and had not a clue as to how to structure a planned experience. At least I was familiar with the student evaluation instrument because I had used the same instrument when I was a student. I had no experience providing a student orientation before and at best had only completed a new employee orientation. In reality, I knew very little about teaching students in the clinic other than my recollections of being a student in the clinic and some classroom lectures that I vaguely remembered on patient education and clinical education. For the next week I tried to informally question more experienced physical therapists about how they taught their students. I did not want them to know that I felt incompetent. I also tried to reflect on what my CIs did during my four clinical experiences by posing questions such as: How did they provide an orientation to the facility and the specific health care environment? What issues were discussed during the first few days of the experience? What were their expectations for my performance? Did I get a schedule on the first day and what was included on that schedule? What did they do to make me feel comfortable or uncomfortable? What did I remember most about my clinical educators that were positive or negative? Based on my limited discussions with professional peers and my personal reflections, I developed a better, albeit limited, understanding of my perceived roles and responsibilities. All too soon it was time for me to teach my first student.

Case Situation 2

After 8 years of clinical practice in three different practice settings with 6 of those years involved in clinical education, I was finally getting my first professional doctor of physical therapy (DPT) student. The student was completing his final (third) year of the program on a 6-month internship. I had certainly had experience with managing, supervising, and evaluating students during their clinical education experiences, but this was my first opportunity to supervise a DPT student for an extended clinical experience of 6 months. My first concern was that I only possessed a baccalaureate degree in physical therapy, with the addition of numerous continuing education courses provided by content experts and master clinicians. Even with my clinical experience and additional training, however, I still had several pressing concerns. Was I adequately prepared to manage a DPT student's clinical experience? Would the knowledge and skills that I possessed be adequate to keep pace with what he had learned in his program? What would I do with a student for 6 months, as the longest clinical education experience that I had managed thus far was only 10 weeks.

In the past, I received excellent comments and feedback from students and academic programs regarding my performance as a CI, but those were different circumstances. Faced with the prospect of supervising a DPT student for a 6-month internship, I found myself questioning my ability and competence as a CI.

The first sketch is all too common in contemporary clinical education, but illustrates a situation that can be prevented or eliminated given adequate training and resources. The second sketch is an emerging situation in physical therapy clinical education, and describes new challenges confronting both experienced and novice clinical educators as a result of a transitioning doctoring profession, with a concomitant lengthening[2] of clinical education experiences. For both case situations, information provided in this chapter assists novice and experienced clinical educators with information and resources about the clinical education milieu; the roles and responsibilities of faculty, clinicians, and students involved in clinical education; preparation to be a successful clinical teacher; and alternative supervisory approaches and models for the delivery of clinical education.

Chapter Objectives

After reading this chapter, the reader will be able to

1. Understand the complexities of and relationships between different contextual frameworks in which students' academic and clinical learning occur.
2. Recognize the dynamic organizational structure of clinical education and the roles and responsibilities of persons functioning within this structure.
3. Define the preferred attributes of clinical educators that contribute to enhanced student learning.
4. Identify qualities of effective clinical education development training programs to enhance clinical teaching abilities.
5. Determine how to collaboratively define realistic student learning expectations and objectives for clinical education experiences to ensure attainment of clinical learning outcomes.
6. Describe alternative cooperative and collaborative approaches to providing supervision and their relative strengths, considerations, and limitations.

Physical Therapy Education

Imagine education for physical therapists and physical therapist assistants occurring solely in an academic milieu or without any student clinical practice as an integral part of the educational process. Since the profession's inception, clinical practice as part of the curriculum has always been and continues to be of paramount importance and at the heart of students' educational experiences. Of significance is clinical practice's role in students' progression through the professional (entry-level) curriculum. This is achieved by bridging the worlds of theory and practice, teaching in a "real-world" laboratory lessons that can only be learned through practice, introducing students to the peculiarities of the practice environment and the profession, and refining knowledge, psychomotor skills, and professional behaviors by managing patients with progressively more complex pathologies.[3] This aspect of the physical therapy professional curriculum is known as *clinical education*. On the one hand, clinical education is not currently constrained by type of practice setting or its geographical location, diversity of persons capable of serving as clinical educators, or the patient populations that clinical educators serve.[4-6] On the other hand, clinical educators are powerful role models for students during their professional education and significantly influence where, how, and with whom students choose to practice after graduation, and whether they choose to become future clinical educators.[7-9] Thus, the outcome of physical therapy education is, in part, a reflection of the quality of clinical educators who help prepare graduates to deliver quality, cost-effective, and evidence-based services to meet the needs and demands of society within an ever-changing health care environment.

Differences between Academic and Clinical Education

The greatest fundamental difference between academic and clinical education lies in their service orientations. Physical therapy academic education, situated within higher education, exists for the primary purpose of educating students to attain core knowledge, skills, and behaviors. In contrast, clinical education, situated within the practice environment, exists first and foremost to provide cost-effective and high-quality care and education for patients, clients, their families, and caregivers. Academic faculty are remunerated for their teaching, scholarship, and community and professional services. Clinical educators are compensated for their services as practitioners by rendering patient/client care and related activities. In most cases, unless as a function of experience or as an employee of an academic institution, clinical educators receive little or no financial compensation for teaching students.[10] Physical therapy clinical educators are placed in a precarious position of trying to effectively balance and respond to two "masters." The first master, the practice setting, requires the practitioner to deliver evidence-based, cost-effective, and high-quality patient services. The second master, higher education, wants the clinical educator to respond to the needs of the student learner and the educational outcomes of the academic program.

Other differences between physical therapy clinical education and academic education relate to the design of the learning experience. Educating students in higher education most often occurs in a predictable classroom environment that is characterized by a beginning and ending of the learning session, and a method (written, oral, practical) of assessing the student's readiness for clinical practice. Student instruction can be provided in numerous formats with varying degrees of structure, including lecture augmented by the use of audiovisuals, laboratory practice, discussion seminars, collaborative peer activities, tutorials, problem-based case discussions, computer-based instruction and simulations, and independent or group work practicums. With advancements in technology, such as distance education, hypermedia, and virtual reality, today's traditional teaching-learning archetype is being challenged, and alternative structures and systems for classroom learning are clearly in our future.[11]

In contrast, the clinical classroom by its very nature is dynamic and flexible. It is a more unpredictable learning laboratory that is constrained by time only as it relates to the length of a patient's visit or the workday schedule. Sometimes, to an observer, delivery of patient care and educating students in the practice environment may seem analogous in that they appear unstructured and at times even chaotic. Remarkably, student learning continues with or without patients and is not constrained by walls or by location (e.g., community-based services or home visits). Learning is not measured by written examination, but rather is assessed based on the quality, efficiency, and outcomes of patient/client care provided by a student when measured against a standard of clinical performance.[12] Resources available to the clinical teacher may include many of those used by academic faculty, such as instruction using audiovisuals, practice on a fellow student or the clinical educator, or discussion and analysis of a journal article. Additional resources available to the clinical educator include collaborative student learning within and between disciplines, video libraries of patient cases, in-service education, grand rounds, surgery observation, special clinics and screenings (e.g., seating clinic, fitness screenings, community-based education to prevent common falls in the elderly), pre-surgical examinations, on-site continuing education course offerings, observation and interactions with other health professionals, and participation in clinical research. Rich learning opportunities are available in practice that complement, clarify, and augment much of what is provided in physical therapy academic education.[13]

Because learning occurs within the context of practice and patient care, the clinical teacher must be characterized as more of "a guide by the side" rather than the "sage on stage" that characterizes the classroom educator.[14] The clinical teacher, primarily through interactions and handling of patients, assumes multiple roles, including facilitator, coach, supervisor, role model, mentor, and performance evaluator.[12] The clinical educator provides opportunities for students to experience safe practice. She or he asks probing questions that encourage the learner to reflect, reinforces students' thinking and clinical decision making, fosters scholarly inquiry and sorting fact from fiction, and, by example, teaches students how to manage ambiguities (e.g., balancing functional and psychosocial needs of the patient with available third-party payment for services).[14–16]

In summary, higher education and health care environments differ in relation to student learning because educators in each assume distinct roles and responsibilities that are circumscribed by the context in which learning occurs and the primary customer is being served. Despite these differences, it is imperative that the two systems communicate and interact on a regular basis to fulfill the curricular outcomes of physical therapy programs. In fact, academic and clinical educators, as partners, must make concerted efforts to consciously bridge their differences. "The frightening prospect is that these forces, if left to run their course without intervention, will likely drive education and practice further apart."[17] To understand how these systems currently interact to ensure graduates can deliver safe and effective quality patient/client care requires an understanding of the organizational structure of clinical education.

Relationship between Clinical and Academic Education

The organization of clinical education is designed to provide a way for academic faculty to share with clinical faculty their respective curricula and student expectations. In return, clinical faculty inform academic faculty of the relevance of the academic curriculum to entry-level practice and the ability of students to translate knowledge and theory into practice as evidenced by their clinical performance.[18] Excluding students, the organizational system is often designed with persons providing three essential positions within clinical education. Persons assuming these roles must continually interact to ensure the provision of quality physical therapy education for students. These three roles are most commonly titled the ACCE (or director of clinical education [DCE]), the CCCE, and the CI. The ACCE/DCE is situated in the academy, whereas the CCCE and CI are based in clinical practice.

Although the three primary players and the students largely manage physical therapy clinical education, it is important to remember that it is every physical therapist and physical therapist assistant educator's responsibility to be vested in clinical education. Clinical education represents approximately 28–30% of the total curriculum and is characterized as that part of the academic experience that allows students to apply theory and didactic knowledge to the real world of clinical practice.[2] As such, all academic faculty contribute to the effectiveness of the clinical learning experience because student performance in the clinic is a direct reflection of how they were educated by faculty during the didactic portion of the curriculum. Faculty must seek to better understand how their classroom experiences relate to student performance in the clinic, and clinicians must comprehend how and what information presented in the classroom relates to the clinical education process and entry-level expectations. This is accomplished when faculty are involved in clinical site visits using established guidelines[19] and when they facilitate continuing education, external funding, and clinical research in collaboration with clinicians.[20] Decisions about student clinical competence should not rest solely with the ACCE/DCE, but should reflect the collective wisdom of academic and clinical faculty assessments,[21] student self-assessments, consumers,[22] and employer assessments.[23] Additionally, the academic program has a responsibility to visibly demonstrate its commitment to clinical education by actively involving clinical educators in relevant aspects of curriculum development, implementation, and assessment of the physical therapy program.

Clinical Education Roles and Responsibilities

Roles and Responsibilities of Students

The true messengers in clinical education are students. Students provide feedback to everyone involved in the clinical education system. Given the various alternative configurations for providing clinical education, students bear a heavy burden, because learning experiences are provided based on information received from academic programs that may be incomplete or inaccurate in relation to individual student learning needs. Only students can articulate their needs to the CI on a daily basis; therefore, they must take responsibility for their learning if they wish to maximize their time in the practice setting.[24] Students must actively participate in the decision-making process of clinical site selection[25,26] and be willing to assume a risk in openly asking for available clinical learning experiences that permit successful progression through the curriculum. This means that ongoing student self-assessment and reflection, which identify the student's knowledge and performance strengths, deficiencies, and inconsistencies, must occur.[15] As part of this responsibility, students must feel comfortable providing constructive feedback to academic and clinical faculty. Faculty must remain open and flexible to student needs and be willing to modify the curriculum when revisions are shown to be necessary.

Self-accountability for behavior and actions is critically important for students as part of their learning contract. However, faculty should guide and model appropriate professional behavior and be willing to confront areas in which the students' professional values and behaviors are considered inappropriate or problematic.[27]

Roles and Responsibilities of the Academic Coordinator/Director of Clinical Education

Since 1982, the roles, responsibilities, and career issues of the ACCE in physical therapy education have been investigated and discussed by several authors.[28–30] Although these studies span more than a decade, the responsibilities assumed by the ACCE have essentially remained consistent, except for those areas in which technology and collaborative initiatives have enhanced administrative efficiency and effectiveness, and those times when the ACCE is on a tenure track rather than a clinical track.

The ACCE functions in a pivotal faculty role in physical therapy education. She or he serves as the liaison between the didactic and clinical components of the program. In some programs, due to the number of students and the resultant number of clinical education sites required, more than one person has assumed ACCE responsibilities (as co-ACCEs or as ACCE/DCE and assistant ACCE). In those cases in which the ACCE is designated as the DCE, responsibilities are considered to be commensurate with managing and directing a program (including budget, personnel, and resources).

The ACCE/DCE of a physical therapist program should be a licensed physical therapist with a postprofessional master's degree and preferably be in the process of or have earned a doctoral degree, and should teach students, engage in research, and provide community and professional service while balancing the many other unique responsibilities associated with the position.[31] The ACCE/DCE of a physical therapist assistant program should be either a physical therapist assistant or physical therapist. The roles and associated responsibilities of an ACCE/DCE[30–32] are found in Table 6-1.

Additional activities that the ACCE/DCE may be involved in include (1) participation in consortia activities (e.g., a group of regional academic programs and clinical educators that sponsor collaborative initiatives); (2) accreditation-related activities; (3) program curriculum and university-based committee activities; (4) clinical education research; (5) management of budget allocations related to clinical education; (6) coordination of clinical education advisory committees; and (7) state, regional, and national activities related to clinical education. In some cases, ACCEs/DCEs have assumed a "broker" role in clinical education by linking clinical educators to facilitate clinical education research, arranging creative student clinical experiences (e.g., forming cooperative relationships for solo or rural practices), and forming collaborative

Table 6-1   Roles and Responsibilities of the Academic Coordinator of
Clinical Education (ACCE) and Director of Clinical Education (DCE)

Primary roles of the ACCE/DCE	Responsibilities associated with each role
Communication between the academic institution and affiliated clinical education sites	Provide clinical sites with current program information (i.e., program philosophy, policy and procedures, clinical education agreements, clinical placement requests, student clinical assignments, required information for accreditation, and federal and state regulations that affect patient/client care provided by students).
	Foster ongoing and reciprocal communication between academic and clinical faculty and students through various mediums (e.g., phone, written, electronic correspondence, on-site visitations).[33]
Clinical education program planning, implementation, and assessment	Perform academic and administrative responsibilities consistent with the Commission on Accreditation in Physical Therapy Education (CAPTE), federal and state regulations, institutional policy, and practice setting requirements.
	Coordinate and teach students about clinical education and related content, including the need to actively participate in the outcome of their clinical learning experiences.
	Remain current regarding issues in health care delivery and higher education that affect the provision of clinical education.
	Coordinate, monitor, and assess the clinical placement of students.
	Develop, maintain, and administer information and education technology systems that support clinical education and the curriculum.
	Coordinate, facilitate, and evaluate clinical education in the academic program, including instruments used for evaluation of the clinical education component of the curriculum, for purposes of curricular assessment and revisions.[5,6,29,30]
	Review student clinical performance evaluations and provide feedback and counsel.[34]
	Determine, in collaboration with program faculty, whether students have successfully met explicit learning objectives for the clinical experience to enable continued progression through the curriculum.

Primary roles of the ACCE/DCE	Responsibilities associated with each role
Clinical education site development	Develop criteria and procedures for maintaining quality clinical sites committed.
	Develop and maintain an adequate number of clinical education sites relative to quality, quantity, and diversity of learning experiences (e.g., continuum of care, lifespan, commonly seen patient/client diagnoses) to meet the educational needs of students and the academic program.
Clinical faculty development	Assess the faculty development needs of clinical educators.
	Develop, provide, and assess clinical faculty development programs that educate and empower clinical educators to effectively fulfill their roles as clinical teachers.[34]

Source: Adapted from Department of Education. An American Physical Therapy Association Model Position Description for the Academic Coordinator for Clinical Education/Director of Clinical Education. Alexandria, VA: American Physical Therapy Association, 1999.

working relationships with other academic institutions, faculty, or professions to increase access to clinical sites.

In 1988, Deusinger and Rose[35] challenged ACCEs to reexamine their role as part of physical therapy education by saying, "Like the dinosaur, the position of the ACCE is certain to become extinct in physical therapy education. The viability of this position is threatened because of the present preoccupation with administrative logistics and student counseling, a preoccupation that prohibits full participation as an academic physical therapist." They go on to suggest that "the role of the ACCE must be redefined for this faculty member to survive the demands of academia and serve the needs of the profession."[35] They expressed the hope that ACCEs would not become extinct in this position but instead would be transformed and emerge as an equal, valued, and respected member of the academic community. Given the growing numbers of doctoral-prepared ACCEs who are on tenure tracks, the possibility that their vision may be realized is closer today than ever before.

Roles and Responsibilities of the Center Coordinator of Clinical Education

The CCCE's primary role is to serve as a liaison between the clinical site and the academic institutions. From the student's perspective, the CCCE functions in a unique but critical capacity. The CCCE is viewed as the neutral party at the clinical site who functions in the role of active listener, problem solver, conflict manager, and negotiator when differences occur between a student's perception of her or his performance and the CI's perception of the performance. In some situations, CCCEs function as mentors for individuals serving as CIs or those potentially interested in becoming CIs.[4]

Because of current pressure in health care settings to maximize human resources, it is as likely that the CCCE may be a physical therapist or physical therapist assistant as it is that the individual may be a non-physical therapy professional (e.g., occupational therapist or speech therapist). Whether the CCCE is a physical therapist or physical therapist assistant or another health care professional, the following characteristics and qualities are considered universal to the role:

1. Knowledge of professional ethics and legal behaviors.
2. Experience in providing clinical education to students in the respective professions.
3. Interest in students and commitment to providing quality learning experiences.
4. Effective interpersonal communication and organizational skills.
5. Knowledge of the clinical education site and its resources.
6. Capability to consult in the evaluation process.
7. Knowledge of contemporary issues in clinical practice and the clinical education program, educational theory, and issues in health care delivery.

If the CCCE is a physical therapist or physical therapist assistant, it is expected that he or she will possess attributes commensurate with that of CIs (see CCCE role responsibilities in the following list). CCCEs can assess their capabilities and competence by completing the American Physical Therapy Association (APTA) self-assessment for CCCEs.[4]

Responsibilities that are considered specific to the CCCE role associated with clinical site development include

1. Obtaining administrative support to develop a clinical education program by providing clinical education site administrators with sound rationale for development.
2. Determining clinical site readiness to accept students.
3. Contacting academic programs to determine if the clinical site's clinical education philosophy and mission are congruent with that of the academic program.
4. Completing the necessary documentation to become an affiliated clinical education program (e.g., negotiated legal contracts that define the roles and responsibilities of the clinical site and the academic institu-

tion; clinical site information form[13] that documents essential information about the clinical site, personnel, and available student learning experiences; policy and procedure manuals; and, in some cases, self-assessments for the clinical education site, the CI, and the CCCE). The CCCE ensures that all required documentation is completed accurately and in a timely manner and is updated as warranted by changes in personnel and the clinical site.[4]

Activities of the CCCE that are associated with preparing for and providing on-site student learning experiences include

1. Coordinating the CI student assignments and assessing the availability of learning experiences for students at the clinical site.
2. Responding to inquiries by the academic program for available student placements and scheduling the number of students that can be reasonably accommodated by the clinical site on an annual basis.
3. Developing guidelines to determine when physical therapists and physical therapist assistants are competent to serve as CIs for students.
4. Providing mechanisms whereby CIs can receive the necessary training to provide quality student clinical instruction.
5. Reviewing student clinical performance assessments to ensure their accuracy and timely completion.
6. Understanding legal risks,[36,37] including the Americans With Disabilities Act[38,39] provisions associated with teaching and supervising students in the clinic.

Although the CCCE position is considered essential to physical therapy clinical education, a word of caution must be provided given the milieu in which contemporary physical therapy clinical education occurs. Because of consolidation and cutbacks that have occurred throughout the health care system, either no CCCE may be designated at a clinical site or individuals serving as CCCEs may lack the appropriate qualifications, clinical teaching experience, or ability to mentor CIs. Of greatest concern is the loss of experienced mentors in clinical practice to educate the next generation of clinical teachers ultimately responsible for ensuring the future quality and effectiveness of physical therapy services.[40]

The profession is aware of the potential implications that could result with the loss of the CCCE. One continuing education development program implemented by APTA, is a voluntary Clinical Instructor Education and Credentialing Program[41] to provide educators (CIs, CCCEs, and academic faculty) in physical therapy with the essential knowledge and skills needed to plan, implement, and evaluate a quality clinical education program.

Roles and Responsibilities of the Clinical Instructor

When asked if they can recall any of their CIs, most health care professionals invariably answer "yes." Many say they remember not only the CIs who were exemplary role models but also those perceived to be poor role models. Likewise, they remember why a particular CI was remarkable or why they were disappointed with their CI's performance. Impressions left by clinical educators are lifelong; a laudable tribute and commentary to the role that a CI plays in the life of every health profession student.

The CI is involved with the daily responsibility and direct provision of high-quality student clinical learning experiences. Students often believe that the success or failure of the clinical learning experience can be attributed to the CI. Other synonyms for the CI include clinical tutor, clinical supervisor, clinical preceptor, clinical teacher, clinical mentor, and clinical educator. Each of these labels can be identified with one or more roles that this individual routinely performs. Much has been written in the literature of health care about the CI's role and responsibilities and the attributes of the CI that enhance student learning.[12,42–46] CIs significantly contribute to students' understanding of and competence in physical therapy clinical practice and serve as strong role models that guide students' visions of how they would like to practice in the future. Thus, the CI is responsible for providing an environment that fosters students' professionalism and encourages the development of an independent problem solver and a reflective, competent entry-level practitioner.

Skills and Qualifications of a Successful Clinical Instructor

In general, CIs' roles are multifaceted and include a range of behaviors, including facilitating, supervising, coaching, guiding, consulting, teaching, evaluating, counseling, advising, career planning, role modeling, mentoring, and socializing. Before serving as a CI for students in physical therapy, competence should be demonstrated by the CI in seven performance dimensions.

1. Clinical competence evidenced through the use of a systematic approach to care using the patient/client management model (i.e., examination, evaluation, diagnosis, prognosis, intervention, outcomes),[47–49] critical thinking skills, and effective time management skills.
2. Adherence to legal practice standards[36,37] and demonstration of ethical behavior that meets or exceeds the expectations of members of the profession of physical therapy.

3. Effective communication skills, including the ability to provide feedback to students, demonstrate skill in active listening, and initiate communication that may be difficult or confrontational.[44,45]
4. Effective behavior, conduct, and interpersonal relationships with patients/clients, students, colleagues, and other health care providers.
5. Effective instructional skills, including organizing, facilitating, implementing, and evaluating planned and unplanned learning experiences that take into consideration student learning needs, level of performance within the curriculum, goals of the clinical education experience, and the available facility resources.
6. Effective supervisory skills that include clarifying goals and student performance expectations, providing timely formal and informal feedback, making periodic adjustments to structured learning experiences, performing constructive and cumulative evaluations of student performance, and fostering reflective practice skills.[50]
7. Effective performance evaluation skills to determine professional competence,[48,49] ineffective or unsafe practices,[51] constructive remedial activities to address specific performance deficits, challenging activities to engage exemplary performers, and the ability to engage students in ongoing self-assessment.

Individuals can evaluate their readiness for or competence in serving as a CI by completing the self-assessment for CIs.[4]

Minimal qualifications for persons serving as CIs include (1) at least 1 year of clinical experience and the ability to perform CI responsibilities; (2) a willingness to work with students by pursuing learning experiences in clinical teaching; (3) a current state license, registration, or both (as required by specific state practice act), or certification or graduation from an accredited physical therapist assistant program; (4) positive representation of the profession by assuming responsibility for career and self-development and demonstrating this responsibility to students; and (5) willingness to act as a professional role model and the ability to recognize the impact of this role on students.[4,41]

Developing skills as a CI begins with an awareness of the parallels that exist between the roles of practitioner and CI. By recognizing these parallels, one can better understand how to transfer knowledge, skill, and behaviors used in delivering patient care to the task of designing a clinical student learning experience. Table 6-2 illustrates parallel relationships between practitioners and their patient/client management roles and CIs and their roles in coordination and implementation of student learning experiences.

Table 6-2   Roles of the Practitioner and Clinical Instructor

Roles of the practitioner	Roles of the clinical instructor
Patient referral and taking patient/client history	Preplanning for the learning experience and providing an orientation to the clinical site
Initial patient examination, diagnosis, and problem identification	Assessing students by identifying their strengths, learning needs, and previous experiences
Determining long-term functional goals mutually with the patient/client	Setting overall student objectives and clarifying learning expectations with the assistance of students and the academic program
Defining short-term patient/client goals	Defining specific student behavioral and learning objectives
Clarifying patient/client plan of care	Designing creative student learning experiences
Performing patient/client reexamination and assessing the level of progression	Providing formative student evaluations and assessing the level of progression toward defined outcomes
Assessing patient/client outcomes and readiness for physical therapy discharge	Providing summative student evaluations and assessing students' readiness for continued progress through the curriculum or entry into practice

Source: Adapted from the American Physical Therapy Association Clinical Instructor Education and Credentialing Program, American Physical Therapy Association. The Clinician and Clinical Educator. Alexandria, VA: 2000;Section I-8.

Clinical Instructor: Communication Skills

Several studies have focused on factors related to affective behaviors that are critical to effective learning experiences.[42,45,52] Affective characteristics of physical therapists found to contribute positively to patient/client care as well as effective clinical teaching include a positive attitude toward work, flexibility, compassion, sense of humor, openness to ideas and suggestions, friendliness, discipline and organization within the setting, and confidence in abilities and knowledge.[52] Students consistently rank communication, interpersonal relations, and teaching behaviors as the most valuable instructor behaviors in the clinical learning process. In a study by Young and Shaw, students rated university faculty as effective teachers when they provided genuine respect for students, motivated students, provided a comfortable learning atmosphere, demonstrated concern for students, demonstrated effective communication, provided course organization, and found value in the course.[53] Similar to that of clinical teachers, the majority of the rated items related to the affective domain.

Not surprisingly, the smallest differences found between "best" and "worst" clinical teachers were demonstrated in professional skills and knowledge.[42,54]

In one study by Emery, students ranked many of the behaviors identified to be necessary for effective clinical teaching as weak in their CIs.[42] Because more CIs are attending clinical education training courses and credentialing programs,[10,41] it might be presumed that these deficiencies would be reported less frequently.

The area of student performance most frequently cited by CIs as lacking is also in the affective domain, specifically interpersonal relations and communication.[55,56] ACCEs previously reported that they are less comfortable failing students for solely affective problems unless they occur in conjunction with safety, psychomotor, or cognitive deficiencies.[57] In the past, physical therapy education did not have adequate mechanisms for clearly defining and assessing those professional, affective behaviors to which students should be held accountable in both classroom and clinic settings. However, instruments were developed in the mid-1990s that can be used in the classroom[58] (e.g., Generic Abilities Assessment) and the clinic[21,59] (e.g., Clinical Performance Instrument and Generic Abilities Assessment) that clearly define performance expectations for student affective behaviors. Longitudinal studies should be conducted to determine if the widespread use of these tools that clearly define expectations for acceptable professional behaviors translates into improved interpersonal relations and communication skills for both students and CIs.

Successful Clinical Instructors: Other Factors

Other factors that contribute to the success of clinical teaching and supervision are (1) the provision of student-centered teaching strategies that encourage activities such as reflection[14–16]; (2) support for increased student autonomy; (3) application of situational leadership theories applied in clinical learning that help students participate more responsibly in their learning experiences[60]; (4) belief in a model of the best clinical practices in physical therapy; and (5) explication of models of problem solving and decision making, which can assist students in making better management decisions with sound clinical judgment, especially under ambiguous situations.[61–63] Clinical teaching has also been shown to be more effective when systematic instructional strategies (e.g., preparation, briefing, planning, practice, debriefing) and repeated learning opportunities are available to students to reinforce learning.[60,64] Enhancement of student learning occurs when the purpose of the learning experience is clearly defined, expectations for student and CI performance are clarified, the level of commitment is determined for all persons involved in the learning experience, and the timing, structure, frequency, and method of formative and summative evaluations are provided.[65] One of the greatest challenges for the CI is to find a balance for learners between nurturance and separateness. This is not unlike the delicate balance needed with patients/clients when providing physical therapy services. Specific techniques for teaching students in the clinical setting are provided in Chapter 7.

Preparation for Clinical Instruction

To develop the requisite knowledge, skills, and behaviors needed to effectively perform their responsibilities as CIs, adequate formal preparation is strongly recommended in the areas of teaching, supervision, interpersonal relations, communication, evaluation, and professional skill competence. Montgomery[66] believes that in addition to lack of formal training, many CIs also lack the "experience, maturity, and wisdom" to serve as mentors to physical therapy students. However, evidence shows the contrary. CIs reported on average between 1 to 2 years of clinical experience before beginning to teach in the clinical setting, and slightly more than half (53.4%) have attended a clinical training course.[10]

Development and publication of voluntary Guidelines and Self-Assessments in Clinical Education[4] have significantly influenced clinical training courses and programs to use the seven performance dimensions, described previously in this chapter under Skills and Qualifications of a Successful Clinical Instructor, as a basis for defining training objectives. In addition, many academic programs, clinical sites, and consortia provide training programs for CIs.

Many CIs believe that they are inadequately prepared for teaching[4] in the areas of (1) application of questioning and problem-solving techniques; (2) application of different levels of questioning in the domains of learning (see Chapter 2); (3) application of behavioral questioning to address affective issues and ways of improving the quality of questions[67]; (4) application of learning theory, including domains of learning and their hierarchies and an understanding of the elements of and methods used to assess learning styles[68]; (5) application of educational methodology, including adult learning and teaching theories and principles[69]; and (6) understanding of the context in which learning occurs.

Training Programs for Clinical Instructors

Training programs for CIs should provide specific information about selecting appropriate, creative, and effective teaching methods that actively involve learners in both self-directed and guided experiences.[69,70] Clinical teaching methods discussed might include demonstration-performance, teacher exposition, seminars, case analyses, case incident studies, role playing and rehearsal, reflective diaries,[71,72] double-entry journals,[73] evidence-based journal clubs,[74] conferences, brainstorming sessions, reflective discussions, and self-directed activities.[75]

Clinical training programs should also address the process of clinical evaluation. Basic concepts of clinical evaluation include (1) feedback, summative, and formative evaluations; (2) methods and techniques of evaluation such as competency-based, outcomes performance assessments, use of portfolios, and student self-assessment; (3) problems in and legal aspects of clinical evaluation[36,37]; and (4) a basic understanding of different evaluation instruments including how to critique their relative strengths and limitations and how to determine the most appropriate evaluation instruments for the specific clinical setting.[41,58,75–78]

Development of effective communication and conflict management skills should be included in clinical training programs. Specific content to be addressed includes components of and barriers to communication, ways of improving interpersonal, professional, and organizational communication, sources of conflict in the clinical setting, and techniques for identifying, managing, and resolving conflict.[75-79]

Fundamental components of clinical training should include an understanding of the roles, characteristics, and responsibilities of the CI and the organizational structure of clinical education within the total curriculum and management of the clinical environment and students' experiences within that environment.[4,80] Management of the environment includes

1. Assessment of available learning resources.
2. Establishment of guidelines for a safe environment for patients/clients and students.
3. Understanding federal regulations related to the Americans with Disabilities Act and state regulations related to physical therapy practice.
4. Creation of a filing system for confidential documents and other forms.
5. Development of a schedule for students.
6. Motivation of students to perform required tasks.
7. Development of a policy and procedure manual (printed or electronic) for students.
8. Selection of student orientation methods that are efficient and comprehensive (e.g., videotape of the clinical site, an established student orienting a new student).
9. Understanding the management of patients/clients with diverse backgrounds.
10. Promotion of positive learning experiences through learning contracts or other approaches.[41,79]

Frequently, as part of the tangible rewards of being a clinical educator, academic programs, clinical education consortia, or other clinical education special interest groups will sponsor 1–2 day continuing education programs for their clinical faculty at little to no cost.[9,81] Continuing education programs are generally identified as "basic or advanced courses" in clinical education. Training issues addressed in this chapter, in general, reflect content found in basic CI training courses.

Some training programs may offer state or regional credentialing or certificates and continuing education units (CEUs). However, most continuing education CI training programs do not have a mechanism for assessing the effectiveness of the training program in relation to knowledge, skills, and competence obtained by the learner.[82] Deusinger et al.[83] report on a 1994–1995 pilot study, funded by APTA and directed by principal investigator Michael Emery in collaboration with Nancy Peatman and Lynn Foord in cooperation with the New England Consortium of ACCEs, Inc., which was conducted to develop a valid and reliable training and assessment system for credentialing clinical educators. A program was designed to ensure that clinical educators who complete the program are able to satisfactorily meet the APTA Guidelines for Clinical Instructors.

As a result of the successful pilot project, in 1997, APTA funded and developed a national voluntary CI Education and Credentialing Program for physical therapist and physical therapist assistant clinical educators. This program is divided into two distinct parts: Part I, CI didactic curriculum via an interactive course format; and Part II, a credentialing process. Parts I and II are designed to be taught together to first provide and then assess the knowledge and skills identified as essential for physical therapist and physical therapist assistant clinical educators.

The didactic program addresses issues of

1. Planning and preparation of clinical educators for students during their clinical education experiences.
2. Developing planned and unplanned learning experiences.
3. Supporting ongoing student learning through questioning and providing effective feedback.
4. Developing knowledge and skills of performance evaluation.
5. Identifying and managing students with exceptional (i.e., demonstrating deficiencies or distinctive performance) situations.
6. Identifying legal implications for clinical educators, including issues presented with Americans with Disabilities Act legislation.

Part II of the program is a credentialing process to assess participants' achievement of curricular outcomes through a six-station assessment center.

Parts I and II of the program are available to both novice (minimum of one year of clinical experience) and experienced physical therapist and physical therapist assistant educators (including ACCEs, CCCEs, CIs, and academic faculty). Successful completion of the program results in the awarding of an APTA CI credential certificate and CEUs (1.5). Today, there are just over 7,000 physical therapist and physical therapist assistant credentialed CIs in the United States.[41]

In November 2000, Part I (didactic component) of the program became available to non-physical therapy providers who are licensed, registered, or certified by their respective discipline, have a minimum of 1 year of clinical experience, and are deemed competent practitioners by their respective discipline. Completion of the didactic component of the program results in the non-physical therapy participant receiving CEUs (1.2).

Only credentialed clinical trainers recognized by the APTA can provide the CI education and credentialing program. To become a credentialed clinical trainer, physical therapists and physical therapist assistants must apply for the Train-the-Trainer course and meet established eligibility criteria to be invited to complete a 3-day intensive training program. By the end of the course, participants are expected to demonstrate mastery of the program content to be taught, ability to manage and coordinate the assessment center, and to competently teach, using active teaching strategies, selected content to audiences of different levels and disciplines. Credentialed clinical trainers are required to renew their credential every 3 years through a portfolio review process by the APTA Clinical Instructor Education Board.

Finally, developing expertise as a CI requires knowledge, skill, and experience with positive and problematic student learning situations. Not unlike the learning experiences designed for students, CIs require opportunities to practice and reinforce knowledge and skills learned in clinical training programs, to learn from their mistakes,[84] and to apply this knowledge to real student situations, preferably with the guidance of a clinical teaching mentor. Thus, the process of learning to become a master clinical teacher is not unlike that of learning to become an expert clinician.[85] Mastery of the subject matter related to providing effective clinical education, understanding the needs of learners and patients/clients to whom care is given, understanding the context in which clinical learning occurs, having competence and confidence in one's ability as a practitioner, and the ability to translate educational theory into the practice using sound principles of teaching and reflective practice as applied to the clinical setting, all contribute to developing qualities of a master clinical teacher.[43,86]

Student Objectives and Expectations for Clinical Learning Experiences

Designing a clinical education program for students requires a structural framework, a road map, for ensuring that each planned learning experience meets the expected performance outcomes. In addition, the academic program must determine how progressive clinical experiences will, in conjunction with the didactic curriculum, accomplish the curricular performance outcomes required of students for entry into practice. Although at times the road may wind and even detour, if students, clinicians, and academic faculty can clearly articulate specific, expected learning and performance outcomes, the program can be adjusted throughout the clinical experience according to the students' needs.

Academic programs determine objectives that students must achieve and those that students can choose for progression through the curriculum. In certain circumstances, students and academic faculty may have curricular gaps and needs that only the clinical education sites can address.

The clinical site must determine what experiences it can offer and the objectives for those experiences that can be accomplished within the specific clinical setting and available time frame. The clinical site must also consider how the academic program's objectives coincide with or differ from the clinical site's learning objectives. Ultimately, the CI's function is to make learning experiences for students coherent.

Students are accountable for setting specific learning objectives for each clinical experience and adjusting them accordingly during the experience. These objectives are based on expected knowledge, skills, and behaviors they hope to acquire within a particular setting. Objectives are influenced by factors such as area of special interest or patient/client care provided, congruence with organizational structure provided for learning, and personal knowledge of the facility and its reputation. Students must actively seek learning experiences in which their knowledge and skills are deficient or with which they have little or no prior exposure.

The literature is consistent in considering the determination of objectives in clinical education as fundamental to planning learning experiences of all lengths. Although several methods can be used to provide objectives, one popular form is the behavioral objective. In this format, the objectives describe the learner, the conditions under which the learner must function, the learner's behavior at the completion of the learning experience, and the evaluation method(s) that will be used to assess the learning. Thus, the CI is aware of the planning and evaluative components required to determine student competence, and students understand precisely what is expected of them during the experience.[48,49]

The four major factors that determine the objectives in health professional programs are (1) the health needs and demands of society, (2) the nature of the subject matter, (3) characteristics of the learners, and (4) professional standards.[87] Obviously, with the changing and expanding need for physical therapy services, dramatic shifts in technology, and fluctuations in health care, it is critical that academic programs continually reassess curricular objectives to ensure their relevancy. In a study of applicants to physical therapist programs in 2000, applicants reported that they are applying to programs because they are more interested in providing patient/client care than employment opportunities.[88] The converse was true of the 1994 applicants to physical therapist programs. Thus, faculty should continually assess learners' values and attitudes about their education given resultant influences on curricular design and performance outcomes. Last, as part of a profession's responsibility, it must, on a regular basis, determine those behavioral outcomes that are believed to be essential for all graduates when entering practice.[48,49]

Behavioral objectives in clinical education should address all domains of learning at multiple hierarchical levels to ensure that learning experiences are incremental and comprehensive (see Chapter 2). As students progress through successive clinical experiences, consideration should be given to defining behavioral objectives that move up the hierarchy within each domain. For example, early student experiences may define behavioral objectives in the cognitive domain at the levels of knowledge, comprehension, and basic application compared to later clinical experiences that expect students to perform in the cognitive domain at the levels of analysis, synthesis, and evaluation.

Well-written objectives should be learner centered rather than teacher centered, be outcome oriented rather than process oriented, be outcome based rather than a statement of the material to be addressed, be a description of only one outcome, be specific rather than general, and be observable and measurable. Table 6-3 illustrates each of these requirements and contrasts correct and incorrect methods of writing an objective.

Effective clinical educators use both global and behavioral objectives. Global objectives describe the broader, more general outcome expectations for student performance, whereas behavioral objectives are more specific and help to further define each incremental learning experience.[87] For example, a global objective in the psychomotor domain might state, "The student will be able to examine a patient." A specific behavioral objective accompanying this global objective might state, "The student will accurately examine a patient with complex shoulder pathology in 30 minutes using a systematic approach substantiated by the literature." The progression of a set of behavioral objectives should lead to the achievement of global objectives. With

Table 6-3   Appropriate and Inappropriate Constructs for Writing Behavioral Objectives

Requirement	Correct example	Inappropriate example
Learner-centered vs. teacher-centered	The student will perform goniometric measurements.	The teacher will show the student how to perform goniometric measurements.
Outcome oriented vs. process oriented	The student will collect five articles on cerebral palsy.	The student will gather information on cerebral palsy.
Outcome oriented vs. merely stating the material to be addressed	The student will examine the biomechanics of the knee.	The student will look at biomechanical knee problems.
Describes only one outcome vs. describing multiple outcomes	The student will conduct a patient/client history.	The student will list the questions to ask in a patient/client history, interview the patient, conduct the history, and identify the appropriate tests and measures to examine.
Specific vs. general	The student will accurately perform manual muscle testing on the ankle.	The student will perform manual muscle testing.
Observable and measurable vs. not observable and quantifiable	The student will provide a rationale for the intervention based on evidence.	The student will know why he or she is providing an intervention.

Source: Adapted from American Physical Therapy Association Clinical Instructor Education and Credentialing Program Manual. Clinician as Clinical Educator. Alexandria, VA: 2000;Section I-11.

subsequent clinical experiences, some global objectives will be cumulative in nature, whereas others may be distinctive. However, the sum total of all global objectives in clinical education, in conjunction with the didactic curriculum, should adequately address those performance aspects that are required of students to satisfactorily progress through the curriculum and be prepared for initial clinical practice.

In summary, behavioral objectives in clinical education are sequenced in light of didactic components that have been completed; are achievable by the specific clinical setting; comprehensive, in that they address all domains of learning and progress students through each of the respective hierarchies; and are congruent with the philosophy, goals, mission, and outcomes of the academic program.

Models of Clinical Education

Although the most prevalent model of clinical education used in physical therapy is currently the integrated model,[2] the four models listed below can be found in selected physical therapist programs. These clinical education models[89] are defined as

1. The integrated model, in which the degree is conferred on completion of both didactic and clinical components with clinical education experiences arranged throughout the curriculum and with shared responsibility between the academic program and clinical education sites.

2. The independent and separate model (e.g., medicine), in which the degree is conferred on completion of the didactic program, followed by a separate and independent clinical education experience that is required to obtain a license to practice. In this model, the clinical education site controls and manages the clinical education program, including readiness to progress through and exit the clinical experience and to be eligible to take the licensure examination.

3. The self-contained model (e.g., nursing), in which the degree is conferred on completion of the didactic and faculty supervised patient/client experiences. Students complete supervised patient contact experiences with academic faculty members (salaries paid for by the academic institution) serving as advisors and clinical supervisors/mentors.

4. The hybrid model, in which clinical education experiences may occur in any combination of the above models and may provide for simulated and real patient care in didactic and clinical environments.

Although the academic program, with consultation from the clinical education community, may elect to use any of the above models, that should not preclude the CI from using any of the alternative supervisory approaches discussed below when providing clinical education programs for students in practice.

Alternative Supervisory Approaches in Clinical Education

To do justice to alternative supervisory approaches in clinical education would require space beyond that which can be allocated in this chapter. Therefore, only salient points are highlighted. An attempt has been made, however, to provide the reader with a table that consolidates the strengths, considerations, and limitations of alternative supervisory approaches into a quick and functional reference (Table 6-4). Nevertheless, the reader is encouraged to explore references cited in this section. Propelled by changes within health care

Table 6-4   Strengths, Considerations, and Limitations of Alternative Supervisory Approaches in Clinical Education

Design	Strengths	Considerations and limitations
One CI to one student (traditional design)	Allows the CI to maintain greater control of the learning experience Can easily monitor student performance Familiar student learning design Can easily provide line-of-sight supervision	Student less likely to learn from other clinicians Limited opportunities for collaborative learning Fosters student dependence on the CI
One CI to two or more students (collaborative-peer design)[73,91–99]	Fosters collaborative learning through peer interactions Enhances clinical competence related to clinical judgment Develops greater self-reliance, independence, and interdependence Teaches students to use and maximize limited resources Allows the CI to facilitate and guide the learning experience Fosters student problem solving and critical thinking skills Makes orientation less costly and time consuming Teaches students group presentation skills by providing collaborative projects or in-services Enhances service productivity in some settings (e.g., acute care)[95–97] Is useful for structured part-time group learning experiences	Initially requires more planning, effort, and organization time Requires that the total patient load is able to accommodate student needs Requires additional time to complete student performance evaluations Presents the possibility that too many patients will remain for the available clinicians after students have completed their training May be more likely used by an experienced CI Requires the CI to be highly flexible Can be problematic for CIs who wish to control learning experiences May be problematic for "needy" students or students requiring remedial work Is most successful when the CI carries a limited or no patient/client caseload

Design	Strengths	Considerations and limitations
One PT and PTA/CI team to one PT and PTA student team (supervisor-director design)[100,101]	Enhances understanding and skills associated with direction and supervision Enhances understanding of the roles and responsibilities of the PTA Provides opportunities for PT students to learn appropriate use of the PTA through role modeling by the PT/PTA CI team Provides for collaboration and sharing of information between PT and PTA students Maximizes clinical site resources and minimizes competition for limited numbers of clinical sites when PT/PTA programs provide student clinical education concurrently	Assumes that a PTA is employed at the clinical site Requires that the PT/PTA/CI team clearly understands the appropriate direction, supervision, and use of the PTA, and role model behaviors that demonstrate this understanding Assumes that the PTA and PT value and respect each other as co-workers Requires that the PT and PTA students are comfortable with their respective roles, strengths, and limitations so that they can learn from each other
One CI to two students paired from the same program at different clinical levels (student-peer mentor design)[102,103]	Same as one CI to two or more students design Allows the experienced student to develop supervisory skills Allows students to use each other as a resource and accept feedback more easily Allows the experienced student to orient the inexperienced student when beginning times are staggered Allows the experienced student to serve as the lead in situations in which the inexperienced student has not completed the didactic content Is useful in situations in which the inexperienced student has a shorter clinical experience	Same as one CI to two or more students design Can be problematic if students are not compatible in their learning styles or interpersonal interactions Requires alternative leadership design situations in which one student is the leader and the other is the aide, and vice versa

Table 6-4   *continued*

Design	Strengths	Considerations and limitations
Two part-time CIs or two CIs on different rotations to one or more students[103]	Maximizes opportunities for part-time personnel to be involved as CIs (often experienced clinicians) Increases opportunities for clinical sites with part-time clinicians to participate in clinical education Exposes students to multiple approaches to care delivery Allows part-time and full-time CIs to show comparable abilities in providing learning experiences Permits students in the same setting to be exposed to different learning experiences with different CIs Allows a clinical site to accommodate more students by using multiple rotations within the same setting Allows for greater variability in length of the clinical experience Increases CI productivity in comparison with clinicians who are not involved Reduces supervisors' direct patient-related responsibilities Decreases the number of superficial questions posed by students	Requires frequent and effective communication between CIs Can confuse students if expectations of the CIs differ Requires additional time for organization and planning Requires greater coordination between CIs in completing student performance evaluations Allows the possibility that students may compare CIs or CIs may compare students Can make it difficult for students to achieve their learning objectives Can decrease the variety and number patients/clients in the student caseload
Two CIs (one more experienced and one less experienced) to two or more students (teacher-mentor design)[103]	Provides a mechanism to mentor and develop an inexperienced CI through role modeling and teaching Allows students to learn to use parallel processes as inexperienced CIs Ensures that the experienced CI's knowledge is passed on to others Allows students to be part of a positive learning CI model that can be emulated	Requires an open and trusting relationship between CIs Requires that the inexperienced CI is comfortable knowing that he or she is inexperienced Confuses students as to which CI they are accountable to Requires excellent communication and clarity of roles between CIs

Design	Strengths	Considerations and limitations
Multiple rural or single practices offering collaborative clinical learning experiences (cooperative-network design)[104–106]	Permits solo practice settings to network with other sites to provide student clinical experiences Provides a support system for clinical teachers in rural settings Networking provides a mechanism to access clinical faculty training Enhances opportunities for students to be exposed to rural and solo practices Augments student learning experiences through interactions with multiple clinicians who provide care in different clinical settings Ensures that a mechanism is available for students to continue their learning experience uninterrupted in case of a CI's absence	Requires coordination and excellent communication between practice settings and CIs May be more difficult to implement because of different practice setting protocols and regulations Requires more complex coordination by the academic program with different legal contracts
One or more CIs from the same or different disciplines to one or more students from different disciplines (interdisciplinary-cooperative design)[106–108]	Provides a learning model that teaches collaborative team learning among different disciplines Gives students a better understanding of the roles and relationships between different disciplines in clinical practice Teaches students team leadership and follower skills Models a more ideal learning environment to learn how to work more effectively together in an interdisciplinary setting Assists in minimizing "turf battles" that affect quality learning Teaches students consultative skills with other professions	Applies only if different disciplines exist at the clinical site Requires excellent communication between and among the different disciplines Requires exceptional planning and organizational skills Requires that CIs trust, respect, and value each other's expertise and contributions to the learning process May cause problematic "turf battles" if interdisciplinary cooperation does not exist or where "turf battles" already exist

CI = clinical instructor.

delivery, this issue has emerged as one of the more expansive areas of clinical education research in the health professions.

Frequently, physical therapy clinical educators will comment that alternative approaches to student supervision were implemented in practice in the 1960s and 1970s and that this issue is not altogether new. However, during that time little or no empirical evidence was reported that described these supervisory approaches, their benefits or limitations, or their outcome effectiveness. In the 1990s, research emerged on the effectiveness of various approaches to student supervision that determined how best to provide student clinical education given limited personnel, patient/client, financial, and space resources. In the 1995 issue of *PT Magazine*, Gandy[90] provides a context for understanding why the profession is confronted with the need to provide more collaborative and interdependent methods for providing high-quality student learning experiences in varied practice settings. The fundamental basis for these changes lies in the need to "adjust our focus—even replace the lens—and explore alternatives that more efficiently use available limited practice and education resources and provide an environment for learning that more closely approximates current and future practice."[90] In the1990s, pervasive changes occurred in the configuration of practice and the delivery of physical therapy services; the breadth, depth, and design of physical therapist curricula to accommodate an expanding body of knowledge in physical therapy; the needs and changing values of students; the fluctuating numbers of students enrolled in physical therapy programs; increasing length of full-time clinical education experiences[2]; and the levels of experience of persons providing on-site student clinical supervision. Collectively, these changes have challenged the profession to rethink the one CI to one student supervisory approach and to consider and evaluate the use of other supervisory designs.

Collaborative and Cooperative Learning

Collaborative and cooperative learning were originally developed for educating persons of different ages, experience, and levels of mastery of interdependence. Cooperative learning was principally designed for primary school education to assist children in becoming more efficient and effective in learning to work together successfully on substantive issues, to hold students accountable for learning collectively rather than in competition with one another, and to provide social integration regardless of issues of diversity. Collaborative learning is similar to cooperative learning in that the goal is to help students work together on substantive issues. However, collaborative learning was developed primarily to make students enrolled in higher education more efficient and effective in aspects of education that are not content driven, to shift the locus of classroom authority from the teacher to student groups, and to facilitate structural reform and conceptual rethinking of higher education.[109]

Although perceived by some to be synonymous and interchangeable terminology, collaborative and cooperative learning within the context of small group learning are markedly dissimilar. Distinctions between collaborative and cooperative learning are generally drawn between the nature and authority of knowledge. The major disadvantage of collaborative learning is that, in attaining rewards of self-directed and peer learning, it sacrifices learner accountability.[109] Cooperative learning's major flaw is that by emphasizing accountability it risks replicating within each small group the more traditional model of teacher autonomy.[110] These two approaches also differ in terms of style, function, and teacher involvement; the extent to which students need to be trained to work together in groups; different outcomes, such as mastery of facts, the development of judgment, and construction of knowledge; the importance of different aspects of personal, social, and/or cognitive growth among students; and implementation concerns (e.g., group formation, task construction, and grading procedures).[111]

However, collaborative and cooperative learning are based on the fundamental assumption that knowledge is a social construct, and open-ended tasks that facilitate collaboration and control by learners restructure the classroom environment.[109] The two philosophies also argue that learning in an active mode is more effective than passive reception—the teacher is a facilitator, coach, or "guide by the side"—teaching and learning are shared experiences between teachers and students, participating in small group activities develops higher-order thinking skills and enhances abilities to use knowledge, accepting responsibility for learning as an individual and as a member of a group enhances intellectual development, articulating one's ideas in a small group setting enhances students' abilities to critically reflect on their thought processes and assumptions, belonging to a small group and supportive community increases student success and retention, and appreciating diversity is essential for survival in a multicultural society.[110] Although there are distinctions between these two types of learning, for the purposes of exploring and implementing alternative supervisory designs in physical therapy clinical education, it is preferable to unite both learning approaches by drawing on each of their strengths to enhance the achievement of desired outcomes.

It is important to note that merely placing two or more students together during a clinical experience does not connote cooperative or collaborative learning. Specific components must be present for small group learning to be truly cooperative and collaborative. As Johnson et al. stated, "[a] group must have clear positive interdependence and members must promote each other's learning and success face to face, hold each other individually accountable to do his or her fair share of the work, appropriately use interpersonal and small group skills needed for cooperative efforts to be successful, and process as a group how effectively members are working together."[112]

Finally, assessment of any learning approach should be considered in light of (1) the context in which learning must occur; (2) the academic program's expectations; (3) the available resources; (4) the availability of patients/clients; (5) the support of administration for clinical education specifically addressing productivity, cost-effectiveness, and reimbursement of care delivery; (6) the expertise, experience, and attributes of persons serving as clinical educators; (7) the relationship between all individuals involved in the teaching-learning process; (8) the characteristics of students; (9) strengths, limitations, and considerations of a particular supervisory approach; (10) the time available for planning and evaluating the alternative supervisory approach; (11) the desired outcomes of the learning experience; and (12) the strategies for ensuring successful implementation.

Summary

This chapter discusses topics perceived as most critical to understanding how to adequately prepare effective physical therapy teachers in clinical settings. It is understandable how situations like the two presented at the beginning of this chapter might readily occur. Today there are resources and professional development opportunities for preparing future clinical educators and enhancing the knowledge and skills of experienced clinical educators. Many aspects of clinical teaching have been shown to be grounded in literature that provides conceptual models and investigative studies that help to define components essential for quality education and training programs for clinical teachers.

The reader is encouraged to explore references provided in the annotated bibliography at the end of this chapter to learn more about clinical instruction. As more clinical educators critically investigate the use of alternative supervisory approaches, the profession will derive greater knowledge and understanding about the evidence-based differences between these designs and their resultant outcomes and effectiveness. Perhaps discussions espousing the benefit of one design over another will be resolved based on empirical evidence rather than intuition, historical precedent, and personal anecdotes.

It is my belief that implementing clinical teaching professional development programs is not sufficient. To ensure the future long-term viability of physical therapy necessitates that the process of becoming a CI should begin when educating students during their professional studies.[113] Students should be oriented as part of their active participation in clinical education to understand the organizational structure and roles and responsibilities of the ACCE/DCE, CCCE, and CI. In addition, students should learn how to give and receive feedback, critically evaluate their learning experiences, and routinely perform self-assessments to monitor their growth and development throughout progressive learning experiences. They should begin to develop an understanding and appreciation for the analogous processes used in providing aspects of classroom teaching, clinical teaching, and physical therapy services. In this way, students will learn to translate the process of service delivery, which is the primary focus of their clinical education and initial practice, to teaching students in clinical settings, which is one of the first roles they will assume as practitioners.

Clinical educators must be held accountable for role modeling those behaviors that they would like future practitioners to aspire to, and for demonstrating effective clinical teaching practices to ensure that students learn the knowledge, skills, and behaviors that are believed to be essential for entry into practice. Understanding one of the principles of pedagogy (i.e., that graduates will often teach in the clinical setting the way they were taught) means that CIs must critically examine their teaching to determine if their current approach is the legacy they wish to pass on. Andragogy, principles of adult learning, applies to physical therapy students and how they learn. Perhaps if CIs can recall their clinical education experiences as students, it will remind them of the pivotal role they play in the lives of all students. If CIs live by this rule, they can reshape clinical education. More important, individuals who serve to benefit most from these changes are the future graduates of physical therapist and physical therapist assistant programs that will deliver quality and cost-effective physical therapy care to patients/clients in an ever-changing health care environment.

References

1. Katzentzakis N. In Canfield J, Hansen MV. A 3rd Serving of Chicken Soup for the Soul. Deerfield Beach, FL: Health Communication Inc., 1996;113.
2. Department of Accreditation. Physical Therapist Program 2000 Fact Sheet. Alexandria, VA: American Physical Therapy Association, 2000;10.
3. Barnes MR. The twenty-sixth Mary McMillan lecture. Phys Ther 1992; 72:817.

4. American Physical Therapy Association. Guidelines and Self-Assessments for Clinical Education. Alexandria, VA: American Physical Therapy Association, 1999.

5. Commission on Accreditation in Physical Therapy Education. Evaluative Criteria for Accreditation of Education Programs for the Preparation of Physical Therapists. Alexandria, VA: American Physical Therapy Association, effective 1998.

6. Commission on Accreditation in Physical Therapy Education. Evaluative Criteria for Accreditation of Education Programs for the Preparation of Physical Therapist Assistants. Alexandria, VA: American Physical Therapy Association, effective 2002.

7. Emery MJ, Gandy JS, Goldstein M. Factors Influencing Career Selection of Students. Presented at American Physical Therapy Association Combined Sections Meeting. Reno, NV: February, 1995.

8. Buchanan CI, Noonan AC, O'Brien ML. Factors influencing job selection of new physical therapy graduates. J Phys Ther Educ 1994;8:39.

9. Gwyer J. Rewards of teaching physical therapy students: clinical instructor's perspective. J Phys Ther Educ 1993;7:63.

10. American Physical Therapy Association, Department of Clinical Education. 1992 Clinical Faculty Survey. Alexandria, VA: American Physical Therapy Association, 1992.

11. Sandroni S. Enhancing clinical teaching with information technologies: what can we do right now? Acad Med 1997;72:770.

12. Scully RM, Shepard KF. Clinical teaching in physical therapy education: an ethnographic study. Phys Ther 1983;63:349.

13. Department of Education. Clinical Site Information Form (CSIF). Alexandria, VA: American Physical Therapy Association, 1999.

14. Schön D. Educating the Reflective Practitioner. San Francisco: Jossey-Bass, 1987;3.

15. Jensen G, Denton B. Teaching physical therapy students to reflect: a suggestion for clinical education. J Phys Ther Educ 1991;5:33.

16. Gandy JS, Jensen G. Groupwork and reflective practicums in physical therapy education: models for professional behavior development. J Phys Ther Educ 1992;6:6.

17. Black JPH. The indispensable link between practice and education. R.E.A.D. Education Division Newsletter. Alexandria, VA: American Physical Therapy Association, 1995;8.

18. Peatman N, Albro R, DeMont M, et al. Survey of center clinical coordinators: format of clinical education and preferred methods of communication. J Phys Ther Educ 1988;2:28.

19. Ebert MS. Guide to Visiting Physical Therapist and Physical Therapist Assistant Students at Clinical Sites for Academic Coordinators of Clinical Education and Other Faculty. New York: Columbia University, 1995.

20. May BJ, Smith HG, Dennis JK. Combined clinical site visits and regional continuing education for clinical instructors. J Phys Ther Educ 1992;6:52.

21. American Physical Therapy Association. Physical Therapy Student Clinical Performance Instruments. Alexandria, VA: American Physical Therapy Association, 1998.

22. Dettman MA, Slaughter DS, Jensen RH. What consumers say about physical therapy program graduates. J Phys Ther Educ 1995;9:7.

23. Mathwig K, Clarke F, Owens T, Gramet P. Selection criteria for employment of entry-level physical therapists: a survey of New York State employers. J Phys Ther Educ 2001;15:65.

24. Higgs J. Managing clinical education: the educator-manager and the self-directed learner. Physiotherapy 1992;78:822.

25. Wojcik B, Rogers J. Enhancing clinical decision making through student self selection of clinical education experiences. J Phys Ther Educ 1992; 6:60.

26. Shoaf LD. Comparison of the student/site computer matching program and manual matching of physical therapy students in clinical education. J Phys Ther Educ 1999;13:39.

27. Ettinger ER. Role modeling for clinical educators. J Optometric Educ 1991;16–60.

28. Harris MJ, Fogel M, Blacconiere M. Job satisfaction among academic coordinators of clinical education in physical therapy. Phys Ther 1987;67:958.

29. Strickler SM. The academic coordinator of clinical education: current status, questions, and challenges for the 1990s and beyond. J Phys Ther Educ 1991;5:3.

30. Clouten N. The academic coordinator of clinical education: career issues. J Phys Ther Educ 1994;8:32.

31. Department of Education. An American Physical Therapy Association Model Position Description for the Academic Coordinator/Director of Clinical Education. Alexandria, VA: American Physical Therapy Association, 1999.

32. Gleeson PB, Utsey C (eds). Manual for the PT and PTA ACCE. Houston: Texas Consortium for Physical Therapy Clinical Education, Inc., 2000.

33. Ingram D, Hanks J. Preferred communication methods for physical therapy clinical experiences. J Phys Ther Educ 2000;14:39.

34. Kondela-Cebulski PM. Counseling function of academic coordinators of clinical education from select entry-level physical therapy educational programs. Phys Ther 1982;62:470.
35. Deusinger SS, Rose SJ. Opinions and comments: the dinosaur of academic physical therapy. Phys Ther 1988;68:412.
36. Smith HG. Introduction to legal risks associated with clinical education. J Phys Ther Educ 1994;8:67.
37. Fein BD. A review of the legal issues surrounding academic dismissal. J Phys Ther Educ 2001;15:21.
38. Americans with Disabilities Act of 1990. PL No 101-336, 42 USC §12101.103 (1990).
39. Ingram D. Essential functions required of physical therapist and physical therapist assistant students. J Phys Ther Educ 1994;6:57.
40. Emery MJ. The impact of the prospective payment system: perceived changes in the nature of practice and clinical education. Phys Ther 1993;73:11.
41. American Physical Therapy Association. Clinical Instructor Education and Credentialing Program and Manual. Alexandria, VA: American Physical Therapy Association, 2000.
42. Emery MJ. Effectiveness of the clinical instructor: students' perspective. Phys Ther 1982;64:1079.
43. Irby M. What clinical teachers in medicine need to know. Acad Med 1994;69:333.
44. Dunlevy CL, Wolf KN. Perceived differences in the importance and frequency of clinical teaching behaviors. J Allied Health 1992;21:175.
45. Emery MJ, Wilkinson CP. Perceived importance and frequency of clinical teaching behaviors: surveys of students, clinical instructors, and center coordinators of clinical education. J Phys Ther Educ 1987;1:29.
46. Jarski RW, Kulig K, Olson RE. Clinical teaching in physical therapy: student and teacher perceptions. Phys Ther 1990;70:173.
47. American Physical Therapy Association. Guide to Physical Therapist Practice (2nd ed). Phys Ther 2001;81:9.
48. American Physical Therapy Association. A Normative Model for Physical Therapist Professional Education, Version 2000. Alexandria, VA: American Physical Therapy Association, 2000.
49. American Physical Therapy Association. A Normative Model for Physical Therapist Assistant Education, Version 99. Alexandria, VA: American Physical Therapy Association, 1999.
50. Hayward LM. Becoming a self-reflective teacher: a meaningful research process. J Phys Ther Educ 2000;14:21.

51. Hayes KW, Huber G, Rogers J, Sanders B. Behaviors that cause clinical instructors to question the clinical competence of physical therapist students. Phys Ther 1999;79:653.

52. Wojcik R. Students' perceptions of the affective characteristics of physical therapists. Master's thesis. University of Illinois, Health Sciences Center, 1984.

53. Young S, Shaw DG. Profiles of effective college and university teachers. J Higher Educ 1999;70:670.

54. Irby DM, Ramsey PG, Gillmore GM, Schaad D. Characteristics of effective clinical teachers of ambulatory care medicine. Acad Med 1991;6:54.

55. Foord L, DeMont M. Teaching students in the clinical setting: managing the problem situation. J Phys Ther Educ 1990;4:61.

56. Ramsborg GC, Holloway R. Congruence of student, faculty, and graduate perceptions of positive and negative learning experiences. J Am Assoc Nurse Anesthetists 1987;55:135.

57. Gandy JS. How academic coordinators of clinical education resolve student problems [abstract]. Phys Ther 1985;65:695.

58. May WW, Morgan BJ, Lemke JC, et al. Model for ability-based assessment in physical therapy education. J Phys Ther Educ 1995;9:3.

59. Ullian JA, Blanc CJ, Simpson DE. An alternative approach to defining the role of the clinical teacher. Acad Med 1994;69:832.

60. Keenan MJ, Hoover PS, Hoover R, et al. Leadership theory lets clinical instructors guide students toward autonomy. Nurs Health Care 1988; 9:82.

61. Denton B. Facilitating clinical judgment across the curriculum. J Phys Ther Educ 1992;6:60.

62. Burnett CN, Mahoney PJ, Chidley MJ, et al. Problem-solving approach to clinical education. Phys Ther 1986;66:1730.

63. Slaughter DS, Brown DS, Gardner DL, et al. Improving physical therapy students' clinical problem-solving skills: an analytical questioning model. Phys Ther 1989;69:441.

64. Allen SS, Bland CJ, Harris IB, et al. Structured clinical teaching strategy. Med Teach 1991;13:177.

65. Anderson DC, Harris IB, Allen S, et al. Comparing students' feedback about clinical instruction with their performances. Acad Med 1991;66:29.

66. Montgomery J. Clinical Faculty: Revitalization for 2001. In Section for Education and Department of Education, Pivotal Issues in Clinical Education Present Status/Future Needs. Washington, DC: American Physical Therapy Association, 1988;7.

67. Schell K. Teaching tools: Promoting student questioning. Nurse Educ 1998;23:8.
68. Claxton CS, Murrell PH. Learning Styles: Implications for Improving Educational Practices. ASHE-ERIC Higher Education Report No. 4. Washington, DC: Association for the Study of Higher Education, 1987.
69. Merriam SB. An Update on Adult Learning Theory. New Directions for Adult and Continuing Education (No. 57). San Francisco: Jossey-Bass, 1993;15.
70. Silberman M. Active Training: A Handbook of Techniques, Designs, Case Examples, and Tips. San Francisco: Jossey-Bass/Pfeiffer, 1998.
71. Mostrom E, Shepard KF. Teaching and learning about patient education in physical therapy professional preparation: academic and clinical considerations. J Phys Ther Educ 1999;13:8.
72. Marland G, McSherry W. The reflective diary: an aid to practice-based learning. Nurs Stand 1997;12:49.
73. Nolinske T, Millis B. Cooperative learning as an approach to pedagogy. Am J Occ Ther 1999;53:31.
74. Elnicki DM, Halperin AK, Shockor WT, Aronoff SC. Multidisciplinary evidence-based medicine journal clubs: curriculum design and participants' reactions. Am J Med Sci 1999;317:243.
75. Watts N. Handbook of Clinical Teaching. New York: Churchill Livingstone, 1990;37.
76. Deusinger SS. Evaluating the effectiveness of clinical education. J Phys Ther Educ 1990;4:66.
77. Henry JN. Using feedback and evaluation effectively in clinical supervision: model for interaction characteristics and strategies. Phys Ther 1985;65:354.
78. Hrachovy J, Clopton N, Baggett K, et al. Use of the Blue MACS: acceptance by clinical instructors and self-reports of adherence. Phys Ther 2000;80:652.
79. Deusinger S (ed). The Clinical Instructor's Handbook (2nd ed). St. Louis: Central ACCE Consortium, Washington University School of Medicine, 2000.
80. Barr JS, Gwyer J, Talmor A. Evaluation of clinical centers in physical therapy. Phys Ther 1982;62:850.
81. Department of Education/Clinical Instructor Education Board. 2000 Credentialed Clinical Instructor Survey. Alexandria, VA: American Physical Therapy Association, 2000.
82. Norcross JC, Stevenson JF. Evaluating Clinical Training: Measurement and Utilization Implications from Three National Studies [abstract]. Pre-

sented at the Annual Meeting of the Evaluation and Research Society. Toronto: October, 1985.

83. Deusinger S, Cornbleet SL, Stith JS. Using assessment centers to promote clinical faculty development. J Phys Ther Educ 1991;5:14.

84. Pinsky LE, Irby DM. "If at first you don't success": using failure to improve teaching. Acad Med 1997;72:973.

85. Jensen GM, Gwyer J, Shepard KF, Hack LM. Expert practice in physical therapy. Phys Ther 2000;80:28.

86. Grossman PL. The Making of a Teacher: Teacher Knowledge and Teacher Education. New York: Columbia University, 1990.

87. Moore ML, Perry JF. Clinical Education in Physical Therapy: Present Status/Future Needs. Washington, DC: Section for Education, American Physical Therapy Association, 1976;3:1.

88. Goldstein M, Gandy J. Survey of 2000 Applicants to Physical Therapist Programs. J Phys Ther Educ 2001;15:9.

89. Education Division, American Physical Therapy Association. "Clinical Education: Dare to Innovate." A consensus conference on alternative models of clinical education. Alexandria VA: American Physical Therapy Association 1998;4.

90. Gandy JS. Clinical education through a new lens: collaboration and interdependence. PT Mag 1995;3:40.

91. Emery MJ, Nalette E. Student staffed clinics: creative clinical education during times of constraint. Clin Manage Phys Ther 1986;6:6.

92. DeClute J, Ladyshewsky R. Enhancing clinical competence using a collaborative clinical education model. Phys Ther 1993;73:683.

93. Nemshick MT, Shepard KF. Physical therapy clinical education in a 2:1 student-instructor education model. Phys Ther 1996;76:968.

94. Haffner Zavadak K, Konccky Dolnack C, Polich S, et al. Clinical education series: 2:1 collaborative models. PT Mag 1995;3:46.

95. Ladyshewsky RK. Enhancing service productivity in acute care inpatient settings using a collaborative clinical education model. Phys Ther 1995;75:503.

96. Ladyshewsky RK, Barrie SC, Drake VM. A comparison of productivity and learning outcome in individual and cooperative physical therapy clinical education models. Phys Ther 1998;78:1288.

97. Dupont L, Roy R, Gauthier-Gagnon C, Lamoureux M. Group supervision and productivity: from myth to reality. J Phys Ther Educ 1997;11:31.

98. Ladyshewsky R. Clinical teaching and the 2:1 student to clinical instructor ratio. J Phys Ther Educ 1995;7:31.

99. Ozga K, Baker B. A Collaborative Clinical Education Model: One Academic Faculty Member and Four Students. Presented at American Physical Therapy Association Combined Sections Meeting. Reno, NV: 1995.

100. Foord L, Kaufman R. Strategies for use of a 2:1 teaching model in physical therapist assistant clinical education [abstract]. Phys Ther 1994;74.

101. Wynn KE. The MPT-PTA collaborative model. PT Mag 1996;4:75.

102. Escovitz ES. Using senior students as clinical skills teaching assistants. Acad Med 1990;65:733.

103. Gerace L, Sibilano H. preparing students for peer collaboration: a clinical teaching model. J Nurs Educ 1984;23:206.

104. Delehanty MJ. Recruitment and retention of physical therapists in rural areas: an interdisciplinary approach [abstract]. Phys Ther 1993;73: 70.

105. Clark SL, Schlachter S. Development of clinical education sites in an area health education system. Phys Ther 1981;61:904.

106. Blakely RL, Jackson-Brownlow V. Interdisciplinary rural health education and training (IRHET) [abstract]. Phys Ther 1993;73:66.

107. Perkins J, Tryssenaar J. Making interdisciplinary education effective for rehabilitation students. J Allied Health 1994;23:133.

108. Betz CL, Raynor O, Turman J. Use of an interdisciplinary team for clinical instruction. Nurse Educ 1998;23:32.

109. Brufee KA. Sharing our toys—cooperative learning versus collaborative learning. Change 1995;27:12.

110. Matthews RS, Cooper JL, Davidson N, et al. Building bridges between cooperative and collaborative learning. Change 1995;27:35.

111. Gamson ZF. Collaborative learning comes of age. Change 1994;26:44.

112. Johnson DW, Johnson RT, Smith KA. Cooperative Learning: Increasing College Faculty and Instructional Productivity. ASHE-ERIC Higher Education Report No. 4. Washington, DC: The George Washington University, School of Education and Human Development, 1991;25.

113. Halcarz PA, Marzouk DK, Avila E, et al. Preparation of entry-level students for future roles as clinical instructors. J Phys Ther Educ 1991;5:78.

Annotated Bibliography

American Physical Therapy Association, Clinical Education: An Anthology (Volumes I, II, and III). Alexandria, VA: American Physical Therapy Association, 1992; 1996; 2000. Taken together, these three publications include a collection of 267 articles compiled from literature in physical therapy as well as other professions. Articles included in these references provide research in seven core dimensions in clinical education. These dimensions include (1) clinical faculty (ACCEs/DCEs, CCCEs, and CIs), (2) clinical environment and resources, (3) design of clinical education, (4) evaluation and research, (5) academic issues associated with clinical education, (6) student issues in clinical education, and the emerging area of (7) technology in clinical education. Overall, these publications span the physical therapy literature in clinical education from the early 1980s through 1999. These three anthologies are an excellent reference for persons involved in clinical education.

American Physical Therapy Association, Guidelines and Self-Assessments for Clinical Education. Alexandria, VA: American Physical Therapy Association, 1999. This reference describes guidelines for clinical education sites, CIs, and CCCEs that were endorsed by the APTA House of Delegates in June 1993. These voluntary guidelines were designed to describe the fundamental and essential performance criteria that should guide the selection and development of clinical sites and individuals who serve as clinical educators. These guidelines are accompanied by three self-assessment documents that allow the clinical education site, CIs, and CCCEs to assess their performance as meeting the guideline, not meeting the guideline, or aspects of their performance being developed. Academic programs and clinical sites wanting to identify targeted areas for clinical faculty and clinical site development can use information gleaned from these self-assessments.

Ladyshewsky R, Healy E. The 2:1 Teaching Model in Clinical Education. A Manual for Clinical Instructors. Toronto. Department of Rehabilitation Medicine, Division of Physical Therapy, University of Toronto, 1990. This manual describes the two-student to one-CI collaborative clinical teaching design and provides the necessary steps to implement this supervisory approach in the clinic. The manual is user friendly, easy to understand, and provides a conceptual framework for understanding some of the issues described in this chapter. This manual assists the CI in organizing, planning, implementing, and evaluating the collaborative learning design. This manual can be purchased through the University of Toronto, Department of Rehabilitation Medicine, Division of Physical Therapy, 256 McCaul Street, Toronto, Ontario, Canada M5T 1W5.

Watts N. Handbook of Clinical Teaching. New York: Churchill Livingstone, 1990. This book provides a practical and user-friendly resource for health professionals to augment their knowledge and skills in providing clinical education for students. For illustrative and teaching purposes, Watts uses a multidisciplinary approach to understanding clinical teaching and encourages the completion of practice exercises in partnerships or collaborative interdisciplinary teams to reinforce learning. She facilitates learning through three essential teaching components—acquiring information, providing practice exercises, and giving immediate feedback. Some of the topics addressed include planning for student practice, performing a learning needs assessment, designing a learning contract, supervising practice of a complex skill, influencing student attitudes and values, giving effective feedback, and analyzing one's teaching style.

Silberman M. Active Training: A Handbook of Techniques, Designs, Case Examples, and Tips. San Francisco: Jossey-Bass/Pfeiffer, 1998. This text is an excellent reference for academic and clinical teachers that provides active training approaches to engage audiences in the learning process. Silberman provides a systematic approach to active teaching that begins with the reflective planning process through design implementation and, finally, instructional and programmatic evaluation. Innovative strategies and case examples are provided to assist the instructor in developing variety in his or her teaching and for assessing which approaches may be best suited for different audiences. This reference is a must for anyone involved in teaching.

Gleeson P, Utsey C (eds). Manual for the PT and PTA ACCE. Houston: Texas Consortium for Physical Therapy Clinical Education, Inc., 2000. This comprehensive manual provides the ACCE with practical and "how-to" tips associated with the ACCE's roles and responsibilities. Some of the topics addressed in this manual include structure of the clinical education program, financial administration of a clinical education program, contractual agreements, academic policies and procedures, legal issues and the ADA, clinical education site development, managing students, and clinical faculty development. Members of the Texas Consortium have provided a rich framework for ACCEs to enable them to thrive in their position while minimizing potential pitfalls along the way. This manual can be purchased through The Texas Consortium, Inc., Texas Woman's University, School of Physical Therapy, 1130 M. D. Anderson Boulevard, Houston, TX 77030.

Deusinger S (ed). The Clinical Instructor's Handbook (2nd ed). St. Louis: Central ACCE Consortium, 1999. This handbook is a foundational resource for novice and experienced clinical educators and reinforces content learned in the APTA Clinical Instructor Education and Credentialing Program. This handbook contains four readable sections that correspond with information contained in Chapters 6 and 7 of this text. The sections include preparing for clinical education, selecting teaching strategies and methods, considering variables that affect learning, and documenting outcomes of clinical education. This handbook can be purchased through the Central ACCE Consortium, Washington University School of Medicine, Program in Physical Therapy, 4444 Forest Park, Campus Box 8502, St. Louis, MO 63108.

Grossman P. The Making of a Teacher: Teacher Knowledge and Teacher Education. New York: Teachers College Press, 1990. This text provides an insightful and deeper understanding of educational practice and how to improve it through a sound conceptual framework and the use of case sketches. Her cutting-edge research provides an understanding of the differences in what teachers believe and value, how those values are actually enacted in the classroom, and how beliefs and values affect content that teachers teach. At first glance, clinical educators may perceive that an examination of six English teachers, as the subjects of this text, have little to no relationship to their roles in clinical practice. However, of great significance is the realization that teacher education programs that provide a coherent vision for teaching and learning do influence the quality of teaching. In addition, these teacher education programs ultimately affect how students construct their emerging and evolving knowledge and understanding of content, which subsequently facilitates the integration of that knowledge into practice.

7

Techniques for Teaching Students in Clinical Settings

Karen A. Paschal

> When you are a Bear of Very Little Brain and you think of things, you find sometimes that a thing which seemed very thingish inside you is quite different when it gets out into the open and has other people looking at it.
> —Winnie-the-Pooh, in A. A. Milne's *The House at Pooh Corner*

Clinical education has long been recognized as a necessary part of physical therapy education. In 1968, Callahan et al. stated that the purpose of clinical education was "to assist the student to correlate clinical practices with basic sciences; to acquire new knowledge, attitudes and skill to develop ability to observe, to evaluate, to develop realistic goals and plan effective treatment programs; to accept professional responsibility; to maintain a spirit of inquiry and to develop a pattern for continuing education."[1] Despite major changes in health care delivery and physical therapy, this purpose reflects the present goal of physical therapy clinical education.

The importance of clinical education is expressed by students when they remind instructors that "real learning" in physical therapy occurs in the clinic. In fact, long after physical therapists forget what was taught in which course during academic preparation, they remember their clinical education experiences. Physical therapists remember not only specific experiences with patients but also remember their clinical teachers. It is not unusual to hear a clinical teacher say, "I remember when I was a student and my clinical instructor (CI). . . ." Whether perceived as outstanding or mediocre, the clinical teacher has a profound effect on how students practice and how they want to teach the next generation of students. Much of what CIs know, do, and value in their positions was learned when they were students. However, as strong as those beliefs and ideas may be, the very "thingish" ideas CIs have about clinical teaching may be perceived quite differently when enacted.

Consider these accounts of a clinical education experience described quite differently by a young CI and a student.

CLINICAL INSTRUCTOR: Jeff is a bright student. He's enthusiastic and eager to learn. I know this is only his second clinical affiliation and he hasn't had all of his classroom work yet, but he's on the right track. I've really tried to spend time teaching him. I wanted that when I was a student. My CI just let me go for it on my own. I mean, I learned, but I would have liked to have had someone there giving me feedback and teaching me more advanced skills. I think this approach has helped Jeff.

JEFF: This is different from my first affiliation. I'm really just watching my CI most of the time. Like with the new patient I saw this morning. I started the history, but she interrupted and just kept asking all the questions. Then, I started the examination, but I guess I wasn't doing something quite right, so she stepped in. It seems like she lectures to me all the time. I know I can't do everything perfectly, but I'd just like to try. I could think of most of the things she did with the patient, but all I got to do was watch her. That's not really true. She let me do the ultrasound.

This CI's intentions are good but quite different when they translate into practice. In trying to improve on her experience as a student, the CI focuses on herself as the teacher rather than the student. How could she restructure her teaching to better facilitate learning? How could she teach and at the same time allow Jeff to learn by doing? This chapter focuses on pragmatic teaching techniques for use in the clinical setting. Avoiding highly specified, technical explanations of what clinical teachers do, this chapter uses an approach that recognizes the judgment of clinical teachers in the use of fundamental, practical, and realistic teaching techniques in typically unique and often ambiguous conditions that are the "real world" of physical therapy practice.

Chapter Objectives

After completing this chapter, the reader will be able to

1. Describe the dynamic environment in which clinical education occurs.
2. Describe the clinical learning process and identify expected outcomes.

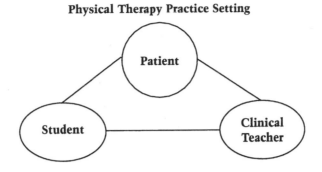

Figure 7-1 Fundamental elements of clinical education.

3. Discuss and give examples of the four roles of a clinical teacher.
4. Identify practical strategies for enhancing clinical teaching methods.
5. Promote the professional development of students to facilitate the transition from clinical education to new graduate.

Context of Clinical Education

Clinical learning is situated in the context of physical therapy practice. It occurs in real practice settings, with real patients, and with real physical therapists as clinical teachers. Figure 7-1 diagrams the essential elements in clinical education that provide context for the learning experience.

Historically, clinical education has occurred in settings in which administrators, directors, and, most important, physical therapy clinical teachers have been willing to provide it. As the treatment of patients with impairments and functional limitations related to human movement and movement dysfunction has moved from inpatient to outpatient settings, physical therapy clinical education has moved from hospitals to a variety of community-based centers, including outpatient health care facilities, schools, retirement centers, health promotion and wellness centers, and preschools. Changes in how and where health care is delivered have affected, for the most part positively, the traditional inpatient basis for students' clinical education. The modern teaching hospital has become a large intensive care unit, where physical therapy students have short-term access to critically ill patients who only represent a small and very ill portion of the total spectrum of physical therapy practice. Students get a fuller view of the quality of life of a patient when the patient is seen not only during acute illness requiring hospitalization, but also in outpatient clinics where patients are treated for movement-related disorders that

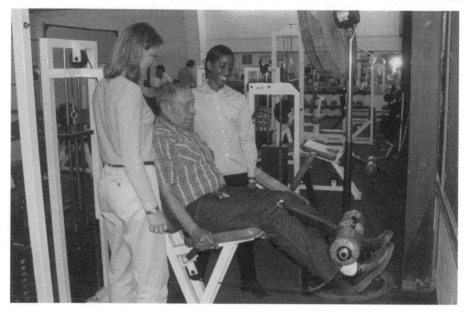

Figure 7-2   Patient, student, and clinical instructor co-participate in an early clinical learning experience.

impact everyday activities. The spectrum of clinical experiences that a student can have is tremendous.

Explicitly defining the desired outcome for each clinical experience dictates the appropriate timing in the curriculum, the duration of the experience, the type of setting, and the qualifications of the clinical teachers. Students' early experiences may be even more critical than experiences that occur after the completion of the didactic curriculum because they are generally short, and the impact of the experience provides the framework for the student to develop patterns of lifelong clinical learning (Figure 7-2). The days of hands-off observation for students are over, although this may be the temptation in a busy clinical practice where productivity standards are high, and there is little time for teaching and practicing basic skills. Students must be ready to enter the clinic setting and interact with patients. They must know where to start. They must come with the expectation that they learn by thinking and doing with a patient.

What does a student need to know on day 1 of a clinical learning experience? What is best taught in the classroom or the laboratory? What is best learned during a clinical education experience? Basic knowledge and skills are prerequisites to clinical learning. Consider the example given in Table 7-1. Muscle performance examinations are routinely provided by physical thera-

Table 7-1 Muscle Performance Examinations Provided by Physical Therapists

Learning environment	*Primary learning activity*
Classroom	Acquisition of knowledge
	• definition of muscle performance
	• characteristics of performance
	• mediators of performance
	• reasons for examination
	• selection of specific tests and measures
	• expected examination outcomes
Laboratory	Acquisition of skill
	• tests and measures for conducting a muscle performance examination, including generation of data
Clinic	Use of knowledge and skill for clinical decision making and patient management in
	• evaluation
	• diagnosis
	• prognosis
	• determination of appropriate intervention

Source: Adapted from American Physical Therapy Association. Guide to Physical Therapist Practice (2nd ed). Phys Ther 2001;81:9.

pists. Knowledge of these examinations, as well as rudimentary skill in performing them, is acquired in the classroom and laboratory. In the clinical setting, the student learns to use this knowledge and skill in clinical decision making and patient management.

Academic and Clinical Teaching: Two Different Realities

The primary difference between academic and clinical teaching is that control of academic teaching lies with the educational system, and control of clinical teaching lies with the health care system and, ultimately, the patient. This fundamental difference underlies all aspects of developing a clinical education program, and it must be recognized and accommodated in clinical education programs. The academic setting has been organized for the efficiency and convenience of the system, its administration and faculty, and technologies, whereas the clinical system is generally organized for the convenience of delivering health care to the patient. Most educational issues flow from this basic difference, including those of appropriate and attainable educational objectives, effective instruction and evaluation methods, effect of clinical education on the patient and patient care, and costs of teaching.

Table 7-2   Ground Rules Framing the Context of the Clinical Education Experience

Sources	Examples
External	University mission and objectives
	Assignment of students
	Time and length of assignment
Internal	Department policies and procedures
	Assignment of the clinical instructor
	Health requirements
Clinical teacher	Preparation and experience
	Value judgments—for example,
	Patient primacy
	Professionalism

Source: Adapted from RM Scully. Clinical Teaching of Physical Therapy Students in Clinical Education [Ph.D. dissertation]. Columbia University, 1974.

Prevailing Conditions in the Clinical Environment

The clinical setting is a unique and complex learning environment. Student performance is based on knowing and doing in a real situation with a real patient or client. The learning situation within the clinic is framed by several factors or ground rules.

Scully[2] suggests that there are three generic sources for the ground rules that frame the clinical learning environment: (1) those originating external to the clinical education facility, (2) those originating internal to the clinical education facility, and (3) those originating from within the clinical teacher. Table 7-2 gives examples of each. Although these delineations are helpful in understanding the origin of factors influencing the context of the clinical experience, examples may not fit exclusively in one category.

Consider the examples of Natasha and Anne. Both are physical therapy students assigned to a pediatric clinical setting by their respective academic programs. Student assignment or placement is an academic prerogative, and the method used varies from program to program. The following descriptions of the placement procedures that affect Natasha and Anne provide an example of external factors that impact the clinical education experience.

NATASHA: A pediatrics rotation is important to me. I don't have much experience with children. But, I volunteered over the summer at a camp for kids with AIDS [acquired immunodeficiency syndrome], and I took the pediatric elective. It was tough, but I'm really excited about learning to do all we talked about. The student who was here last year said this was a great place!

ANNE: I'm not planning to get a job in pediatrics or anything. I just sort of got sent here—I was at the end of the lottery. I mean, I want to be well rounded and everything, but I don't want to work with kids. I just want to get the basics. You know, so if kids ever come into my office I'll know what to do with them.

On closer examination, however, the effect of this external factor, the placement procedures, may not be so clear cut. Consider values held by two physical therapists who could be assigned as Anne's CI:

CLINICAL INSTRUCTOR A: It's going to be a long 8 weeks. Anne doesn't want to be here. You can't just learn the basics and expect to be a good physical therapist. Where do I even begin with her?

CLINICAL INSTRUCTOR B: I appreciate Anne's honesty, and I hope I can work with her to become more diplomatic. I think there are many aspects of pediatric practice that apply to all patients. I think we can work together to create an excellent experience. I want to start by learning more about her interests.

The attitudes held by each of these therapists would greatly influence Anne's clinical education experience. Think of other external and internal constraints imposed on the clinical education process. In almost every case, the CI's knowledge, skill, values, and attitudes could reframe the learning context in a way that would dramatically change the outcome of the clinical experience.

Consider the demands imposed by the changing health care delivery system. Although addressed by academic programs in the curriculum, students often express the reality as follows:

ROBERTO: This hospital isn't a very good place right now. There's a lot of change going on. The patients are all seen in their rooms or in little satellite departments on the floors. It seems like all we do is get them out of bed. I don't have time for a complete examination before they're discharged. The biggest job the therapists have is deciding where to refer the patients when they're discharged from the hospital. I want to do real physical therapy.

The CI, Mariah, has the ability to reframe this response and challenge Roberto to make the most of his learning experience by expressing something like the following:

MARIAH: You're absolutely right. I think we sometimes get the notion that physical therapy means using our hands all the time. Sometimes, though, the emphasis is on using our heads to think and plan. We can learn about the patient's functional status before admission; we know what's happened here, and then it's our job to make the best possible guess about the future and make recommendations based on that. What a challenge! Discharge planning is a focus from the beginning, and even our treatments need to take that into consideration. What do you think about Mr. Baird, whom we saw this morning?

After the context of the clinical education experience is understood, physical therapists can develop ways to mold it as Clinical Instructor B and Mariah did. CIs can often reframe the circumstances if they view the ground rules as defining opportunities and challenges that allow them to better enable student clinical learning.

Given these prevailing conditions, it is important to ask the following: How do students learn in the clinic? What is helpful for clinical teachers to know and understand about the clinical learning process?

Clinical Learning

The purpose of this section is neither to review the work of learning theorists[3–8] nor to examine the literature related to student physical therapists' learning.[9–14] Rather, this section provides a contextual basis of clinical learning to use in the upcoming section Roles of the Clinical Teacher: Diagnosing Readiness, Planning, Teaching, and Evaluating. John Dewey provided key descriptors of the clinical learning process when he stated, "education is not an affair of 'telling' and being told, but an active and constructive process."[15] Successful clinical learning requires the student to make meaning of knowledge in a clinical sense and then to enact that meaning when providing physical therapy services.

Student Ownership and Responsibility

The clinical education experience belongs to the student, despite the fact that it occurs in the CI's clinic. It involves patients to whom the CI has legal and ethical responsibilities. It requires the CI's time, energy, and creativity. It is imperative, however, that the student accepts ownership and responsibility for the experience. Clinical education is an opportunity for a student to learn not only the knowledge, skills, values, and attitudes of the profession, but it is also the first experience in a lifelong pattern of learn-

Table 7-3　Principles That Dampen or Motivate Students to Enhance Competence and Encourage Self-Determination in Actions

	Dampeners	*Motivators*
Focus of goal orientation	Judgment	Development and learning
Performance expectations	Low	High
Learning opportunities	Governed by rules and regulations	Self-directed
	Prescriptive, mandatory experiences	Multiple opportunities with recommendations
Instructional strategies	Routine	Challenging
	Extrinsic rewards and incentives	Encourage deep and rich thinking processes
Feedback/evaluation	Dominate and control behavior	Available but infrequent from external sources
Institutional/personal premiums	Emphasize conformity	Emphasize creativity, innovation, and alternative perspectives

Source: Adapted from R Lewthwaite, JM Burnfield, L Tompson, et al. Education and development principles. Presented at: Seventh National Physical Therapy Clinical Education Conference; April, 1995; Buffalo, NY.

ing and continual development as a physical therapist. Table 7-3 summarizes principles that enhance competence and encourage self-determination in actions. It is important that students assume responsibility for learning what they need to know and how to go about learning it.

There are several learning experiences that can be used to encourage student ownership for clinical learning. The student should prepare for each experience by becoming familiar with the Clinical Site Information Form and any orientation materials sent before the student's arrival. Based on this information, the CI may wish to ask students to prepare specific personal goals and learning objectives they would like to meet during their time at the facility. This student-specific information provides an excellent basis for discussion during orientation, at which time the CI can affirm or revise student goals and plan relevant learning experiences. It is important to revisit these goals and objectives periodically. The CI can use them in weekly planning or as a part of the midterm evaluation by asking what the student has accomplished, what activities still need to be undertaken, or if further revisions or additions need to be made. Having the student develop objectives within the context of practice enables the student to further develop professional identity and mission as a physical therapist or physical therapist assistant. In doing so, the student acquires a framework for establishing lifelong learning habits.

Process of Clinical Learning

Clinical learning is a process of mutual inquiry conducted by the student and CI during the provision of patient care services. It is a process during which the student co-participates in clinical decision making with a skilled practitioner, the CI. As such, it is a situated learning experience in which teaching and learning occur around the patient in a series of complex interactions. Contrary to what CIs may think, *it doesn't just happen*. Consider Katie's experience as she and her CI described it to the Director of Clinical Education (DCE) for her academic program during his on-site visit:

CLINICAL INSTRUCTOR: She's doing fine. I don't have any complaints. You know, she's right where she should be. I don't mean that she's perfect, but time and more experience help. She just has the usual student problems. She asks questions. She fits in here, and she'll be a good physical therapist someday.

KATIE: I don't know. It's not bad, but I'm not sure that I'm learning. I mean, I know I'm learning, but I think I could be doing more. I sort of feel like a junior therapist. I come in, treat my patients with some help, and go home.

Katie is participating in the third of four clinical education experiences. She performs adequately but seems stuck. She thinks that she isn't learning as much as she is capable of, but she does not seem to know where to go from here. Consider steps the DCE might take, the CI's responsibilities, and what Katie needs to do to continue the learning process.

Bridging Theory with Practice

A primary goal of clinical teaching is to enable the student to build bridges between theory and practice. Theoretical knowledge and fundamental skills taught in the physical therapy classroom and laboratory may be embedded in a patient problem orientation, but students rarely, if ever, learn in the clinical context until their first clinical education experience. The need for bridging theory and practice is made clear by example in this statement by Becky, a student in her first clinical education experience:

BECKY: I was doing okay until the patient threw me off track by giving the wrong answer to my question. I mean, she isn't supposed to have pain in her shoulder all night long, unless she has cancer or something bad like that. I was pretty sure she had a frozen shoulder.

Clinical practice is all about patient responses that don't fit with textbook diagnoses. There are no multiple choice patients for whom a circle around the best answer restores function. Academic knowledge needs to be reformatted in the contextual basis of patient care. Clinical wisdom is based on far more than building on the facts. It is a transformation of knowledge done by integrating reflective experience. This is illustrated in the following example:

STUDENT: My CI is so smart. How did she learn all she knows? Yesterday a patient tried to refuse treatment, but she just didn't take "no" for an answer. The patient ended up doing better during the treatment session than I had ever seen him do. Then, this morning, Mr. Jones said that he wasn't up to physical therapy. She just said, "Okay, we'll check back later." An hour later, they called a code. I looked at his chart and everything. There was nothing to predict that. How did she know?

Physical therapists practice with a tacit knowledge not found in books and rarely described in the literature. Consider how this knowledge is conveyed to students.

The bridge between theory and practice is not a one-way street. Students often co-participate in practice and generate questions based on their experiences. These questions lead them back to the literature for increased knowledge and deeper understanding. Clinical education is all about transforming and putting knowledge to use. The role of the CI is to scaffold student performance to greater sophistication. Consider the learning experience Moriam describes:

MORIAM: I evaluated my first patient yesterday. I had done parts of several exams with my CI, but this was the first in which I was responsible for the whole thing. My CI made suggestions, and I implemented them as I went along. It went pretty well. The patient will be back tomorrow, and I'm anxious to see how he's doing. After I finished the note (with revisions), I thought I was done. But my CI asked me to go home and compare what I had done with the *Guide to Physical Therapist Practice*. We'd used it at school, but I never thought about using it here in the clinic. Anyway, I had to find the practice pattern, and then I was surprised that it helped me think of things I hadn't thought of. With this CI, there's always more to learn. . . .

Moriam's CI challenged her to move beyond "good enough." By suggesting a framework for reflecting on her actions, the CI fostered what Mentkowski and Associates called "learning that lasts."[16]

Ability to Perform Effective Actions

Knowing is not enough. Students must learn to put their knowledge to work and, in doing so, practice and perform fundamental skills to enhance movement. Physical therapists examine, assess, evaluate, plan, and intervene. They palpate, stabilize, mobilize, facilitate, and inhibit. They teach, motivate, simplify, and modify. Skilled performance of these actions comes only with practice, development, and refinement. Rhonda, a second-year student, describes her struggle with learning palpation:

RHONDA: I know anatomy, and I got 100% on the functional anatomy practical. But here I'm only positive that I differentiate skin and bone. There're layers of soft tissue in between! I touch every patient that comes in, and I still don't think I'm always feeling what my CI feels.

Rhonda appears to be working hard to practice and develop her palpation skills. Consider what her CI's role is in helping her to perform effective actions.

Acculturation

Acculturation is the process by which a student is socialized into the profession of physical therapy. The socialization process is an account of how a new person is added to the group and becomes a member capable of meeting the traditional expectations of the profession. Physical therapy is a service-oriented profession. Clinical education occurs in settings where patients come to receive care. Patients are not exhibits who give time and money to come to a clinic to provide an example of a diagnosis for a student. They are real people with movement dysfunctions that limit their ability to live their lives the way they would choose. Students must learn what it means to provide service.

The majority of students use their own lives as the primary example for the way others live and may assume that their own beliefs, values, and socioeconomic status are those of the people whom they serve. Consider Cindy's comment. She is a 21-year-old student from a Midwestern farming community. She has been assigned to the liver transplant service of a metropolitan teaching hospital on the East Coast.

CINDY: Can you believe it? We are waiting to discharge this woman until her maid flies in from the Middle East. Her husband is too lazy to help her at the family house. I can't believe it. She doesn't even need that much help anymore.

Cindy's narrow norms of culture indicate a need for learning. Consider suggestions you could give her CI that would help Cindy enlarge her view.

Although most students have experienced physical therapy as a patient or have a friend or relative that has, they often fail to realize the broad scope of physical therapy practice, even after class work. Difficulties in learning within this very broad context of practice may not be evident until the clinical education experience. For example, consider the challenge Joe faced as you read about his experience, beginning with a phone call from his CI to the DCE in the third week of an 8-week affiliation on a trauma unit:

CLINICAL INSTRUCTOR: I'm sorry to bother you, but Joe's not back from lunch. I probably should have called about everything earlier, but things just kept getting worse slowly. Now I've had it! I don't even know where to begin. He's late all the time. He doesn't seem interested. I just can't engage him. It's almost as if he's avoiding the patients. He's smart enough and has good ideas about what to do, but I just can't get him to do anything. Sometimes up on the unit he just disappears. It's like he's hiding from me.

Joe's behavior was atypical in relation to his academic performance and previous clinical education experiences. During an on-site conference with the DCE the next morning, when Joe was asked how the affiliation was progressing, he focused exclusively on Jeff, a 24-year-old patient with a traumatic brain injury at Rancho Level I who had been injured in a motor vehicle accident when he was thrown from his car. He shared that Jeff's parents, siblings, and girlfriend were devastated, and Joe kept repeating, "Jeff is never going to be the same." As the conversation progressed, the DCE commented that Joe's CI had expressed her concern that Joe might be avoiding her. "What are you hiding from?" the DCE asked. He very honestly answered, "Life."

Experienced physical therapists may forget their initial reactions to the complexities of specialized practice settings, such as the trauma unit, skilled nursing facility, preschool program for children with developmental disabilities, athletic training room, neonatal intensive care unit, and hospice. Consider techniques a CI can use to explore personal feelings and reactions to difficult issues within professional practice and whether it is possible to validate a student's feelings while the student develops the ability to practice professionally in the challenging and sometimes overwhelming context of practice.

Critical Analysis of Clinical Competence

Accurate self-assessment is a critical ability for professional practice. Students acquire expectations about their own abilities from several sources. Successful experiences provide a foundation on which to build from observing role models or receiving verbal feedback provided by a clinical teacher or a patient.[17] Consider how a CI contributes to a student's ability to accurately self-assess performance and judge the outcome of professional actions, and how a student learns to evaluate his or her capabilities compared with entry-level competence or the performance of an expert clinician.[18]

Outcomes of the Clinical Learning Process

The academic program formally defines the expected outcome for any clinical education experience. Ultimately, however, the goal of clinical learning is for the student to progress from other-assisted to self-assisted learning while developing patterns of learning that form the basis for a lifelong, reflective practice.[19,20]

Other-Assisted to Self-Assisted Learning

When students begin the clinical education process, their learning is directed by the academic faculty, CIs, and physical therapist role models. As they progress through their clinical learning experiences, however, each student assumes more responsibility for her or his learning. Selected statements from students at various stages in an academic program demonstrate this progress:

CLAUDIA: I wanted to show you this schedule that I received from my clinical site. Each of the 4 weeks has particular things I'm going to focus on. During the first week, I get an in-service on "overview of patient examination" and by the end, I'll do all of the peripheral joints.

Compare the assistance Claudia accepts from others with the initiative in self-assisted learning that Brad demonstrates:

BRAD: I kept thinking about this patient and his problem. I just had to devise a way to gain more mobility. I came up with a mobilization we hadn't learned in class and one that probably wouldn't even be possible on a normal elbow. I had the patient sit on a stool next to the treatment table and place his forearm on the table. I stood next to him and palpated for the displaced radial head. Then, I placed my thumbs on the head and directed a force caudally. At the beginning of treatment, only minimal displacement was possible. By the end, I believe 4 or 5 millimeters might have been possible. It was very interesting to think about this problem and satisfying to come up with a unique solution. I felt very good about being successful with it.

Consider how a CI interacts with each of these students to enable them to progress in self-assisted learning, and how the teacher knows when students are ready to assume more responsibility for their learning.

Lifelong, Reflective Practice

Lifelong, reflective practice is a hallmark of professional behavior. With so much to learn in the brief periods of clinical education, how does a student begin this endeavor? Students are often required to keep a journal or may be asked to present a case report as an in-service educational program during their clinical experiences. In addition to ongoing conversations with their CIs, these reflective activities encourage students to think about and question their actions. But these activities end at the conclusion of the clinical experience. Consider what might guarantee that the reflective process becomes lifelong, and what responsibility the clinical teacher assumes for this during the clinical education experience. One tool that is being used across disciplines is the portfolio.

The development of a portfolio offers an opportunity for students to reflect on their learning and professional development. By gathering and sorting examples of their professional work, defining moments of success and failure, and reflecting on the evidence they have presented, students are placed in a position of authority to assess and validate their personal development as professionals.[21] Portfolios should be structured and coached by the CI, academic faculty, or both for the purpose of guidance and feedback. They are often organized thematically. For example, a student might provide evidence of entry-level competence in the components of patient management. Beyond the selection of good examples of clinical work, the student must reflect on the content. If the student presented evidence of a patient examination, the student might ask herself or himself, "What is entry-level competence when performing this patient examination? What components are present or absent? How does my work differ from expert practice?"[18] By placing emphasis on judgment and meaning making, the student is encouraged to investigate her or his own learning experience. Consider Mark's example:

MARK: I needed to provide evidence that I could demonstrate mastery of entry-level professional clinical skills based on physical therapy examination, evaluation, diagnosis, prognosis, intervention, and appropriate health care use. I wrote a case study on a patient and included the literature I had used when I worked with the patient. I compared my patient care with the *Guide to Physical Therapist Practice*.[22] Then my CI and I discussed what I had discovered and the ideas I had to improve. He was especially helpful in prioritizing parts of the practice pattern to meet my patient's needs.

Writing the case study and comparing his practice to the *Guide* allowed Mark to reflect on his actions. His CI provided a further opportunity for learning by reflecting with Mark and offering his clinical wisdom. By including this example in his portfolio, Mark has provided evidence of his learning process, as well as created an opportunity for further reflection and learning in the future. The portfolio provides a vehicle for students to record and celebrate their professional growth and offers many opportunities for thoughtful deliberation and discourse. In addition, a portfolio may provide the student with a basis for planning in the crucial transition from student to new graduate.

Roles of the Clinical Teacher: Diagnosing Readiness, Planning, Teaching, and Evaluating

Good clinical teachers enable student learning. They begin by inviting students to participate in the community of physical therapy practice and, then they plan, model, coach, question, encourage, instruct, supervise, and evaluate to optimize the learning experience. Table 7-4 highlights specific enabling acts used by good teachers. These are incorporated throughout this discussion.

Scully describes the role of the clinical teacher as "pacing the student to professional competency," which involves diagnosis of readiness, selection of clinical problems, supervision, and evaluation.[2] These categories, although not exhaustive or exclusive, provide a useful framework for considering the functions of the clinical teacher.

Diagnosis of Student Readiness

Traditionally, the clinical teacher has limited knowledge of a specific student's background before the student's arrival. It is incumbent on the academic institution to provide information about the educational program and the didactic curriculum for review. The clinical teacher needs to gain an understanding of the school's mission and the goals and objectives of the academic program because these frame the context in which the curriculum is presented. A list of completed classes and course descriptions provide the content to which a student has been exposed and suggest curricular themes around which the academic faculty have chosen to instruct. Recalling previous clinical education experiences of students from a particular program at your clinical practice may also be helpful.

Knowing the student's academic preparation to date, however, provides little information about the implicit curriculum, the personal context in

Table 7-4   Thirty-Five Enabling Acts for Clinical Teachers

---

1. Invite students to participate in a community of practice where good work has been done by former students.
2. Demonstrate the power truth telling exerts on learning.
3. Get students doing good work that counts for them and their patients.
4. Along with the students, start good work of your own.
5. Begin to know your students as people rather than as students.
6. Make it clear that you believe in the students' abilities to work at high levels of excellence.
7. Sit on the same physical level as your students when conversing with them, and speak in simple, clear language. Expect that they will do the same.
8. Avoid didactic monologues. Don't expect a given answer in discussions.
9. Encourage dialogues between the experiences and ideas of students and the experiences and ideas of experts.
10. Work from experience into theory and vice versa.
11. Move students from success to success, yet prepare them to accept occasional failure.
12. Help students view mistakes as opportunities.
13. Exercise imagination.
14. Capitalize on storytelling.
15. Provide opportunities for responsible decision making.
16. Enable students to think about learning as "finding" in addition to "receiving."
17. Enable understanding of the "whole" instead of "bits and pieces."
18. Become vulnerable to students by sharing feelings with them about the good work you are doing with and alongside them.
19. Arrange that students see, do, and remember in the context of practice.
20. Encourage humor and spontaneity.
21. Plan so that no learning experience is useless.
22. Enable students to own the knowledge, skills, and values of professional practice.
23. Cultivate rigor and joy in practice.
24. Help students refine their uses of emotion.
25. Make practice an act with meaning—always.
26. Avoid badgering and cruelty.
27. Avoid excessive praise of students' works.
28. Test the work of the student against work in the world outside.
29. Find ways of making public the good works of the students.
30. Show students that working habits taken on in the clinic will prove valuable in the future.
31. Provide evaluations of students' work when the evaluation least interferes with learning.
32. Give students ample time to complete their work.
33. Help students polish and refine work as they bring it to completion.
34. Sense the moments for letting go of students.
35. Never deny students their lives.

Source: Adapted from K Macrorie. 20 Teachers. New York: Oxford University Press, 1984.

which knowledge, skills, and values were learned and developed, or the clinical competency the student is able to demonstrate. Consider the cases of Natalie and Beth, classmates who are in the second week of their first clinical learning experience:

NATALIE'S CLINICAL INSTRUCTOR: Natalie has progressed much more quickly than most students during a first affiliation. Her 3 years of work as a physical therapist assistant are evident in her interaction with patients and other members of the health care team, as well as her fundamental handling skills. She observed me the first day, and then we began coevaluating and cotreating on day 2. We still work together, but she has assumed more and more responsibility for the patient. She is working hard to take our findings from the examination, make clinical judgments, and then work with the patient to set functional goals and think of creative ways to meet those goals. Because she's competent in so many of the "pieces," she's been able to focus on higher-level objectives.

BETH'S CLINICAL INSTRUCTOR: Beth was tentative the first week, and I felt I needed to push her to get involved. She was very apprehensive. She did say that this was really her first experience working with patients. They're never quite like your lab partner! She's doing well, though. After several days of observing, we're working with the patients together. She's participating in aspects of examination and intervention. This morning, for example, she re-evaluated the range of motion of a young man we're seeing following multiple fractures received in a motorcycle accident. She had planned a routine to minimize the need for the patient to change positions and practiced on her roommate last night. She's also going to be responsible for the subjective exam with an outpatient coming in today for the first time after a total knee replacement.

Life experiences, particularly those in health care, can alter a student's starting point in the clinic. Other, less definitive, factors can affect fundamental skills in communication, management, teaching, and a host of components of professional practice. Information specific to each student is essential to accurately diagnose readiness for learning experiences.

Pre-Experience Planning for the Clinical Education Experience

Preparation for the clinical education experience is a key component that begins after a student is assigned to a CI. The CI should introduce herself or himself and begin to exchange information as soon as possible. The time and energy spent in this process allow the clinical teacher and the student to reap rich rewards during the experience. The instructor

Dear Student's First Name,

I was delighted to learn that you will be affiliating at ABCD Medical Center, in City, State. My name is Susannah Perez, and I will be your clinical instructor for the 12 weeks you are with us. I have been at ABCD Medical Center for 2 years; before that I worked for a private outpatient PT practice here in the city. My primary responsibilities include patient care at a Satellite clinic 4 miles west of the Medical Center where we see patients with a wide range of neuromusculoskeletal problems and management related to outpatient rehab services at all of our sites. I also see patients in Osteoporosis Clinic at the center one afternoon per week. My working hours are 7:00 a.m. to 3:30 p.m. I do work one weekend at the center every 6–8 weeks and that's an opportunity you may want to consider.

This is an exciting time at the Medical Center. We recently consolidated with several other health care facilities and are in the process of restructuring the management of physical therapy services at all the sites. Although change can be a bit disconcerting at times, I think this will be a wonderful opportunity to experience first hand what changes in the health care delivery really mean! In addition, we'll work as a team with a physical therapist assistant, Ken, and another student who will be joining us for the last 6 weeks of your affiliation.

I enjoyed working with a student from your University 2 years ago and I'm anxious to learn about any changes that have taken place since then. From looking at your curriculum, I know that you've had three short-term affiliations during your academic preparation and this is your first of three, 12-week affiliations prior to graduation. I'm enclosing a copy of our updated Clinical Center Information Form, a copy of brochures about the Medical Center and the city, and a list of additional clinical learning opportunities for students at our facility. I hope these will begin to answer some of the questions you may have and help you prepare for this affiliation.

I want to involve you in planning this experience so we can work together to meet your needs as well as the goals and objectives of your academic program. After you've had an opportunity to review the enclosed materials, please write down your goals and objectives for this experience. Please send them to me at least 2 weeks before you arrive. We'll devote 2 hours of your first morning to orientation, discussion, and planning for the 12 weeks, and getting you off to a good start.

In the meantime, if you have any questions or need additional information, please let me know. I can be reached at 123-456-7890. If I'm not available, please leave a message on my voicemail and a telephone number where I can reach you. If it's better to call you at home during the evening, just let me know. I look forward to meeting you in person!

Sincerely,
Susannah Perez, PT, DPT, OCS

Figure 7-3 Sample letter of welcome from a clinical instructor.

should communicate directly with the student. This can be done in person, by telephone, by mail, or by e-mail. See Figure 7-3 for a sample letter welcoming a student. This letter contains key elements important to any type of initial contact. It does the following:

- Welcomes
- Introduces the clinical teacher and facility

- Demonstrates *truth telling*, or telling the truth in a candid, forthright, honest, frank, and open manner
- Conveys expectations
- Encourages student's active participation

The combination of information provided and requested allows the student and clinical teacher to begin thinking and planning.

Student Orientation to the Clinical Setting and the Clinical Education Program

The first day of any new experience can be overwhelming. A well-planned orientation session can handle administrative details, introduce the student to key members of the health care delivery team, and provide pragmatic information that the student needs. The fact that, for example, the hand-held dynamometers in the clinic are in the third drawer to the left of the hydrocollator packs between examination rooms three and four is probably not essential. These three questions may guide your planning: What does the student need to know before beginning to learn in the context of patient care? What can wait until later? What is best learned along the way?

Orientation is the time for the CI to begin assessing the student by verbal exchange. What can the student tell about herself or himself? Encourage the students to talk about physical therapy, and listen to what physical therapy means to them. Share experiences and describe your expectations and standards. If you are able to share less-than-perfect performances and what you learned from them, you give the student permission to take risks, make mistakes, and learn from them. Review the student's goals and objectives. They may not be realistic at this point, at your facility, or for a variety of reasons. Help students determine what they really want from this experience. Determine whether students' revised goals and objectives can be measured with the evaluation instrument required by the academic program. Review clinical education materials that the student may have from the academic program, and determine whether there are additional assignments for the student to complete.

Orientation is also the time to begin joint planning. Include in this planning expectations for yourself and the student. The verbal exchange and planning that occur during orientation set the tone for conversations and learning activities that continue throughout the clinical experience. It is essential for the instructor to convey the importance of open truth telling and create an environment that encourages it.

Student Self-Assessment versus Demonstrated Abilities

Self-insight and the ability to self-assess are skills based on knowledge and values. The student's self-assessment and the accuracy of that assessment are important components of the diagnosis of readiness. It is critical to evaluate whether a student's self-assessment matches the student's demonstrated abilities. The first days of any experience allow the instructor to assess the student's abilities. Ask yourself, "Is the information that has been shared congruent with what I'm seeing?"

Performance testing is an ongoing piece of clinical teaching that must be done in a manner that allows the student to focus on learning and development, rather than the adequacy of performance. Thad's CI did it in the following way:

THAD: At first, we talked about the patient before he came. If the patient had a preliminary diagnosis, I told Cassie, my CI, what I knew, and we figured out what I didn't know. Sometimes Cassie didn't know either, and then we looked it up. And then we planned where I'd start. I thought you started with the history, but you really start by watching the patient walk back from the waiting room. She helped me plan the history based on what we knew from the referral. I'd go in to the examination room with the patient and take the history. Cassie would knock and come in later, and I'd tell her what I knew, and we'd get the patient to chime in. Sometimes, Cassie asked questions if she didn't understand. That helped remind me of important things I might have forgotten to ask. Then it was up to me to tell the patient what I was going to do in the examination and do it. Cassie might say something like, "You might want to check _____ to see if _____," which would clue me in. Then I'd do it, and Cassie would help if I got stuck or seemed to be headed in the wrong way. It's hard to explain, but it's like the three of us are all working together to figure out the best way for the patient to get better. Now I do more on my own. I know Cassie won't let me really mess up, but I also know that I'm the one in charge, and she's not going to let me off the hook. I'm starting to feel like a real physical therapist!

Cassie is able to determine Thad's performance capabilities by working and conversing with him over the patient right in the context of practice. She uses questioning to assist in assessing the congruency between self-assessment and demonstrated abilities. Abrams[23] describes four types of questions: (1) knowledge questions, (2) translation questions, (3) excogitative questions, and (4) evaluation questions. Each can be an effective tool to gain understanding of the student's abilities, as well as an effective teaching tool. See Table 7-5 for a brief description of each type of question.

1. *Knowledge questions* are directed to guide the student to recall facts or principles. This information may have been learned in a classroom lec-

Table 7-5   Questions to Enhance Clinical Learning

Types of questions	Purpose
Knowledge	Recall facts or principles
Translation	Demonstrate understanding of knowledge
Excogitative	Challenge problem-solving and clinical decision-making skills
Evaluation	Require the student to make judgments about the value of ideas, solutions, and methods

Source: Adapted from RG Abrams. Questioning in preclinical and clinical instruction. J Dent Educ 1983;47:599.

ture, a text, or a previous clinical education experience. Never presume that a student has the prerequisite knowledge needed to examine or treat a patient with a particular disease, impairment, or disability, particularly during early clinical education experiences. Knowledge questions provide the clinical teacher with an understanding of the gaps in the essential knowledge of the student, confusions the student may have (i.e., the student has ideas that are fuzzy or not clearly differentiated), or errors in the student's perceptions. These questions should not be viewed as a test or an examination, but as a tool to aid in diagnosing a student's readiness for a particular learning experience. Knowledge questions need to be asked in a manner that encourages verbal exchange and provides the student with an opportunity to support and reinforce basic information or correct misconceptions. The following are examples of knowledge questions:

- Why does maintaining a moist wound bed facilitate re-epithelialization? (This question may lead to a discussion of wound dressings, their application, and the choice of dressing that a therapist might recommend for the patient being treated.)
- What motions are contraindicated for this patient immediately after a total hip replacement? (This question may serve to cue the student as he or she proceeds to the functional application of knowledge and begins to transfer the patient from a wheelchair to a mat table.)

2. *Translation questions* require a student to demonstrate understanding of knowledge. They may require the student to perform a simple transformation (e.g., translating medical terminology to lay language for patient and family education) or to interpret the functional meaning of a laboratory test (e.g., the effect a low hematocrit may have on endurance). True learning in the clinical setting may not occur until the learner becomes the teacher—

that is, until the student is able to translate her or his knowledge for a patient, a peer, the CI, or another health care practitioner. Translation questions enable the student to use knowledge. The following are examples of translation questions:

- How would you explain ultrasound to a 72-year-old patient? (This question provides an opportunity for the student to practice translating her or his classroom and laboratory knowledge into clear, concise, and understandable terms for a patient.)
- After observing the total knee arthroplasty in the operating room yesterday, what functional limitations might you expect this patient to have? (This question directs the student to consider the physical therapy meaning of a supplemental learning experience. The passive experience of observing a surgical procedure becomes active as the student is required to make meaning of it.)

3. *Excogitative questions* challenge the student's problem-solving and clinical decision-making abilities. They require a student to reorganize knowledge, apply principles, and predict outcomes. These questions may be especially appropriate after a student has taken the patient's history and performed the objective examination. They may guide the development of goals as well as the treatment plan. The following are examples of excogitative questions:

- What is the patient's functional limitation? Based on your findings, what can you recommend to this patient? (These questions require that the student think about function related to the impairments found on examination. The student must then decide what can be done to improve function.)

4. *Evaluation questions* "use all of the previous thought processes to judge the value of ideas, solutions, methods, or materials."[23] The process of self-assessment is a critical component of the lifelong learning process. Phrased properly, evaluation questions reinforce self-assisted learning and encourage critical analysis. The following are examples of evaluative questions:

- What criteria do you use to determine whether the patient is independent in transfers?
- How do you determine whether the patient is ready to return to work?
- After working with this patient for a week, how successful do you think the rehabilitation program will be? (These questions, used within the context of patient examination, evaluation, and intervention, can enable a clinical teacher to gain a better understanding of what a student knows, what the student is doing, and why it is being done.)

Ongoing Reevaluation of Student Performance

Thad's depiction of his clinical learning experience, presented above, describes the opportunity his CI created for reevaluating his performance on an ongoing basis. The context of patient care provides a unique environment in which the CI can evaluate student performance and teach, monitor and reinforce, and question and answer almost simultaneously. Ongoing reevaluation is critical to ensure that selection of clinical learning experiences matches the student's readiness.

A note of caution: Accurate diagnosis of readiness can be a challenging endeavor. Just as in physical therapy patient care, assessment does not always lead to an accurate diagnosis. Consider the case of Daneen, a student in her first clinical experience, as she evaluated José, a 22-year-old man who was referred with shoulder pain:

DANEEN: José, I'm going to do your upper quarter screen. This is to rule out any problems with your cervical region, elbow, wrist, and hand so we can concentrate on your shoulder. Good. Now abduct your shoulder. That means bringing it out like this. That's to test your deltoid. It's innervated by the axillary nerve. That's C-5. Don't let me push it down. Good. Now I want you to . . .

Daneen's CI is concerned about her ability to provide patient education at an appropriate level for her patient. It could be argued that Daneen is not providing patient education at all. Rather, she is self-talking aloud. She is performing examination techniques that she has not mastered, and she needs to talk herself through the procedure, explaining to herself what she is doing and why. She has not yet reached a competency level that allows her to demonstrate proficiency in the skill while instructing the patient with appropriate patient-oriented language. An accurate diagnosis of readiness would lead the CI, in this case, to allow Daneen to practice the techniques until they were automatic; then, she would be able to orient her focus to the patient rather than use a scripted performance. Daneen needs to be able to perform an upper quarter screen without thinking about each step. This allows her to listen and talk with the patient.

Selection of Clinical Problems

Clinical learning experiences or problems need to be selected based on the potential they provide for useful learning. The CI may be able to choose between patients, but this may not be possible in the real world of practice. More than likely, the CI needs to identify learning opportunities within the context of practice that day or even at that moment.

General guidelines for the selection of clinical learning experiences must acknowledge that students need to learn routines and standards before they develop creative alternatives. Students are searching for a right way to think and perform, and their tolerance for ambiguity, unexpected events, or variation is relatively low. Once confidence develops, students can discern when routine approaches fit and when they do not. Routines are rare when comparing patients, but there may be many similarities when considering "pieces" of physical therapy examination or intervention. For example, you may want to have the student work with patients with similar diagnoses to establish confidence in procedural reasoning and technical skills. Repeated actions over time enable students to look for patterns, develop hypotheses, and learn to respond to the unexpected. Once the pattern of learning is established, challenge the known and dare the student to stretch beyond his or her comfort zone.

Consider the following example: Mary has worked with Joe for the first 2 days of his first full-time experience after completion of the didactic curriculum in his educational program. So far he has been observing. He seems comfortable conversing with patients, asks appropriate questions, and demonstrates adequate fundamental handling skills when he participates in cotreating. Mary suggests the following:

MARY: Joe, you observed me evaluate Sam Jones, Dr. Stevenson's patient, who was 1-day post-op [postoperative] ACL [anterior cruciate ligament] reconstruction. It looks like Diane Reeves, a new patient coming in at 1:00 this afternoon, may have a similar diagnosis. I'd like you to see her. I'll be there if you have questions or need assistance, but I'd like you to take the lead. Why don't you take the next 20 minutes and outline how you would proceed? We can discuss your plans at 12:30, and then you'll be ready to go.

Mary selected this learning opportunity to extend Joe's experience from the previous day, when he had observed an examination of a patient with a similar diagnosis. This time, however, Mary can evaluate Joe's ability to plan the examination and his skill in performing it. By discussing his plans and participating in a supporting role during the examination, she can monitor his actions, protect the patient (if necessary), and instruct throughout the process as needed.

A student with more advanced knowledge and skills may be asked to focus on a different learning experience with the same patient, as in the following example:

CLINICAL INSTRUCTOR: I know that you've been working with several patients who have had ACL reconstructions. What would you think about treating them at the same time in more of a group approach? The staff has discussed this off and on. After an initial evaluation and setting up patients' treatment programs, could a group of five or six be scheduled at the same time? Are there activities they could do as a group? What effect would this have on outcomes? Could you help in developing a proposal for the staff meeting next month, considering this with factors such as time, cost, and outcome? Denise, our director, has gathered the data we have that might be relevant and suggested meeting with you tomorrow to share her ideas and begin discussing this project with you. Your knowledge and skills in working with patients with this diagnosis are good, beyond entry level, and I think you're ready to view the delivery of physical therapy service in a broader scope.

The selection of clinical problems and learning experiences progresses throughout the clinical experience with consideration of the student's readiness, types of patients, numbers of patients, and level of student responsibility. Choose clinical problems to challenge the student to learn. It is not so much a choice of patients, but what you choose to have the student do with them in the context of patient-centered service. Students should progress from self-centered to patient-centered learning in preparation for real-world practice. Specific clinical learning experiences are site dependent but should build on past experiences. *Clinical education is not intended to be a sampler in which each diagnosis is seen once and each technique is tried. There is no evidence that variety makes a better practitioner.* If a student can problem solve with a new patient of an unknown diagnosis and learn to improve the patient's function, the student should be able to use these problem-solving tools and generalize from one case to the next with increasing skill.

Supervision of Student Performance

Supervision includes monitoring a student's performances, providing supportive guidance, and directing instruction. Refer again to Thad's description of his learning experience presented earlier. Cassie, Thad's CI, works alongside Thad and observes his performance on an ongoing basis. However, at a more advanced level, ongoing, direct observation may be less frequent, with information derived from written documentation or even patient outcomes. Most important, Cassie conveys to Thad her strong belief in his present and future clinical capabilities.

While providing supportive guidance to students, a clinical teacher must also provide targeted instruction. In the beginning of this chapter, Jeff's CI describes the instruction she provides to him. Her teaching is not focused and is perceived as a didactic monologue that got in the way of Jeff's learning. It is important to move beyond the book knowledge and laboratory skills a student brings to the clinic, but it is essential to listen to the student and teach in response to the student's questions—when asked or when you think the student should be asking. It is important to teach over the patient and enable the student to build the bridge between theory and practice. Make your reasoning process explicit while providing a safe environment for the student to develop an understanding of her or his own reasoning process while working with you. Students should be encouraged to question their own practice, and they should be given permission to question the instructor's. The instructor should teach students to take effective actions.

Good clinical teachers do not have to know everything. One hopes that the student generates questions that the instructor can't answer. A vital component of clinical education is learning where to find those answers. The instructor should model and teach the student to use the resources available by looking in references, asking another therapist, asking the patient, or asking other health care practitioners.

Experienced clinical teachers admit that the most difficult part of working with students is giving up their own patients. Physical therapists value the relationships they develop with their patients and take pride in their ability to help them. Giving up ownership of that responsibility isn't easy for the therapist. Likewise, it is difficult to give up control of the student as the student moves from other-assisted to self-assisted learning. Supervision should focus on encouraging independence and professional initiative in the broadest sense of patient care while minimizing risk to the patient and student.

Evaluation of Student Performance

The purpose of evaluation is to measure performance, enhance attainment of goals, and minimize risk to patients. Evaluation begins in the pre-experience planning phase and continues throughout the clinical learning experience, concluding with a summative evaluation at the end of the experience. This summative evaluation incorporates multiple sources of information to make the decision about the student's readiness to practice by assessing the student's cognitive, psychomotor, and affective behaviors.[24] The evaluation is used by the academic institution to determine the success or failure of the student's clinical performance. Specific information and training regarding the use of the evaluation instrument used by a particular academic program are provided by the program. Summative evaluations are necessary to minimize risk to the consumer and determine entry-level competence. For the student, they represent an evaluation of his or her capabilities at a given moment and provide the opportunity for the clinical teacher to give input regarding the next phase of education or learning. Most important, they should encompass an element of self-assessment. Physical therapists occupy the role of clinical teachers and evaluators for only a brief period of time. It is imperative that the student learns to accurately self-assess his or her capabilities and areas that need improvement.

Formative evaluations need to occur throughout the learning experience as a continuous part of clinical teaching. Assess, with the student, where she or he is and where he or she is going. Students need to understand that clinical education is a learning experience. Yes, the student is expected to perform. But based on this performance, clinical problems are selected to provide opportunities for teaching and learning to enable the student to progress to competent professional practice. This is synonymous with the ongoing reevaluation that occurs as a part of diagnosing a student's readiness.

Students often need assistance in distinguishing between their performance and their feelings about that performance. A student who lacks confidence may feel uncertain and judge his or her competencies to be lower than those observed by the clinical teacher. Another student, feeling satisfied with a patient's progress, might fail to consider aspects of his or her intervention in which improvement is needed. It is helpful for teachers to reflect on their own performance out loud. This includes acknowledgment of their limitations in knowledge and skill and errors in judgment, as well as their abilities to rethink and plan for improvement. Modeling is an effective teaching technique to encourage students to develop skill in accurate self-assessment. Students are able to self-assess based on their experiences. These experiences need to be designed to prepare them to self-assess objectively in the context of entry-level professional practice.

CIs rarely fail to identify significant problems that place a student at risk for not successfully completing a clinical education experience. Timing, however, is a key factor. If the instructor has concerns or suspects difficulty, it should be addressed immediately with the student. If the instructor is unable to resolve the problem, she or he should seek advice from the Center Coordinator of Clinical Education or the student's DCE. These are appropriate people from whom to seek information. Questions or concerns are best addressed before they become problems. Clinical educators at all levels are involved in the process of learning to provide better clinical education.

Often, a student is progressing satisfactorily, and then learning plateaus or stalls. In such a case, the instructor must give the student a jump start. If the student has been able to accomplish the program's goals and objectives and his or her personal goals, or is progressing toward that end, can the goals be extended or new goals set that move beyond entry-level competence to mastery? It is important for students to learn that professional development includes ongoing self-assessment and reevaluation, followed by defining new goals targeted at enhancing knowledge and skills. Learning is a lifelong process that continues throughout clinical practice.

Conclusion

This chapter attempts to deal simply with a complex subject. The answers to questions about clinical teaching are dependent on the context in which they are asked. Teaching techniques used by one CI must be molded and modified before they can be applied in another situation. Each topic addressed suggests many more questions. It is my hope that as we continue to plan, develop, and deliver clinical learning experiences that enable the transition from student to practitioner, the desires of physical therapists to continue learning will be reflected in self-directed efforts to know, understand, and become more able and skilled in the clinical education process.

References

1. Callahan M, Decker R, Hirt S, Tappan F. Physical Therapy Education Theory and Practice. New York: Council of Physical Therapy School Directors, 1968;35.
2. Scully RM. Clinical Teaching of Physical Therapy Students in Clinical Education [Ph.D. dissertation]. Columbia University, 1974.
3. Skinner BF. About Behaviorism. New York: Knopf, 1974.
4. Bruner JS. Beyond Information Given: Studies in the Psychology of Knowing. New York: Norton, 1973.
5. Guba EG, Lincoln YS. Fourth Generation Evaluation. Newbury Park, CA: Sage, 1989.
6. Poplin MS. Holistic/constructivist principles of the teaching/learning process: implications for the field of learning disabilities. J Learn Disab 1988:21:93.
7. Vygotsky LS. Mind in Society. Cambridge, MA: Harvard University Press, 1978.
8. Lave J, Wenger E. Situated Learning: Legitimate Peripheral Participation. New York: Cambridge University Press, 1991.
9. Van Langenberghe HVK. Evaluation of students' approaches to studying in a problem-based physical therapy curriculum. Phys Ther 1988;68:522.
10. Graham CL. Conceptual learning processes in physical therapy students. Phys Ther 1996;76:856.
11. Ladyshewsky RK, Barrie SC, Drake VM. A comparison of productivity and learning outcome in individual and cooperative physical therapy clinical education models. Phys Ther 1998;78:1288.

12. Solomon PE, Binkley J, Stratford PW. A descriptive study of learning processes and outcomes in two problem-based curriculum designs. J Phys Ther Educ 1996:10(2):72.

13. Hayward LM, Cairns MA. Physical therapist students' perceptions of and strategic approaches to case-based instruction: suggestions for curriculum design. J Phys Ther Educ 1998;12(2):33.

14. Ladyshewsky RK. Peer-assisted learning in clinical education: a review of terms and learning principles. J Phys Ther Educ 2000;14(2):15.

15. Dewey J. Democracy and Education. New York: Macmillan, 1916;38.

16. Mentkowski M and Associates. Learning That Lasts: Integrating Learning, Development, and Performance in College and Beyond. San Francisco: Jossey-Bass, 2000.

17. Gagne RM, Driscoll MP. Essentials of Learning for Instruction. Englewood Cliffs, NJ: Prentice Hall, 1988.

18. Jensen GM, Gwyer J, Hack LM, et al. Expertise in Physical Therapy Practice. Boston: Butterworth–Heinemann, 1999.

19. Schön DA. The Reflective Practitioner: How Professionals Think in Action. New York: Basic Books, 1983.

20. Jensen GM, Paschal KA. Habits of mind: student transition toward virtuous practice. J Phys Ther Educ 2000;14(3):42.

21. Lyons N (ed). With Portfolio in Hand: Validating the New Teacher Professionalism. New York: Teachers College, 1998.

22. American Physical Therapy Association. Guide to Physical Therapist Practice (2nd ed). Phys Ther 2001;81:9.

23. Abrams RG. Questioning in preclinical and clinical instruction. J Dent Educ 1983;47:599.

24. American Physical Therapy Association. Physical Therapist Student Clinical Performance Instrument. Alexandria, VA: American Physical Therapy Association, 1997.

Annotated Bibliography

Brown LT, Collins A, Duguid P. Situated cognition and the culture of learning. Educ Res 1989;18:32. The authors describe knowledge as resulting from complex, social interactions of the activity, context, and culture in which it is developed. This work is consistent with constructivist learning theory and emphasizes the socially constructed nature of knowledge.

Graham CL. Conceptual learning processes in physical therapy students. Phys Ther 1996;76:856. This author investigated processes used by physical therapy students in developing conceptual knowledge in physical therapy. Graham describes a model of conceptual development that depicts conceptual learning as an active, evolving process that is applicable to the clinical learning situation.

Jensen GM, Gwyer J, Hack LM, Shepard KF. Expertise in Physical Therapy Practice. Boston: Butterworth–Heinemann, 1999. Based on observations and interviews with expert therapists, the authors describe a model of expertise in physical therapy practice and discuss how expert practitioners develop, think, reason, make decisions, and perform in practice. An excellent resource to compare with established performance behaviors expected for entry-level competence.

Lave J, Wenger E. Situated Learning: Legitimate Peripheral Participation. New York: Cambridge University Press, 1991. Lave and Wenger locate learning in the processes of coparticipation and explore how practice grounds learning. They describe cases of Yucatec midwives, Vai and Gola tailors, naval quartermasters, meat cutters, and nondrinking alcoholics in which the learner participates in the actual practice of an expert to a limited degree and with limited responsibility for the product as a whole. This text is highly recommended to broaden the reader's perspective on situated learning beyond the realm of health care.

Lyons N (ed). With Portfolio in Hand: Validating the New Teacher Professionalism. New York: Teachers College, 1998. This book provides a rich description of the possibilities, potentials, and problems of portfolios in the practice and assessment of teaching. Helpful information is presented to guide the preparation of useful portfolios.

Mentkowski M and Associates. Learning That Lasts: Integrating Learning, Development, and Performance in College and Beyond. San Francisco: Jossey-Bass, 2000. The authors define *learning that lasts* as the successful integration of learning, development, and performance. Based on work at Alverno College, this text proposes a theory of learning with practical strategies for teaching.

Scully RM, Shepard KF. Clinical teaching in physical therapy education. Phys Ther 1983;63:349. This ethnographic study examines the process of clinical education from the viewpoint of clinical teachers.

Watts NT. Handbook of Clinical Teaching. New York: Churchill Livingstone, 1990. Watts has contributed a practical handbook with sensible advice to enable clinical teachers to build bridges between the theory and practice of clinical teaching. Each chapter includes exercises and feedback that provide an opportunity for the reader to reflect on the information presented and begin to develop skill in application.

8

Teaching and Learning about Patient Education

Elizabeth Mostrom and Katherine F. Shepard

One of my patients was a 34-year-old woman with multiple sclerosis. This case affected me the most of any other cases so far. I was most affected by her family; what they were going through, how they were coping, and what they shared with me as her physical therapist.

First, her husband shared with me how her disease had progressed. He told me what his wife's functional capabilities were just a few years ago in comparison to what they are now. He shared with me how she had become more and more dependent on him. Before she would only need his assistance for functional activities; now he has to do everything for her.

Then I spoke to her grandmother. She gave me a different perspective on how her granddaughter's illness is affecting the family. She told me how her granddaughter's children were being affected. She told me how sad they had been since their mother went in to the hospital and that every night the youngest child sleeps in his mother's favorite chair, hugging her favorite pillow.

> As I listened to my patient's family, I realized that there is so much more to treating patients than simply treating their illness. As a physical therapist, I must also address the concerns of my patients' families as well as those of my patients. I need to comfort and reassure them when I am able. I need to teach them and give them advice and information from a physical therapy perspective. Most of all, however, I need to listen to them and show genuine concern for what they say and for what matters most to them—their family member, the patient.

The above excerpt from a student reflective journal written about experiences during a clinical internship illustrates some of the powerful lessons learned from patients, families, and clinical instructors (CIs) about the relational foundations of patient and caregiver education. Such experiences are rich resources for students learning about who and what they want to be as a clinician and patient educator—and who and what they don't want to be. In this chapter, we discuss opportunities and strategies for enhancing student learning about both the science and art of patient education in academic and clinical settings.

Chapter Objectives

After completing this chapter, the reader will be able to

1. Identify barriers and facilitators to student learning about patient education in academic and clinical settings.
2. Recognize and describe the role and importance of health belief systems and therapeutic alliances as essential to effective patient education.
3. Discuss how knowledge of cognitive learning theories, motor learning principles, and individual learning styles can enhance one's ability to teach patients and families.
4. Identify and incorporate five specific tips for creating effective home exercise programs (HEPs) for patients.
5. Describe and implement several teaching strategies that can link classroom instruction about patient education with experiential learning in clinical settings.
6. Identify and discuss the primary sources and content of learning about patient education for students during clinical experiences.
7. Describe, design, and implement instructional/learning activities that provide opportunities for dialogue and reflection about patient education during clinical experiences.

Centrality of Patient Education to Clinical Practice

As a large body of literature attests, the role of the physical therapist as a patient educator is central to everyday practice as a clinician.[1-8] Some investigators and the master therapists they studied have gone so far as to characterize therapy as a collaborative, educative endeavor with clinical encounters consisting largely of reciprocal teaching and learning between therapist and client.[9-13] There is little doubt that the effectiveness of therapy can most certainly hinge on the therapist's ability to establish therapeutic relationships with clients and his or her skill as a teacher.

In today's health care environment in which the frequency of patient encounters in therapy has been diminishing, the need for clinicians to be competent patient educators is even more essential. The importance of patient education has been underscored by the Joint Commission on Accreditation of Healthcare Organizations (JCAHO), which requires that inpatient facilities have a comprehensive multidisciplinary program for patient and family education.[14] The JCAHO accreditation manual states, "Education promotes healthy behaviors, supports recovery and a speedy return to function, and enables patients to be involved in decisions about their own care."[14(pPF-3)] The JCAHO standards for patient and family education are shown in Table 8-1. Think about which of these standards physical therapists and physical therapist assistants would be involved in implementing.

The importance of becoming a skilled patient educator for developing and practicing therapists is also reflected in many of the American Physical Therapy Association's core documents, such as the *Guide to Physical Therapy Practice*,[15] the *Normative Model of Physical Therapist Professional Education*,[16] the *Evaluative Criteria for Accreditation of Education Programs for the Preparation of Physical Therapists*,[17] and the *Clinical Performance Instrument*.[18] For example, in the *Guide to Physical Therapy Practice*,[15(p47)] one of the primary interventions carried out by physical therapists is identified as *patient/client related instruction* and is defined as follows:

> The process of informing, educating, or training patients/clients, families, significant others, and caregivers is intended to promote and optimize physical therapy services. Instruction may be related to the current condition; specific impairments, functional limitations, or disabilities; plan of care; need for enhanced performance; transition to a different role or setting;

Table 8-1   Joint Commission on Accreditation of Healthcare Organizations Standards for Patient and Family Education

Patient and Family Education and Responsibilities

- The hospital plans for and supports the provision and coordination of patient education activities.
- The hospital identifies and provides the resources necessary for achieving educational objectives.
- The patient education process is coordinated among appropriate staff or disciplines who are providing care or services.
- The patient receives education and training specific to the patient's assessed needs, abilities, learning preferences, and readiness to learn as appropriate to the care and services provided by the hospital.
- Based on assessed needs, the patient is educated about how to safely and effectively use medications, according to law and regulation, and the hospital's scope of services, as appropriate.
- The patient is educated about nutrition interventions, modified diets, or oral health when applicable.
- The hospital assures that the patient is educated about how to safely and effectively use medical equipment or supplies, as appropriate.
- Patients are educated about pain and managing pain as part of treatment, as appropriate.
- Patients are educated about habilitation or rehabilitation techniques to help them be more functionally independent, as appropriate.
- The patient is educated about other available resources, and when necessary, how to obtain further care, services, or treatment to meet his or her identified needs.
- Education includes information about patient responsibilities in the patient's care.
- Education includes self-care activities, as appropriate.
- Discharge instructions are given to the patient and those responsible for providing continuing care.
- Academic education is provided to children and adolescents either directly by the hospital or through other arrangement, when appropriate.

Source: Reprinted with permission from Joint Commission on Accreditation of Healthcare Organizations. Comprehensive Accreditation Manual for Hospitals. Oakbrook Terrace, IL: JCAHO, 2000;PF1–PF16.

risk factors for developing a problem or dysfunction; or need for health, wellness, or fitness programs. *Physical therapists are responsible for patient/client-related instruction across all settings for all patients/clients.*

Given this wide-ranging and important responsibility, a key question for physical therapist and physical therapist assistant educators is how to best teach and help students learn about patient education in the context of the professional curriculum. How can we foster the development of effective patient-family educators?

Physical therapist and physical therapist assistant professional preparation occurs in two primary environments—academic or classroom settings and clinical settings—each of which has unique physical, social, interpersonal, and cultural characteristics that create the milieu in which learning occurs. In this chapter, we discuss teaching and learning about patient education in each of these environments and consider what aspects of experience in these settings might enhance or impede the development of competent patient educators. We do not wish, however, to create an artificial separation between these two environments with respect to what can be taught and learned about patient education. There is much to be learned in both settings, although there may be some differences in (1) the form and nature of what is taught and learned, and (2) the circumstances in which the teaching and learning occur. Both academic and clinical educators bear responsibility for creating opportunities for linking classroom instruction and clinical experiences so that students can navigate between these two environments with an ever-increasing understanding and valuing of the centrality and artistry of effective patient education in clinical practice.

One ubiquitous challenge to teaching students about patient education has been a commonly held student belief that establishing therapeutic relationships with clients and becoming a skilled patient educator is "common sense" and not the stuff of professional curricula or classroom instruction (nor is it perceived as the stuff of theory and research!). In addition, learning about patient education is not valued by some students because it is not viewed as a hands-on skill requiring the application of their extensive biomedical knowledge in anatomy, neuroanatomy, physiology, kinesiology, and biomechanics. Throughout this chapter, we share some ways that educators might address some of these impediments to motivation and learning.

In our discussion, we draw on theory and research as it relates to teaching and learning about patient education in the classroom and the clinic. We also draw liberally on our collective experience and that of others—academic and clinical educators, clinicians, and students—who have shared their insights and understandings about this topic with us. Finally, we ground our discussion in a belief that teaching is a core activity in physical therapy practice and that the development of therapeutic alliances and collaboration with patients serve as the medium through which client *and* clinician learning occurs.

Teaching and Learning about Patient Education in the Classroom

Introducing Students to Patient Education

We start with the assumption that until students are familiar and at least somewhat comfortable with applying therapeutic techniques, their receptivity to learning about how to teach these techniques to patients is low. In addition, students often perceive themselves as adept when teaching motor skills, to patients on a one-to-one basis. From their own experience of being taught motor skills they follow the traditional sequence of telling the patient what he or she is about to do, then demonstrating the activity and then having the patient perform the activity with guided feedback. Lack of success in patient education, however, begins when students forget that forming a therapeutic alliance with the patient (i.e., carefully listening to the patient and focusing on the patient's life experiences and current goals) is a necessary prerequisite to teaching patients. Lack of success also occurs when students fail to identify the patient and family beliefs that might motivate (or impede) their learning about new ways of functioning.

In the classroom setting students can be introduced to the necessity for and power of the Patient-Practitioner Collaborative Model presented in Chapter 9, and the Health Belief Model of Behavior Change presented in Chapter 10. These models, which are grounded in theory and extensive research, undergird effective patient and family education. Even so, they can be difficult for students to transform into practice while in academic settings. Laboratory work with student peers in no way simulates the critical necessity for establishing therapeutic alliances with patients and families or identifying patient beliefs that will illuminate avenues for receptivity to learning and change. These skills can be taught and are learned during the clinical education portion of the curriculum. (See the later section in this chapter, Lessons Learned from Patients.) So what can the classroom teacher do to foster the development of patient education skills?

One way to introduce students to the notion that patient and family education skills are embedded in all types of clinical practice is for faculty in each course in the curriculum to present the knowledge and skills they are teaching as information students will be teaching to patients and families. For example, the faculty member might discuss with students (or model) how low back pain prevention strategies could be taught to patients or how practice variables that optimize motor learning could be taught to family members. Written examination questions could be phrased in terms of what salient information would need to be taught to patients, and practical examinations could include patient-teaching segments. Once students have been socialized to their role as teachers by this kind of subtle but persistent presentation throughout the curriculum, they tend to be more receptive to learning about specific patient-family education strategies that clearly enhance their success as health care providers.

Telling Is Not Necessarily Teaching

When we teach people something, the expected outcome is for a change to occur in what they know, how they perform, or in their attitudes, beliefs, or ways of understanding. If change were not the desired outcome of teaching, there would be no reason to teach. Understanding that change is the goal may help students see that simply telling a patient what to do may have little effect on the desired outcome of sustained change.

A particular blind spot for students is to approach teaching patients and families as students themselves have been taught most of their lives in athletic endeavors or in academic settings. This means there is an emphasis on repetitive movement ("practice makes perfect") or on cognition and language, especially the written and spoken word. Thus, students should be introduced to ways of teaching and learning that blend and further the teaching and learning behaviors they have observed and acquired in the classroom or on the athletic field.

In many instances, patients will be learning, and thus changing, in at least three domains of learning—cognitive, affective, and psychomotor (and perhaps even in the perceptual and spiritual domains). As students first encounter patient education while immersed in academic programs, it is in the cognitive or thinking domain that students tend to excel, and thus the domain they often overemphasize in their teaching approaches with patients and families. Witness patients looking dazed after long-winded explanations of anatomy and physiology accompanied by the student enthusiastically flipping through illustrations in her or his anatomy textbook. This approach is particularly problematic when the general or specific culture of the patient is ignored,[19] especially when working with the increasing number of patients in our society whose first language is not that of the health care provider. In addition, disease and disability states, as well as pain and psychoemotional states (such as anxiety or depression) can pose formidable barriers to receptivity to and understanding of written and verbal information.

Teaching about Movement

As it is often movement that is being taught, we suggest that students approach patient education first from the psychomotor domain.

Students are familiar with this approach, not only because of their past athletic endeavors, but because much of their own learning in physical therapy about body mechanics and manual diagnosis and treatment skills comes about first through sensing and feeling.[20] In the classroom, students gradually become increasingly kinesthetically aware of what they are feeling and doing with their hands and then link this tactile and movement information with complex biomechanical concepts.[20] Likewise, patients can be assisted to move in ways that will facilitate their kinesthetic awareness. Kinesthetic awareness is often best taught quietly, allowing the patients time to feel correct and incorrect movements and express what they are feeling. The ability to feel correct movement patterns and sequences will go a long way toward helping patients to remember the movement and be able to perform it correctly when the therapist is not present. Once the kinesthetic sense of a movement is learned, students can enhance patient motor learning by using motor learning principles and manipulating practice variables. (See Chapter 11.)

Teaching about Learning Theories

Subsequent to learning to teach patients kinesthetic awareness and how to thoughtfully manipulate motor learning practice variables, students can be exposed to various well-documented learning theories about how people learn in general. Learning theories typically embrace learning simultaneously in cognitive, affective, and psychomotor domains.

Experienced clinicians who are skilled in patient-family education move easily from using one learning theory to another depending on patient receptivity and situational need. Learning theories are essentially perspectives on how people learn. (See the section Learning Theories in Chapter 2.) The following examples of two different learning theories illustrate why students need to be introduced to a variety of learning theories.

Behaviorism is one of the most familiar and traditional theories of learning.[21] Therapists use behaviorism quite naturally when they decide to focus with patients on attaining a specific goal, such as performing an independent bed-to-wheelchair transfer. Breaking a task down into skill components, giving clear directions to the patient regarding how to perform each component, and then positively reinforcing the patient immediately contingent on success is one example of the use of behaviorist learning theory in clinical teaching. The development of behavioral learning contracts is another example of the use of this theory (Figure 8-1). A behavioral learning contract is particularly useful when working with patients who have severe cognitive and perceptual deficits that may lead them to be physically unsafe.

BEHAVIORAL LEARNING CONTRACT

This is a contract between John Yu, MPT, and Susan Abernathy

Goals: Susan will always ask to be helped before she begins walking and WAIT until a staff or family member helps her. Susan agrees this will help prevent further injuries.

Plan of Action: Susan will be monitored from 5 pm to 10 pm by the hospital staff and by her family. She will ring for assistance before she gets up to walk and wait until the staff or a family member assists her. The staff and family member who witness the behavior will document it in Susan's log book.

Mr. Yu will practice this procedure and discuss the safety component of this behavior with Susan on a daily basis during her physical therapy session.

Reward: If Susan follows through with this procedure for a 5-hour period, she may rent a movie of her choice the following evening.

Target Date: _____   **Date Completed:** _____

Both Susan and Mr. Yu have set and agreed to these goals. They agree to work TOGETHER toward the goals.

_____   _____

John Yu, MPT   Susan Abernathy

Figure 8-1   Behavioral learning contract. (Adapted from MT Nemshick. Designing Educational Interventions for Patients and Families. In KF Shepard, GM Jensen [eds]. Handbook of Teaching for Physical Therapists. Boston: Butterworth–Heinemann, 1997.)

Gestalt–Problem Solving

Other patients learn better using a gestalt–problem solving type of learning theory such as that proposed by John Dewey.[22–24] The focus of this theory is on engagement in purposeful activities performed in realistic settings as a condition for learning. The task of the teacher is to provide conditions and tasks that stimulate thinking and then to participate in joint problem solving with the learner. A therapist using this theory might provide opportunities for patients to try out different approaches to movement to see what will and what won't work to allow them to accomplish a personally or socially meaningful task. In using this approach to teaching and learning, the therapist is not telling the patient what to do but rather creating opportunities in a safe and supportive environment for the patient to explore and discuss options—that is, participating in joint problem solving with the patient.

Learning Theory Use

An important issue for students to understand about learning theories is that they must be consciously aware of which learning theory they are using and why they are using it at any point in time. This is no different than being consciously aware of which therapeutic intervention one is using and being able to justify the use of that intervention. In either case, it becomes very difficult to evaluate the effectiveness of an intervention or to select a different approach when one is not clear about the current approach she or he is using.

Teaching about Learning Styles

Another concept that students can learn about patient education in the academic setting is that people tend to teach in a way that mirrors how they learn best. For example, some people learn best by watching and listening, some like to actively experiment with hands-on tasks, and still others like to gather, read, and muse over journal articles or books. Thus, some therapists instinctively demonstrate to the patient who is watching and listening, others may insist on having patients experiment with ways of performing movements, and still others come to treatment sessions loaded down with written and pictorial information. Having students take a learning style inventory and then relating their predominant styles to their prior positive and negative learning experiences can be eye opening. Some commonly used learning style inventories in professional education include the Kolb Learning Styles Inventory,[25] the Canfield Learning Style Inventory,[26] and the Myers-Briggs Type Indicator.[27] Learning styles are more fully discussed in Chapter 2 in the section Student Learning Styles.

One suggestion to enhance student understanding of the importance and usefulness of learning styles is to have student groups work together on an in-depth activity that has the potential to engage many different learning styles. For example, student groups might create a research proposal or present a complex patient case study. After the activity is completed, have the students share their learning styles. This activity may help clarify why feelings of irritation or frustration may have arisen when some students wanted to spend more time in the library and others were off tinkering with methods or arguing about therapeutic interventions.

Once students experience and reflect on how their preferred learning style clearly relates to their interest and success in learning, as well as their preference for certain teaching approaches, a bridge can be made to patient education. Students can then realize that tapping into the patient's own learning style can clearly save time and enhance patient learning and clinical teaching success.

Creating Home Exercise Programs

It is almost impossible to conceive of a patient being discharged from a therapist's care without receiving a HEP. The widespread use of home exercises led the editors of this book to devote an entire chapter (Chapter 12) to identifying educational materials that can be used when designing patient HEPs. In this chapter, we briefly outline some aspects of HEPs that students can be taught in classroom settings. Factors that affect patient learning were discussed earlier in this chapter. In addition to all these factors, students should be aware that

1. Forty-seven percent of the adult population in the United States has deficient literacy skill.[28]
2. Health care providers are prone to give too much information at a vocabulary level too high for many patients and family members to understand.[29]

The possibility and probability of this potential communication gap between therapists and patients may increase as physical therapists are increasingly being educated at the doctorate (DPT) level.

In the academic setting, students can be taught the basics of preparing home programs that are understandable to all patients and family members. These basics include

- Developing home programs with simple figures and a few key words about the type and direction of movement along with the number of repetitions. Lengthy wordy explanations about movements, no matter how carefully written, will not be as helpful as a few key words (preferably the patient's descriptors) that focus the patient's recall on his or her own kinesthetic memories.
- Illustrating home program exercise routines can be done using a number of commercially prepared materials or computer programs useful in rapidly individualizing each home program. (Refer to Chapter 12 for explicit information about computerized patient education materials.) However, no commercial product can take the place of the therapist working side-by-side with the patient explaining exercises[30] and producing a few stick figures to illustrate a point quickly, yet understandably, to a patient who is being discharged right after an initial evaluation. Instead of accepting at face value student comments such as "I can't draw" (they could draw in first grade!), urge them to purchase a step-by-step stick figure drawing book available in most art and book stores. Being able to successfully draw stick figures that include major body joints and direction of movement will enhance the student's interest and

• When assisting someone with increasing or maintaining range of motion, be sure that you read the instructions carefully and follow the pictures for proper hand placement. For instance, when you are helping the person to stretch out his or her shoulder, first, support the upper extremity at the elbow and wrist joints. Turn the hand so that the thumb is facing forward and raise the arm slowly over the person's head until you reach the point of resistance. Once you have reached resistance, hold the arm in that position for 10–15 seconds and then return to its starting position. Repeat this exercise 10 times.	• To Stretch the Shoulder: This exercise will be helpful to keep a person's shoulder from getting stiff. It should be done three times a day until the person can do it alone. Hold the person's arm at the wrist and elbow. Turn their hand so that the thumb is facing toward you. Raise the arm slowly up to the point where it feels tight. Hold the arm in that position for 10 seconds. Lower it back to the person's side. Repeat this 10 times. If you have any questions, please call me or ask me at the next therapy session.
• Grade level = 11	• Grade level = 5

Figure 8-2   Comparison of written instructions at grade levels 11 and 5 using a Fog formula. (Adapted from MT Nemshick. Designing Educational Interventions for Patients and Families. In KF Shepard, GM Jensen [eds]. Handbook of Teaching for Physical Therapists. Boston: Butterworth–Heinemann, 1997.)

skill in on-the-spot patient education. Furthermore, this skill enables students to respond immediately, yet simply, to patients' needs for a form of communication that doesn't rely on spoken or written language.

- When written explanations are given to patients, a Fog assessment should be performed on the written material to ensure that the information presented can be read by someone with no more than a sixth grade education.[31] Fog (or Smog) formulas are based on the premise that the more three syllable words and the longer the sentences, the more difficult the material is to read. Thus, even without a Fog formula, teaching students to write home programs in short sentences using one or two syllable words will facilitate their ability to prepare useful materials for patients (Figure 8-2).

  - Present information in LARGE, EASY-TO-READ TYPE.
  - Use a variety of simple, culturally sensitive pictures.
  - Use a lot of white space between short paragraphs. This is less threatening to people with low literacy levels.[32]

Finally, what can intrigue students when they are learning about patient education in the academic setting is drawing on the many parallels from their own lifetimes of being involved in teaching and learning experiences both in academic environments and other life situations. Once the student's awareness and insights about her or his own teaching-learning experiences have been explored and captured, she or he is ready to be exposed to and learn more from the fascinating but complex world of teaching patients and families—no two of whom will ever be alike.

Teaching and Learning about Patient Education in the Clinic

Clinical education experiences embedded in physical therapy professional curricula offer fertile ground for teaching and learning about patient education. A large body of theory and research on learning and development suggests that learning is most accurately conceived of as an active and social process that involves constructing understandings ("making sense") of self, others, and experience in the context of authentic activities in communities of practice. Variously referred to as *social constructivism, sociohistorical/sociocultural theory,* or *situative views of learning,* these perspectives on learning and development draw on philosophies of education and theories of learning first put forth in the early twentieth century by giants such as John Dewey[23,24] and Soviet psychologist Lev Vygotsky,[33,34] whose influential works were not translated into English until the latter half of the century. Many contemporary researchers and authors have subsequently explored and elaborated on these perspectives through investigations of learning, development, and cognition in a variety of contexts.[35–40] Collectively, this body of work points to the importance of apprenticeship types of experiences, which provide for participation in authentic, social, and situated environments and communities of practice, as essential to learning.

Clinical practice settings are certainly one type of authentic environment. Clinical experiences integrated in physical therapy professional curricula clearly offer great opportunities for learning as students actively engage in joint problem solving and co-constructing understandings with patients, families, and professionals on a day-to-day basis. But it is not just these characteristics that assure learning and professional growth, nor do they guarantee what type of learning occurs—it is the nature of the interactions among participants and the type of engagement in activity in the social milieu that have more to do with what is learned.

Some key questions arise about the nature of teaching and learning about patient education in clinical settings: What lessons do students learn about patient education and their role as a teacher in the course of their clinical experiences? How do they construct new insights and understandings (learn) about patient education? From whom do they learn about patient education? In what ways can physical therapist academic and clinical educators guide and shape the experiences of students in the clinic in such a way that they become sensitive practitioners, skilled relationship builders, and good teachers and collaborators with their patients? Or can we? These questions have been of interest to me (E.M.) and several of my colleagues for the past few years. We have attempted to explore and begin to answer some of these questions by carefully listening to the words and stories of students and clinicians involved in clinical education experiences as shared through (1) regional dialogue groups that meet on a monthly basis during clinical internships[41] and (2) student reflective journals written during clinical experiences.

In our clinical education model,[41,42] students completing two semester-length internships during the final year of the physical therapy program meet on a monthly basis with an academic faculty member (regional clinical coordinator [RCC]) and fellow students in their geographic region. These meetings provide opportunities for (1) discussion among students about their clinical experiences, (2) joint problem solving about perplexing patients or other clinical practice situations, (3) peer teaching about new skills or knowledge gained through clinical internships, and (4) connecting academic course work with clinical learning and experience. Conversations in group meetings often echo the content of student reflective journals that are written throughout the internship experience. Together, regular student group meetings and journal writing are practical strategies for enhancing and extending student learning and development through active engagement in reflection and dialogue during clinical internships.

Importance of Dialogue and Reflection in Learning and Professional Development

Drawing on the seminal works of Dewey,[43] Gadamer,[44] and Schön,[45,46] many authors have emphasized the importance of engaging in dialogue and reflection in and on action to the learning and development of professionals in a variety of disciplines.[47–52] Furthermore, recent investigations of expertise in physical therapy suggest that a common attribute of master therapists is their continual reflection on and about their experience as they seek deeper understandings of themselves, their patients, and their practice.[9–13]

How does an individual become reflective? More specifically, how can physical therapist educators provide opportunities for the development of skillful and thoughtful reflection that becomes educative and growth enhancing? Several authors from physical therapy and other disciplines have suggested a variety of ways to build reflective practica into professional curricula.[47–49,51,53–58] Among these are opportunities for engaging in (1) open dialogue or conversation with others about lived experiences and the ideas, questions, and insights that emerge out of those experiences[23,54,55,59,60]; and

(2) various forms of reflective writing such as journals, diaries, logs, or reflective summaries.[53,56–58,61,62] With respect to the power of writing as a tool for reflection, the words of vanManen[63] and Clark[54] capture the essence of the aim of reflective writing regardless of the form it takes:

> Writing teaches us what we know, and in what way we know what we know. As we commit ourselves to paper, we see ourselves mirrored in the text. Now the text confronts us. . . . Writing gives appearance and body to thought.[63(p127)]

> There is something special about writing. It forces me toward clarity in my thinking. . . . It demands my full attention to the content of the ideas I am trying to express. . . .Writing moves me to remember, reinterpret, and reorganize what I know. . . . Even with self as sole audience, writing often makes for uncomfortable confrontations with logical inconsistencies, confusions, and contradictions that were otherwise quiescent and unconscious. Writing shines light into corners of the mind easier left in darkness.[54(p98)]

Thus, writing about experience can help to push the writer to examine an experience more deeply and make thoughts and feelings about the experience visible and palpable to themselves or others. It can urge them to make sense of some of the exigencies, complexities, and uncertainties that so often accompany experience, especially in the unpredictable world of the clinic. It is the activity of "making sense" of experience that many say constitutes learning.

The reflective journal data presented in this chapter are drawn from journals written by students during the third and final year of a physical therapist professional preparation program leading to the master of science degree. Reflective journals were a requirement of two 14-week clinical internships that comprised the entire concluding year of the program. Students were given guidelines for their journal writing during clinical experiences as shown in Appendix 8-A.

Reflective journals written during final year internships were submitted to one of four RCCs at monthly, regionally based, dialogue group meetings with fellow students during the internships (three meetings per internship). As mentioned earlier, many reflective journal entries served as a stimulus to discussion among students at these meetings, and conversation in groups often mirrored content in journals. Other entries, however, remained a topic of reflection shared only in writing. Journals were read by the RCCs, analyzed for content categories and themes according to an initial coding scheme modified from Jensen and Denton,[56] and returned to students with the reader's reflections on their reflections. In this way it was hoped that a conversation on paper would develop between the RCC and student. To encourage open dialogue between students and faculty, journals were not graded but were a requirement for successful completion of the internships.

Analysis of reflective journal content is ongoing and is focused on gaining insight and understanding about student learning and development during clinical internships and the transition from classroom to clinic. One common theme that has emerged, however, has been that of student experiences and learning about patient education and relationship building with clients and families. These two aspects of achieving therapeutic aims are usually tightly interwoven in student reflections and stories about teaching and learning in the clinic as expressed in journals.

What Students Say about Teaching and Learning in the Clinic

Journal entries about teaching and learning in the clinic often focus on lessons learned from patients and their caregivers and lessons learned from a student's CI or other professional staff members. Learning from patients is frequently reflected in stories about mistakes, challenges, and successes students encounter as they seek to (1) establish partnerships with their patients, and (2) teach patients or caregivers in the context of therapy. Deliberate exploration of the reasons for such challenges or successes, either through writing in journals or through discussion with CIs, RCCs or fellow students, is one way that students often link what they have learned in the classroom with their evolving understandings of the patient collaboration-teaching-learning process in the clinic. Journal entries on learning from CIs highlight the importance of the instructor as a "sounding board," joint problem solver, and model for students as they learn about the complexity of interaction with patients. Some models are powerfully positive influences for students as they think about what they wish to become as a therapist and teacher; others, less so.

Lessons Learned from Patients

Patients are perhaps the most influential teachers for students in the clinic. Numerous encounters with patients from all walks of life with a variety of problems force students to reconsider what they bring to the therapist-patient encounter as well as focus on what the patient brings. They must learn to adapt approaches and improvise moment to moment as they work to create a framework for progress and learning in therapy. Such improvisation does not always come easily, and many students learn a great deal from their most challenging encounters.

One student, writing during her first 14-week internship, expressed a phenomenon observed in much of the journal data—that the ability to learn from patients can be a developmental phenomenon—one that requires a shift in focus from the student's own performance to full attention to the patient.

> One of the most important lessons I have learned . . . is that I am not the center of the relationship between me and my patient. . . . Once I learned this, I stopped being so worried about my performance, or worried that I was missing some vital piece of information. I stopped thinking about myself, and started thinking about my patient first. This seems late in the game to have learned this, but alas, it is true. I stopped feeling so nervous, too. This helped immensely in learning to really listen, or to really feel or see what the patient was trying to show me.

Several investigators studying the professional development of physical therapists have noted shifts from therapist-centered practice to patient-centered practice as one hallmark of growth into clinical mastery.[9,10–13,64] Perhaps this student's insight describes one early and necessary step on the way to such a transition. For clinical and academic faculty, this information urges consideration of ways to decrease students' worry or anxiety about their performance so they can more fully attend to their patients.

Indeed, many students at first express simple frustration about some of their more challenging patients and their mistakes or failures. Later in their clinical experiences, they spend more time writing about how they sought to identify and overcome barriers that could impede success in therapy and what they had learned from such experiences. A few examples of such entries follow.

One student working in a diverse community in a large metropolitan area wrote about her learning about working with individuals of Russian Orthodox Jewish background. Therapists and students alike in this clinic keep a Russian dictionary on hand and work hard to understand some of the language and beliefs of their clients, but much is learned about this in the course of therapy.

> The other day I had my first experience working with a patient who was of Russian Orthodox Jewish background. When I went to introduce myself to this very pleasant gentleman

> dressed in black with a beard and black hat, I held out my hand
> to shake his. I quickly learned, by him informing me, that he
> does not shake women's hands. He is widowed and that is part
> of their religion. Then I had to ultrasound his shoulder so he
> had to take his jacket, shirt, prayer cloth (which I hadn't seen
> before), and undershirt off. Everything was fine but it just made
> me wonder if I couldn't shake his hand, how did he feel sitting
> there without a shirt on and having me work on his shoulder?

The student went on to further study cultural and gender issues in therapy as a result of this encounter. In the context of this experience, she committed herself to (1) exploring more deeply her own cultural autobiography
and beliefs, and (2) learning more about the beliefs and practices of this particular cultural group and how those might influence perceptions and outcomes in therapy. Numerous authors writing from the perspectives of
medical anthropology and sociology have suggested that these activities are
essential to the development of culturally sensitive practice in health
care.[65–68] Furthermore, this reflection (which became a topic of discussion at
a group meeting) provides an exceptional opportunity for reactivating and
reinforcing information previously presented in the classroom on the importance of exploring belief systems and the development of patient-practitioner
collaborations (see Chapters 9 and 10). In the context of this encounter,
explicit ties between theory and research in these areas and actual practice
can be drawn.

Many students wrote about their struggles to establish positive working
relationships with and to teach patients who (1) had cognitive and communi-
cative impairments as a result of their conditions (e.g., traumatic brain
injury, stroke, Alzheimer's disease), (2) were experiencing clinical depression
or lack of motivation to participate in therapy, and (3) were children. In such
cases, students often discovered how important careful listening to the
patients and attention to their past life experiences, illness experience, and
personal needs were in the development of therapist-patient partnerships
and in laying the groundwork for teaching and learning to occur (Figure 8-3).

One student described a breakthrough with a patient who was initially
an unwilling and angry participant in therapy:

> The patient had lots of medical problems, an old injury to his
> left knee and was in [the hospital] for a dislocated right hip. He
> was very depressed. I asked him once about the old knee injury
> and he opened up—told me about playing football and getting
> injured in high school—then he talked about going to dances

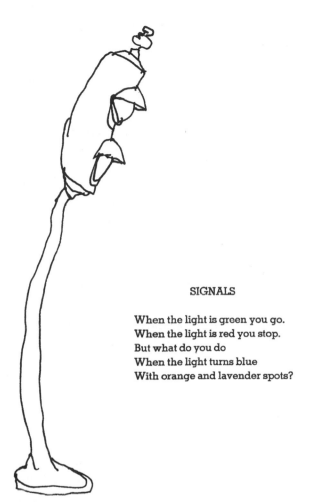

SIGNALS

When the light is green you go.
When the light is red you stop.
But what do you do
When the light turns blue
With orange and lavender spots?

Figure 8-3   Signals. (Reprinted with permission from S Silverstein. A Light in the Attic. New York: Harper Collins Publishers; Copyright 1981 by Evil Eye Music, Inc.)

with his wife—talked about his career in sales. After that, he was very cooperative when exercising with me. In subsequent days, I used that [information] to bring up things to talk about and he would exercise instead of yelling at everyone like he had done the first day.

Another student wrote about a motivational strategy that drew on a patient's past career as a teacher to help her through frightening therapy sessions. This patient had perceptual and visual problems, balance deficits, and some mild confusion as a result of a stroke.

> It was very strange to have a patient look at me with absolute terror in her eyes, begging me not to let her fall, while lying flat on her back on the treatment mat. . . . I found out that Jill [pseudonym] was a teacher and was able to use that to motivate her to try more difficult treatments. I asked her if she gave her students easy or hard homework. She said that she always gave them hard homework because they would learn more. Then I asked her if I should give her easy or hard things to do. She would answer that she should work on hard skills so that she would learn more.

Finally, another student wrote about how learning about a patient's past as a worker on the third shift helped her become an advocate for the patient and suggest an alteration in therapy schedules as a solution to a problem previously ascribed to poor motivation and possible depression. The patient was in an extended care facility and was being seen by the rehabilitation team because of a recent total knee arthroplasty. When therapists worked with her, she repeatedly complained of fatigue and often fell asleep while doing supine exercises.

> . . .this was affecting her progress on the rehab unit. In talking with her, I found out that she worked a third shift job most of her life and simply is not used to the schedule that has been forced on her. She said that if she could even sleep until 9:00 or 9:30 a.m., she would feel much better. Later on at the team meeting, someone raised the issue of this patient's fatigue limiting her progress. The physician immediately began to suggest medications (mostly linked to depression) that would improve her "motivation." Although this was not "my" patient, I cautiously spoke up and told the little tidbit of information I knew about her life pattern. The physician said, "Oh, so we let her sleep late." It has been a week now and the problem seems to be solved. I am slightly afraid that had I not spoken with her, or had I not spoken up, she might be taking medication she simply did not need.

In all of the journal segments, students' stories and reflections converge on an important insight and theme that appear in many journal entries. Students learn that listening to clients, exploring and respecting their life experiences, and gaining information about their current needs, goals, and beliefs facilitate the creation of therapeutic alliances and foster therapist-patient collaboration in therapy. The knowledge gained through carefully listening to patients, when used in the development of an individualized plan of care and determining a personal approach to the patient, can lay the groundwork for successful teaching and learning in therapy.

Many students, experiencing the complexity of establishing relationships and partnerships with patients built on caring, trust, and respect, write about their learning about the many ways these components of therapeutic relationships are interactionally negotiated and conveyed. Some wrote about how, in pediatric encounters, they had to work to respect both the needs and autonomy of the child and the parent concurrently. Others wrote about modifying their previous definitions of what is or is not respectful and caring interaction based on situational demands and personal needs. In the following excerpt, a student discusses his struggle with having to raise his voice in therapy because of a patient's severe loss of hearing.

> I'm learning some things about communication. Past experience has taught me a few things; for example, the importance of body language and gestures beyond verbal language. However, there is always more to know. My latest patient is extremely hard of hearing. . . . In essence, what I learned is that it is okay to yell if the need arises. I suppose I can be timid in some areas and one is raising my voice. I feel that doing so is somehow disrespectful to the person on the receiving end. That may be so in most cases, but there are exceptions. My CI told me simply that if you are doing only what the situation requires, then you are not breaking respectful limits. It took me a while to get used to this, but it makes sense and I have been able to communicate much better with my patient.

In the following excerpt, a student reexamines a policy he held about addressing patients by name.

> My policy, both personally and professionally, is always to address individuals formally unless told to do otherwise. My CI informed me that in certain situations this may need to be altered. For example, I've been working with a patient who had experienced a stroke and was not very responsive to the environment or to people. I hadn't been very successful addressing

> her as Mrs. "X," but when Joan [pseudonym] called her by her
> first name she opened her eyes and turned her head to the
> sound. I never realized the importance or power a single word
> can hold. It is still difficult for me to address any patient by
> their first name, especially older individuals, but I see that in
> certain instances it can be important to do so.

Here students transform previous understandings of respectful interaction in clinical encounters as they reflect on their learning about the dynamic, situational, and individual nature of respect in patient-therapist exchanges. They learn that being respectful is not just one way of being or acting in all situations and that what being respectful means for one person may vary for another.

Beyond the work of establishing relationships with patients that can serve as a foundation for teaching and learning in therapy, many students write specifically about lessons learned about the importance of patient and family education in the clinic. They write about their failures or disappointments as teachers and their successes. A common refrain in journals and in dialogue groups is echoed in the following excerpt:

> I had this one patient with neck and arm pain and she seemed
> really stressed out about the problem and worried that she
> might get worse with therapy. So I decided to keep her initial
> home exercise program really simple at first and I gave her only
> three very mild stretching exercises to do. Well, the next session she came back and I asked her to show me her exercises
> like she was doing them at home. I couldn't believe what I
> saw!! I could hardly recognize what she was doing! From now
> on, I am going to go very slowly when teaching exercises—I am
> going to have the patient show me the exercises several times
> in therapy and make sure that they have written home programs with pictures and simple explanations on them. I think I
> rushed my teaching with this patient and was too timid in my
> instructions because she was so worried about getting worse.

Many students were forced to carefully examine their teaching approaches with patients after encountering such problems with performance of or cooperation with home programs. It is in such situations that classroom content on learning styles, Fog assessments, simplicity in figures and instructions, and teaching for kinesthetic awareness come into clear focus for students as they seek mutual understandings with clients around HEPs.

Furthermore, students are often pushed to explore possible reasons for poor program adherence that go beyond the use of appropriate and effective teaching strategies. One student, after an encounter with poor adherence to a home program, considered what some of the difficulties might be for children and parents doing exercise programs at home.

> If I have a hard time finding time to do trunk strengthening exercises [that I need to do], then don't my patients have a hard time finding time to do a HEP? I think that therapists, including me, forget that parents who have a child who needs to do a HEP have busy lives and may not have time to do the program with their child. If I can keep this in mind, I think I will have better success when it comes to designing a HEP and having the patient actually do it. Also, when I ask a parent or child if they have been doing the HEP, I have to be prepared for the "no's" and armed with the "why's" to do the program and the "how's" to fit it in.

Here, drawing on her own problems with adherence and motivation, the student recognizes the importance of (1) educating both children and parents about *why* certain exercises are important for the child, and (2) consideration of when and *how* home programs might best be integrated into what are already busy days for families. Knowledge of the why's of therapy programs, with special attention to the patient's (or parent's) needs, goals, and health belief systems can make programs more meaningful to clients. Consideration of the when and how of home programs recognizes that patients have lives beyond therapy. These components of teaching with patients and their caregivers move an exchange from one that is therapist centered to one that is more patient focused.

Although these excerpts describe lessons learned about teaching based on perceived failures, many more journal entries detail successes and the excitement of recognizing effective teaching and patient learning.

> Another time I felt good was when I was describing to the patient what was happening with her. I got out the model of the spine and showed her the area from which the problem stemmed. I educated her on the discs and nerve roots. She really seemed to benefit from the discussion and learned a lot. She said it made her understand the purpose of her exercise program and of the treatments we were doing with her. It made me feel good because I felt effective.

Students frequently describe the expression of gratitude from patients or families as moments when they most appreciated the importance of listening to patients' questions and taking time to teach them about their condition and what they could do about it. When students have such experiences and realizations, this is another opportunity for clinical or academic faculty to tie information learned in the classroom on learning theories and learning styles to clinical teaching situations. Asking questions such as "How did you determine what teaching method would be best for this patient?" or "Why do you feel you were so effective in your teaching with this patient?" invites discussion about learning styles and the application of learning theory in the immediate context of a particular patient case.

In the following excerpt, a student describes an experience with a young man who sustained a severe lower-extremity fracture, underwent open reduction and internal fixation and a bone grafting procedure, and also had a peroneal nerve palsy.

> I was able to go to this patient's physician appointments with the family. They had many questions about the surgery, but the doctor was in and out so fast they never seemed to get them answered. I was able to get a copy of the operative report and using a model and picture, explain to them to a limited extent what the physician did. They were happy to know and I was glad for the experience. . . . Today, the patient and parents gave me a small basket of flowers that said "Just wanted to let you know we appreciated all your hard work." I assured them that I appreciated theirs as well. . . .

The explicit valuing of teaching and patient education in therapy was a theme that emerged more often in later versus early journal entries during the course of clinical internships. Perhaps a certain level or repertoire of experience in the clinic is necessary before students come to view teaching and facilitating patient learning as one of their primary roles and responsibilities as a therapist.

Lessons Learned from Clinical Instructors

Another common theme that emerged in reflective journals was student learning about patient-therapist relationships and patient education through observation and side-by-side work with their CIs or other professionals. These individuals are important and powerful models for students as they guide and mediate student participation with patients during their clinical experiences. Virtually all students wrote at some time in their journals about their CI's "style" with patients. These entries often focused on descriptions of the therapist's approach to relationship building and teaching in therapy and the need for adaptability in approaches according to patient needs. Students sometimes sought to emulate their CI's approach to patients; other times they reflected on differences between their preferred style and that of their CIs. Regardless, their reflections suggest they learned a great deal about patient education by observing others' work with patients.

The following are some examples of student entries typical of students' writing about their learning from CIs.

> The depth and breadth of knowledge that Susan has amazes me. . . . Her intuition and grace are priceless. I am very aware of my limitations. Fortunately, I know that each moment I spend with patients and Susan has the potential to teach me something.

> One thing that Mark does model very well is dealing with [difficult] patients. . . . Many of our patients are from the inner city and have limited education and poor communication skills, many are also workman's compensation cases which can complicate things a bit. I feel that I tend to get frustrated easily and this only makes it harder for me to communicate with my patients. Mark is really able to remain very calm and sympathetic and really able to demonstrate this to our patients, and because of this, I feel that he is able to get through to them effectively. I have observed this and I am really working on trying to model this behavior.

Students recognize patterns of effective interaction and teaching by CIs and, often, as stated by this student, actively appropriate and try to emulate the behaviors of their CIs. Others, however, explore differences between CI and student beliefs and approaches to patients as described in the following entry.

> My CI told me I had to stop being so soft-hearted because I was asking if my moving the patient in this way or that way was hurting them. I was commended [on my last internship] . . . for my compassion for the patient. And I had a lot of really difficult patients do anything I wanted them to because I was nice to them. Now I hear . . . that I am too soft. A big lesson: we are all different in our interactions with patients. . . . I know that pain needs to be worked through to an extent. But there also

> needs to be some trust established with people in pain to make
> them want to work through the pain. . . . If I charge into a room
> and put this person into great pain on the first day, they will be
> less likely to work with me in the future. I suppose as I said
> before we are all different.

This student, who was just beginning an acute care internship at the
time of this entry, struggled not only with differences between the CI's
approach to patients and her own approach, but also with adapting to the
reality of needing to progress patients quickly in this setting due to short
lengths of stay in the hospital. Past learning and successes in an outpatient
clinic setting now had to be reconsidered in an entirely new situation with
different demands and constraints.

As students encounter CIs across and within internships, they have the
opportunity to observe various approaches to patient interaction and education. It is in clinical education that students get the chance to observe and
directly experience many different types of teaching-learning styles and consider the impact of their own preferences and those of others on learning outcomes with patients and themselves. In the end, students begin to create a
vision—a unique collage—of what they hope or wish to become as a patient
educator and professional based on these encounters and their own style,
beliefs, and values. Commonly, they selectively appropriate CI behaviors and
values along the way. In the following excerpt, one student summarizes her
observations of several CIs and details what she learned from each of them
about interaction and teaching with patients as well as what she learned
about herself.

> Cindy is a great example for me. She goes with the flow and
> always thinks about five steps ahead of herself and puts
> patients absolutely first as her priority, no matter how much
> messing around and rearranging [of the room] it takes. It is all
> worth it for one tiny step. . . . I worked with Emily (a near mas-
> ter at what she does) . . . as much as I admired Emily and the
> way she placed her hands on patients, there are a handful of
> lessons I learned from myself that actually differed from the
> way she would do things. I'm as proud of these as those I
> learned directly from her. For example, I prefer to be less of a
> therapy director, and more of a therapy facilitator. I feel this
> helps them [patients] take on the responsibility for their well-
> ness more effectively. . . . I worked with Janis (a young PT just
> getting the hang of things). Janis taught me the people lessons,
> how to really engage your patients and treat them personally

PRIMARY SOURCES of LEARNING

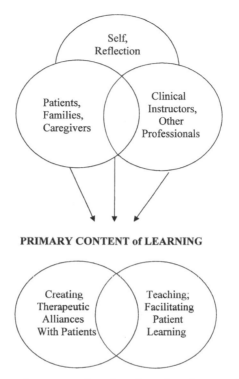

PRIMARY CONTENT of LEARNING

Figure 8-4   Sources and content of student learning about patient education in clinical settings. (Reprinted with permission from E Mostrom, K Shepard. Teaching and learning about patient education in physical therapy professional preparation: academic and clinical considerations. J Phys Ther Educ 1999;13[3]:8–17.)

> and with great care. . . . I also learned from Janis not to be intimidated by co-workers (with more skills and experience) and to accept your rank/position in stride and to do your best to advance yourself (through learning opportunities), but never to discount your authenticity and membership in the profession of physical therapy.

These examples of student reflections during internships make it clear that clinical experiences in professional curricula are powerful and important sites for teaching and learning about patient education and creating and sustaining therapeutic alliances with clients. Figure 8-4 summarizes the sources and content of learning about patient education in clinical settings as suggested by entries in journals and discussion in student dialogue groups.

An important resource for learning for the students described in this chapter was deliberate self-reflection on their experiences as patient educators and their development as a professional across the course of their internships. Reflection can be a valuable vehicle for linking past experience, current understandings, and classroom knowledge with unfolding experience; in the process, students may reconsider and reinterpret their knowledge and experience, thus opening the door for transformed understandings and new insights (see Figure 8-4).

In their writing, students describe lessons learned about patient education and begin to give us glimpses of emergent beliefs about patient-therapist interaction that some investigators have found to be characteristic of expert therapists; most come to recognize the importance and value of active listening to and learning from patients, developing therapeutic and collaborative relationships with clients, and teaching in their work with patients. The students described in this chapter also cultivate the habit of reflection through journal writing and regular dialogue about clinical experiences with fellow students and faculty. These are no small lessons. Academic and clinical faculty must continue to consider how we can amplify and extend these lessons and all opportunities for reflection and learning about thoughtful and effective patient education in clinical and academic settings.

Summary

Teaching students about patient-family education is clearly a joint endeavor between academic and clinical educators in physical therapist and physical therapist assistant professional preparation. As we have suggested in this chapter, experiences in both academic and clinical environments can make unique contributions to student learning about key components of the process of patient education. Not the least of these is the importance of creating and sustaining therapeutic alliances with patients and seeking understandings of their health beliefs as the relational foundation from which reciprocal teaching and learning is fostered in clinical encounters.

Early and explicit dialogue with students about the centrality of patient education to the practice of physical therapy and modeling of the role of therapist as teacher can begin this essential process. Helping students to understand that their ways of knowing may not be how others come to know can sensitize them to the need to learn about learning theories and styles and a variety of pedagogical strategies that can be adapted to individual patient needs. Creating opportunities for self-reflection on experience in both academic and clinical environments can help students to expand, deepen, and transform lessons learned through past experience into future action. Finally, structuring experiences for students to learn from their successes and failures with patients and families in clinical settings can set them on a lifelong journey of reflecting on and learning from each patient encounter. It is this continuous learning that will contribute most to their ongoing development as effective patient educators. Clinical instructors are in a position to be powerful role models and teachers for students regarding patient and family education as they work side-by-side with students in the clinic. The explicit and implicit messages they deliver to students about patient-professional relationships, creating therapeutic alliances, and selecting patient education strategies specific to patient-family needs can have a long-lasting impact on the development of future practitioners and, most important, on the patients they will ultimately serve.

References

1. Avers DL, Gardner DL. Patient Education as a Treatment Modality. In Guccione AA (ed). Geriatric Physical Therapy. St. Louis: CV Mosby, 1993;331–349.
2. Chase L, Elkins J, Readinger JF, Shepard KF. Perceptions of physical therapists toward patient education. Phys Ther 1993;73(11):787–796.
3. Gahimer JE, Domholdt E. Amount of patient education in physical therapy and perceived effects. Phys Ther 1996;76(10):1089–1096.
4. Martin PC, Fell DW. Beyond treatment: patient education for health promotion and disease prevention. J Phys Ther Educ 1999;13(3):49–56.
5. May BJ. Patient education: past and present. J Phys Ther Educ 1999;13(3): 3–7.
6. Sluijs EM. A checklist to assess patient education in physical therapy practice: development and reliability. Phys Ther 1991;71(8):561–569.
7. Sluijs EM. Patient education in physiotherapy: toward a planned approach. Physiotherapy 1991;77:503–508.
8. Stenmar L, Nordholm L. Swedish physical therapists' beliefs on what makes therapy work. Phys Ther 1994;74(11):1034–1039.
9. Jensen GM, Gwyer J, Shepard KF, Hack LM. Expert practice in physical therapy. Phys Ther 2000;80:28–43.
10. Jensen GM, Shepard KF, Gwyer J, Hack LM. Expertise in Physical Therapy Practice. Boston: Butterworth–Heinemann, 1999.
11. Martin C, Siosteen A, Shepard K. The professional development of expert physical therapists in four areas of clinical practice. Nordic Physio 1998;1(1):4–11.
12. Mostrom E. Reciprocal Teaching and Learning in Therapeutic Encounters. In The Wisdom of Practice: Situated Expertise, Teaching, and Learning in

a Transdisciplinary Rehabilitation Clinic. Unpublished Doctoral Dissertation. East Lansing, MI: Michigan State University, 1996;270–373.

13. Mostrom E. Wisdom of Practice in a Transdisciplinary Rehabilitation Clinic: Situated Expertise and Client Centering. In Jensen G, Gwyer J, Hack L, Shepard K (eds). Expertise in Physical Therapy Practice. Boston: Butterworth–Heinemann, 1999;207–230.

14. Joint Commission on Accreditation of Healthcare Organizations. Comprehensive Accreditation Manual for Hospitals. Oakbrook Terrace, IL: JCAHO, 2000;PF1–PF16.

15. American Physical Therapy Association. Guide to Physical Therapy Practice (2nd ed). Alexandria, VA: American Physical Therapy Association, 2001.

16. American Physical Therapy Association. Normative Model of Physical Therapist Professional Education: Version 2000. Alexandria, VA: American Physical Therapy Association, 2000.

17. Commission on Accreditation in Physical Therapy Education. Evaluative Criteria for Accreditation of Education Programs for the Preparation of Physical Therapists. Alexandria, VA: American Physical Therapy Association, Commission on Accreditation in Physical Therapy Education, 1996.

18. American Physical Therapy Association. Physical Therapist Clinical Performance Instrument. Alexandria, VA: American Physical Therapy Association, 1997.

19. Padilla R, Brown K. Culture and patient education: challenges and opportunities. J Phys Ther Educ 1999;13:23–30.

20. Rose M. "Our hands will know": the development of tactile diagnostic skill—teaching, learning, and situated cognition in a physical therapy program. Anthropol Educ Q 1999:30(2):133–160.

21. Phillips DC, Soltis JF. Perspectives on Learning (2nd ed). New York: Teachers College Press, 1991;21–32.

22. Archambault RD. John Dewey on Education: Selected Writings. Chicago: University of Chicago Press, 1974;427–439.

23. Dewey J. Democracy and Education. New York: Free Press, 1916.

24. Dewey J. Experience and Education. New York: Macmillan, 1938.

25. Kolb DA. Learning Styles Inventory. Boston: McBer and Company, 1985.

26. Canfield AA. Learning Style Inventory. Birmingham, MI: Humanics Media, 1980.

27. DiTiberio JK. Education, Learning Styles and Cognitive Styles. In Hammer AL (ed). MBTI Applications: A Decade of Research on the Myers-Briggs Type Indicator. Palo Alto, CA: Consulting Psychologists Press, 1996;123–166.

28. Adult Literacy in America: A First Look at the Results of the National Adult Literacy Survey (2nd ed). Washington, DC: Office of Educational Research and Improvement, Department of Education, 1993.

29. Mayeaux EJ, Murphy DW, Arnold C, et al. Improving patient education for patients with low literacy levels. Am Fam Phys 1996;53:205–211.
30. Friedrick M, Cermak T, Maderbacher P. The effect of brochure use versus therapist teaching on patients performing therapeutic exercises and on changes in impairment status. Phys Ther 1996;76:1082–1088.
31. Doak C, Doak L, Root J. Teaching Patients with Low Literacy Skills. Philadelphia: Lippincott, 1996.
32. Clear and Simple. Developing Effective Print Materials for Low Literate Readers. Bethesda, MD: National Institutes of Health, National Cancer Institute, 1993. NIH Publication No. 95–3594.
33. Vygotsky LS. Thought and Language. Cambridge, MA: MIT Press, 1962.
34. Vygotsky LS. Mind in Society: The Development of Higher Psychological Processes. Cambridge, MA: Harvard University Press, 1978.
35. Brown JS, Collins A, Duguid P. Situated cognition and the culture of learning. Educ Res 1989;18(1):34–41.
36. Cobb P, Bowers J. Cognition and situated learning perspectives in theory and practice. Educ Res 1999;28(2):4–15.
37. Lave J. Cognition in Practice. Cambridge, UK: Cambridge University Press, 1988.
38. Lave J. The Practice of Learning. In Chaiklin S, Lave J (eds). Understanding Practice: Perspectives on Activity and Context. Cambridge, UK: Cambridge University Press, 1993;3–32.
39. Lave J, Wenger E. Situated Learning: Legitimate Peripheral Participation. Cambridge, UK: Cambridge University Press, 1991.
40. Rogoff B. Apprenticeship in Thinking: Cognitive Development in Social Context. New York: Oxford University Press, 1990.
41. Mostrom E, Epstein N, Capehart G, Woods-Reynolds J. Use of a regional clinical coordinator model and clinical education dialogue groups in a physical therapy professional preparation program. Paper presented at: American Physical Therapy Association Combined Sections Meeting, February 6, 1999, Seattle.
42. Woods-Reynolds J, Mostrom E, Capehart G, Epstein N. Use of a final year clinical internship model in a physical therapy preparatory program. Paper presented at: American Physical Therapy Association Combined Sections Meeting, February 14, 1998, Boston.
43. Dewey J. How We Think: A Restatement of the Relation of Reflective Thinking to the Educative Process. Lexington, MA: DC Heath, 1933.
44. Gadamer HG. Truth and Method. New York: Crossroad, 1982.
45. Schön DA. The Reflective Practitioner: How Professionals Think in Action. New York: Basic Books, 1983.
46. Schön DA. Educating the Reflective Practitioner. San Francisco: Jossey-Bass, 1987.

47. Burbules NC. Dialogue in Teaching. New York: Teachers College Press, 1993.

48. Davis C. Professional Socialization: Process That Empowers. In Leadership for Change in Physical Therapy Clinical Education. Alexandria, VA: American Physical Therapy Association, 1986;53–70.

49. Harris IB. New Expectations for Professional competence. In Curry L, Wergin JF and Associates (eds). Educating Professionals. San Francisco: Jossey-Bass, 1993;17–52.

50. Saylor CR. Reflection and professional education: art, science, and competency. Nurse Educ 1990;15(2):8–11.

51. Shepard KF, Jensen GM. Physical therapist curricula for the 1990s: educating the reflective practitioner. Phys Ther 1990;70(9):566–577.

52. Zeichner KM, Liston DP. Teaching student teachers to reflect. Harvard Educ Rev 1987;57(1):23–48.

53. Callister LC. The use of student journals in nursing education: making meaning out of clinical experience. J Nurs Educ 1993;32(4):185–186.

54. Clark CM. Hello learners: living social constructivism. Teaching Educ 1998;10(1):89–110.

55. Gandy J, Jensen GM. Group work and reflective practicums in physical therapy education: models for professional behavior development. J Phys Ther Educ 1992;6(1):6–10.

56. Jensen GM, Denton B. Teaching physical therapy students to reflect: a suggestion for clinical education. J Phys Ther Educ 1991;5(1):33–38.

57. Patton JG, Woods SJ, Agarenzo T, et al. Enhancing the clinical practicum experience through journal writing. J Nurs Educ 1997;36(5):238–240.

58. Perkins, J. Reflective journals: suggestions for educators. J Phys Ther Educ 1996;10(1):8–13.

59. Florio-Ruane S, Clark CM. Authentic conversation: a medium for research on teachers knowledge and a context for professional development. Paper presented at: International Association on Teacher Thinking, September 1993, Goteberg, Sweden.

60. vanManen M. Linking ways of knowing with ways of being practical. Curric Inquiry 1977;6:205–228.

61. Tryssenaar J, Perkins J. From student to therapist: exploring the first year of practice. Am J Occup Ther 2001;55(1):19–27.

62. Tryssenaar J. Interactive journals: an educational strategy to promote reflection. Am J Occup Ther 1996;49(7):695–702.

63. vanManen M. Researching Lived Experience: Human Science for an Action Sensitive Pedagogy. London, Ontario, Canada: Althouse Press, 1990.

64. Dahlgren MA. Learning physiotherapy: student's ways of experiencing the patient encounter. Physiother Res Intl 1998;3(4):257–273.
65. Kleinman A. Patients and Healers in the Context of Culture. Berkeley, CA: University of California Press, 1991.
66. Kleinman A, Eisenberg L, Good B. Culture, illness, and care: clinical lessons from anthropologic and cross-cultural research. Ann Intern Med 1978;88:251–258.
67. Hahn RA. Sickness and Healing: An Anthropological Perspective. New Haven, CT: Yale University Press, 1995.
68. Hellman CG. Culture, Health, and Illness (3rd ed). Oxford, UK: Butterworth–Heinemann, 1994.

Annotated Bibliography

Redman BC. The Process of Patient Education (8th ed). St. Louis: Mosby, 1996. A classic text on patient education revised and updated seven times since 1968. Comprehensive and very readable, with practical clinical ideas clearly illustrating documented pedagogical theory. Most of the clinical illustrations are taken from nursing or general health education situations and can be readily understood by any health care provider. Extensive suggestions are given for planning, presenting, and evaluating educational materials related to health care. The Appendix includes study questions for each chapter.

Lorig K. Patient Education: A Practical Approach. St. Louis: Mosby, 1992. A perfect book for the health care professional who desires to gain knowledge about teaching groups of people. Logically presented practical ideas for conceiving, designing, and evaluating patient education programs. Ideas presented come primarily from the author's work with an extensive arthritis patient education research program that involved thousands of people. In the beginning of the book, the author directs the reader to chapters that will answer problems such as "doctors won't participate," "patients aren't motivated," and "how do I deal with talkative, quiet, belligerent, etc., patients?" The quiet practical wisdom in this book will carry you well beyond patient education.

Davis CM. Patient Practitioner Interaction: An Experiential Manual for Developing the Art of Health Care (3rd ed). Thorofare, NJ: Slack Inc, 1998. The aim of this book is to facilitate the development of health care professionals who are skilled in the establishment of the relational foundations for effective patient-practitioner interaction and education. The author provides numerous individual and group activities designed to help students and practitioners better understand themselves, patients, and the complex and varied situations in which they will find themselves in everyday clinical practice. The first section of the book focuses on expanding awareness of self and exploring personal beliefs and values that one brings into patient-practitioner encounters. The second section focuses on interactions with others and includes chapters on establishing helping relationships, identifying appropriate communication strategies for use with a variety of types of patients, and developing effective approaches to patient education.

Guidelines for Reflective Journal Writing during Clinical Experiences

By now you are familiar with the process of writing reflective journals through your experiences in PT Seminar and other courses. During your clinical education experiences, you will continue this process of reflective journal writing. In addition, you will have other opportunities for reflection and critical analysis of practice (yours and others) as you engage in dialogue with your clinical instructor and other staff members, students, and your regional clinical coordinator while you are completing your internships.

The following are some guidelines for your journal writing during clinical experiences:

- Make at least one journal entry every 2 weeks during your 14-week experiences. Feel free to write more if you wish. At least seven journal entries should be written and submitted to your regional clinical coordinator during the semester.
- Do not make your journals merely documentary (i.e., don't just catalog what you did or saw on a particular day or during the week). Your activity logs are for that purpose. Instead, use your journal writing for the following kinds of reflection that may focus on yourself, your patients and/or their caregivers, the clinical setting and professional interactions in that setting, professional roles, etc.:

    Thought work—puzzling over a situation; re-enacting and reconstructing what happened so you can gain a deeper understanding.

    Writing about a "lesson learned"—What did you learn? How did you learn it? Why was this a good learning experience? Or was it?

Writing about your feelings about people (self, patient, others) or situations that arise in the clinical setting.

Writing about how you see yourself changing during the course of the affiliation (i.e., your personal and professional development over time). Where are you at the beginning of the internship? Where are you at the end? Have you changed? How? In what ways?

This list is not necessarily all inclusive—just something to get you started.

9

Understanding and Influencing Patient Receptivity to Change: The Patient-Practitioner Collaborative Model

Gail M. Jensen, Christopher D. Lorish, and Katherine F. Shepard

This is a brief story of a physical therapist resident who works in a clinical residency program with an expert clinical tutor.

A resident with 5 years of clinical experience is working hard to be more systematic in musculoskeletal assessment. He is evaluating a woman with persistent neck and arm pain following a long course with upper quarter problems after a car accident 2 years ago. The patient has not worked since the accident. The resident sees this patient as a potentially tough case and performs an initial evaluation, which takes the resident more than the allotted 45 minutes. After three visits with the patient, the resident is stumped and frustrated. He cannot isolate any problems and is convinced that perhaps this patient has another agenda and, after any litigation is completed, the symptoms will disappear.

The resident decides to consult his mentor about this difficult case. The mentor skillfully does a quick reassessment by getting the patient to distinguish between the major areas of pain. She asks questions that focus not just on the patient's report of symptoms relative to where they are on the body chart, but also on how they relate to activities in the patient's life. The mentor then has the patient identify what valued activities she has lost because of this accident. The most important activity becomes a major goal for the patient and therapist to work toward with the intervention and exercise program. As the mentor performs the physical assessment, she assists the patient with her movements, carefully monitoring the patient's report of change in symptoms, and encouraging slow and steady movements. As the resident observes, it appears as if the patient is fully cooperative with the mentor. Together, resident and mentor work out a contract with the patient to begin a slow-paced exercise program based on simple movements aimed at giving the patient control over the pain. This program is connected to activities in the patient's daily life.

What does this story tell about understanding and teaching patients? Therapists identify the role of educator, teacher, or facilitator as part of their overall role. When asked about their approach to evaluation and intervention, therapists are likely to focus on identifying the problem(s), the patient's goals, their working hypotheses, their plan for intervention, their diagnosis, and trying to manage the patient within a limited number of visits. Although they mention considering patient goals, physical therapists are unlikely to talk about doing any specific assessment of the patient's beliefs and health behaviors as they relate to a fundamental aspect of most physical therapy interventions—exercise. Not talking about exercise with a patient is like specifying a trip destination without examining a map to identify possible routes. On the other hand, experienced therapists may talk about "reading patients" or "connecting with patients." But what does that mean? Are such things aspects of evaluation and intervention that are part of communicating well and being nice to the patient, or is there more to it?

Chapter Objectives

After completing this chapter, the reader will be able to

1. Discuss the central role of patient-practitioner interactions as part of the therapeutic process.
2. Identify the primary factors that affect adherence, including patient characteristics, disease variables, treatment variables, and patient-practitioner relationship variables.
3. Discuss and apply explanatory models for patient behavior in physical therapy practice.

4. Describe the four-step model for patient-practitioner collaboration that can be integrated into clinical practice.
5. Demonstrate several practical strategies for enhancing patient self-efficacy.
6. Give examples of patient cases that demonstrate application of the patient-practitioner collaboration approach as contrasted with the "professional as expert approach."

The goal of this chapter, in conjunction with Chapter 10, is to provide therapists with practical ideas based on sound theoretical concepts of strategies to enhance patient learning and motivation to follow treatment. The patient-therapist interaction, which is a fundamental aspect of the therapeutic process, is the focus of many of the practical approaches discussed in the chapter. It is out of this interaction that patient and therapist learn about each other, which helps when deciding what actions to take. The therapeutic process is more than assessment and treatment of musculoskeletal impairment. It involves the therapist in understanding and mediating the patient's belief system with the therapist's own. A process of collaborative problem solving and negotiation between the therapist and the patient is necessary to find mutually acceptable treatment goals and treatments. This process may seem unimportant to those comfortable prescribing treatment and expecting the patient's dutiful adherence, but treatment adherence data suggest that patients are frequently not dutiful. Patients often do more or less than prescribed, which puts them at risk for treatment side effects, slow progress, or no progress. By involving patients in the treatment decision making, patient learning becomes self-interested.

In his writing on the role of behavioral diagnosis in medicine, Bartlett[1] says the following:

> Few physicians would think of prescribing a medication without first diagnosing the probable cause of the illness. Yet the same clinicians, when confronted with the problem of behavior change, frequently do not realize that the influences of behavior are multiple and complex. Instead, when confronted with patient non-adherence, they tend to assume that the patient either does not understand or is not motivated. They do not realize that knowledge and motivation are only two of many variables that can influence behavior.

Therapists are involved on a daily basis in teaching or facilitating patient learning, whether by demonstrating the use of proper body mechanics, improving posture, teaching exercise, or providing advice on more efficient movement.[2] A core aspect of teaching patients involves helping them assume responsibility for their health.[3,4] The need for such responsibility on the part of patients is one of the reasons that the use of the term *adherence* or *cooperation* has been suggested over the use of the term *compliance* because of the connotation of patients as passive recipients of professionals' advice.[5] Enhancing patient cooperation or motivating patients is an essential aspect of the therapist's intervention in assisting patients to return to maximal function in their daily lives.[2] Because therapists often take for granted that the patient will do what he or she recommends, they tend to label the patient as unmotivated, lazy, noncompliant, or malingering if the treatment regimen is not followed. Such labels have pejorative connotations that are not helpful, because they remove responsibility from the therapist and provide little guidance for helping the patient overcome barriers to exercising.

Low patient compliance or noncooperation is a significant problem in a wide range of diseases, in all socioeconomic groups, and in various practice settings. Compliance ranges are generally from 30% to 60% for most medical regimens.[5–7] Factors related to non-adherence include patient personal and disease factors as well as treatment and patient-practitioner relationship variables (Table 9-1).[6] There are very little data in physical therapy about patient adherence to exercise regimens.[8–10] A study of physiotherapists and patients in the Netherlands reported that primary factors related to non-adherence were barriers that a patient perceives and encounters, lack of positive feedback, and degree of the patient's perceived helplessness.[9] Turk, a well-known researcher in the area of adherence, summarizes the need for physical therapists to attend to adherence:

> Physical therapists must become as concerned about facilitating compliance as they are about developing an optimal exercise regimen. They need to focus on fostering motivation by influencing the patient's beliefs and attitudes and ultimately their behavior.[11]

Physical therapists know that they are more likely to achieve patient cooperation or adherence when they try to understand the patient's perspective about the condition and its effects. This perspective is the patient's unique interpretation that incorporates sociocultural, emotional, and cognitive factors, which determine the patient's response to the illness.[5–7] The patient's perspective and the process of trying to understand it can be likened to the teacher-student model, in which the student (or patient) is the "empty vessel" into which the teacher (or therapist) pours his or her wisdom and knowledge. For example, exercise is a common health behavior in which therapists often want

Table 9-1   Thirty-Six Factors Related to Treatment Non-Adherence

---

Personal variables (patient)
  Characteristics of the individual
  Sensory disturbance
  Forgetfulness
  Lack of understanding
  Conflicting health benefits
  Competing sociocultural concepts of disease and treatment
  Apathy and pessimism
  Previous history of non-adherence
  Failure to recognize need for treatment
  Health beliefs
  Dissatisfaction with practitioner
  Lack of social support
  Family instability
  Environment that supports non-adherence
  Conflicting demands (e.g., poverty, unemployment)
  Lack of resources
Disease variables
  Chronicity of condition
  Stability of symptoms
  Characteristics of the disorder
Treatment variables
  Characteristics of treatment setting
  Absence of continuity of care
  Long waiting time
  Long time between referral and appointment
  Timing of referral
  Absence of individual appointment
  Inconvenience
  Inadequate supervision by professionals
  Characteristics of treatment
  Complexity of treatment
  Duration of treatment
  Expense
Relationship variables (patient-practitioner)
  Inadequate communication
  Poor rapport
  Attitudinal and behavioral conflicts
  Failure of practitioner to elicit feedback from patient
  Patient dissatisfaction

Source: Reprinted with permission from D Meichenbaum, DC Turk. Facilitating Treatment Adherence. New York: Plenum, 1987.

their patients and clients to engage. Using the empty vessel metaphor as the model of the patient's learning, the therapist who provides knowledge (i.e., gives the patient information through teaching, written materials, or classes about his or her condition or problem) may conclude that if a patient does not improve, he or she should be taught more until the vessel is filled with the right information. However, more knowledge does not necessarily lead to a change in a patient's health behavior.[3,12] Following a treatment plan requires that the patient (1) chooses to do so, (2) knows when to enact the plan, (3) has the psychomotor skills to perform the plan, and (4) remain motivated to follow through until the problem resolves. Thus, although treatment and knowledge of the condition are important, the patient's initial and long-term motivation are critical elements. To understand them, therapists must understand the patient's perspective. Therapists are more likely to facilitate change in the patient's health behaviors by understanding the patient's belief system, which is usually rational and based on culture, past experiences, and support systems.[3,5,12]

This ability to effectively understand the patient's perspective will be increasingly important as the changes in health care affect practice. Because of shrinking health care resources, therapists will be under increased pressure to set priorities and maximize resources. There will be increased pressure to demonstrate that the treatment is effective in improving health outcomes.[13] The pressure on therapists to teach patients and families in a smaller number of visits will increase. Designing therapeutic interventions with the highest likelihood of patient follow-through and adherence will be an essential factor in assessing patient outcomes.[3,8,13] In response to societal needs and demands, increased emphasis on patient education, prevention, and health promotion is found in federal guidelines and in the policies and guidelines of the American Physical Therapy Association (Table 9-2).[2,14–17]

Explanatory Models of Practice

Every therapist has one or more explanatory models in mind when she or he works with patients. These models usually develop by thinking about the patient's wants and needs, how to understand more about a patient's receptivity to change, and how to help a patient do more exercises at home. Just as a patient comes to the clinic with ideas about his or her condition, its immediate and long-term consequences, and the types of treatment that have and have not helped, therapists have their own beliefs for explaining the cause of the patient's condition and the patient's response to treatment. The therapist uses this explanatory framework, or model, to guide patient evaluation and treatment decision making. These models may reflect beliefs about teaching and learning or motivation and behavioral

Table 9-2 Examples of Guidelines for Patient Education, Health Promotion, and Prevention

Source	Examples
U.S. Department of Health and Human Services. Healthy People 2010 (2nd ed). 2 vols. Washington, DC: GPO, 2000. http://www.health.gov/healthypeople	**Overall aim** Improving the health of each individual, the health of communities, and the health of the nation through promoting health and preventing illness, disability, and premature death. **Priority areas** Broad categories, such as health promotion (changes in behavioral choices), health protection (changes in the physical and social environment), access to health care, and clinical preventive services (access to screening, immunization, and counseling).
Commission on Accreditation in Physical Therapy Education, American Physical Therapy Association. Evaluative Criteria for Accreditation of Education Programs for the Preparation of Physical Therapists. Alexandria, VA: American Physical Therapy Association, 2000.	**Graduates of the program** Identify and assess the health needs of individuals, groups, and communities, including screening, prevention, and wellness programs that are appropriate to physical therapy.
Evaluative Criteria for Accreditation of Education Programs for the Preparation of Physical Therapist Assistants. Alexandria, VA: American Physical Therapy Association, 2000.	**Graduates of the program** Interact with patients and families in a manner that provides the desired psychosocial support, including the recognition of cultural and socioeconomic differences. Participate in the teaching of other health care providers, patients, and families.
American Physical Therapy Association Education Division. Normative Model of Physical Therapist Professional Education. Alexandria, VA: American Physical Therapy Association, 2000.	**Practice management expectations for physical therapists in the areas of prevention, health promotion, fitness, and wellness** Provide culturally competent physical therapy services for prevention, health promotion, fitness, and wellness to individuals, groups, and communities. Promote health and quality of life by providing information on health promotion, fitness, wellness, disease, impairment, functional limitation, disability, and health risks related to age, gender, culture, and lifestyle, within the scope of physical therapy practice.

Table 9-2 *continued*

Source	Examples
American Physical Therapy Association Guide to Physical Therapist Practice. Phys Ther 2001;81.	**Goal:** Patient management through prevention in promoting health, wellness, and fitness, and in performing screening activities. **Examples of roles in prevention and in promotion of health, wellness, and fitness:** *Primary prevention*: preventing a target condition in a susceptible population through specific measures as general health promotion. *Prevention screening activities*: identification of lifestyle factors that may lead to increased risk for health problems. *Tertiary prevention and providing information* limiting the degree of disability and promoting rehabilitation and restoration of function in patients with chronic and irreversible diseases.

change. The patient also comes with certain beliefs and expectations about what he or she wants from the provider about the sources and consequences of the illness.

Kleinman[18] initiated the concept of explanatory models to analyze problems that may arise during the clinical encounter between the patient and the provider. Kleinman defined *explanatory models* as "the notions patients, families, and practitioners have about a specific illness episode."[18] These explanatory models represent the patient's attempt to make sense out of the change from "ease" to "disease." These beliefs often incorporate an attempt by the patient to self-disprove and ascribe a course to the condition. The patient's diagnosis and causal beliefs bring into play beliefs about the likely consequences of the condition, the time before the condition resolves, and treatments (home remedies and prescribed). Kleinman[18] and others[12,19] speculate that the effectiveness of clinical communication and the patient's health care outcome may be a function of the extent of discrepancy between the patient's explanatory model and the provider's explanatory model. For example, if a patient comes to physical therapy with the expectation that the therapist will fix his or her problem and will provide lots of massage for his or her sore muscles, but the therapist expects to get this patient on a home exercise program in one visit, there is likely to be a conflict in their interactions, or disappointment when either realizes that she or he is not getting what was expected.

The dominant explanatory model shared by many practitioners is the biomedical model, which focuses on pathology and the disease process, physical symptoms that are a result of the disease process, and the medical intervention that will fix those physical symptoms and the problem.[20] Although useful, the deficiencies of this model as a way of thinking about practice are becoming increasingly apparent. Because of recent discussions in physical therapy about the critical importance of patient outcomes, more emphasis is being placed on addressing the patient's functional needs and health status, rather than just documenting changes in physical impairment measures (e.g., range of motion or strength) and assuming that those changes will result in a positive functional outcome in patients' lives.[21,22] Such emphasis puts the therapist in touch with part of the patient's perspective, because it requires that the therapist know the patient's functional goals. However, this emphasis ignores the other elements of the patient's explanatory model that may affect treatment adherence.

Another example of an explanatory model is a disablement schema, such as the International Classification of Impairments, Disabilities, and Handicaps.[21] A model like this provides therapists with common terms used to think more deeply about the fundamental elements of practice. For example, a patient who has a disease like diabetes, which results in peripheral vascular disease and a subsequent lower extremity amputation, has several areas of *impairment* as a result of the pathology and medical intervention. Impairments, such as loss of range of motion, strength, and endurance, are likely to be measured and documented. In turn, these measures lead to certain *functional limitations* in the patient's daily life, such as limitations in ambulation or in self-care activities. Over time, these changes in the patient's function may, in turn, lead to changes in his or her ability to work or care for himself or herself; such a condition would be considered a *handicap*. As seen in Figure 9-1, a disablement process affects individuals not only at the organ and body level, but also on personal and social levels. Physical therapists' primary role in facilitating patient movement and enhancing function has to do with all of these areas—physical, personal, and social.[21] Achieving these goals requires that the therapist explore the patient's treatment goals and explanatory model to determine possible treatment barriers.

There is increased discussion about the need for health care providers to be more patient centered than provider centered.[12,20] This patient-centered focus places increased emphasis on the quality of the therapeutic encounter between the patient and provider; therefore, therapeutic intervention must be skillfully implemented from the initial contact.

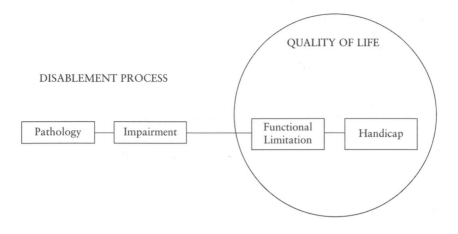

Figure 9-1 Disablement concepts. Use of a conceptual model, such as the model displayed, assists the therapist in attending to and understanding how the disease affects the patient's body, as well as the patient's life. (Adapted from A Jette. Physical disablement concepts for physical therapy research and practice. Phys Ther 1994;74:380.)

Patient-Practitioner Collaborative Model

We propose that a patient-practitioner collaborative model can be used to help physical therapists and physical therapist assistants focus their interventions on the patient's needs and improve the patient's adherence to treatment. This model integrates concepts from several other models in medicine and physical therapy (Figure 9-2).[6,8,12,20,23] At the center of the model is the patient in the context of his or her life. This includes the patient's beliefs, attitudes, skills, and feelings, shaped by a lifetime of his or her diseases, others' diseases and illnesses, and his or her support system. It is useful to distinguish two conceptualizations of ill health—*disease* and *illness*. *Disease* represents what went wrong with the body as a machine, whereas *illness* represents the person's experience of a disease on his or her life. Patients come to physical therapists with many beliefs about their illness experiences. Such beliefs may or may not be scientifically correct. Diseases, on the other hand, are diagnosed by the therapist using the biomedical model. The focus of most practitioners' evaluative processes is finding out the diagnosis or diagnoses; the patient's illness experience may not be explicitly understood by the practitioner. As a consequence, the patient's and therapist's goals and explanations are disconnected. Connecting with the patient means developing a relationship that allows probing

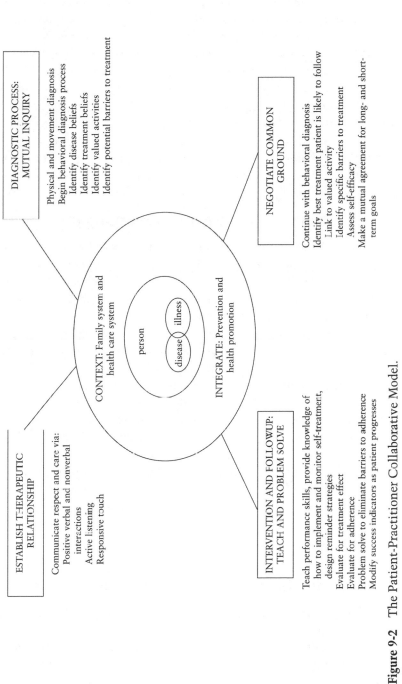

Figure 9-2 The Patient-Practitioner Collaborative Model.

the patient's beliefs as the first step of negotiating a treatment. We argue here that understanding disease and illness is a critical aspect of therapeutic intervention. Essential to the therapist's role as a professional is understanding not only the context of the patient's life and the health care system, but also how these contexts influence manifestations of the patient's disease and illness. Finally, through the process of persuasion, education, and support, therapists need to teach patients how to prevent disease or relapse and promote health. The model we propose has four phases: (1) establishing the therapeutic relationship, (2) diagnosing through mutual inquiry, (3) finding common ground through negotiation, and (4) intervening and following up. This model can easily be integrated into the physical therapy evaluation process. Table 9-3 provides an example of a patient-centered approach, compared to a provider-centered approach, to evaluation and treatment.

Establish the Therapeutic Relationship

The concept of the patient as a person is central to all aspects of therapeutic evaluation and intervention. The evaluative process begins with establishing a therapeutic relationship or connecting with a patient during the interview. Doing so is crucial for making the patient feel comfortable revealing her or his beliefs and feelings about the evaluation and treatment. Verbal and nonverbal behaviors contribute to this therapeutic relationship. Although some may think that these behaviors are common sense, when practitioners are focused on gathering evaluative data regarding clinical signs and symptoms, they are often unaware of their verbal and nonverbal interactions. For example, when under pressure to get the needed evaluative data, a busy therapist may not make eye contact, or she or he may cut off a patient's story and gather only disease data without asking about the patient's concerns. The message to the patient is that the condition is important, not the patient. The patient is reduced to the facts about his or her symptoms. Table 9-4 provides an overview of key behaviors that facilitate or impede the therapist's connection with the patient.[8,24] Consistent and timely use of behaviors that facilitate connection has a great deal to do with whether the patient reveals her or his beliefs and becomes a willing partner in treatment.

Diagnostic Process as Mutual Inquiry

Some form of the diagnostic process is usually at the heart of a physical therapy evaluation. This process begins the second the patient and therapist meet. The process usually intensifies as the therapist interviews the patient and begins the physical examination. We advocate that, along

Table 9-3 Contrasting Approaches to Patient Evaluation and Management

Patient case: Mrs. Olsen is an 86-year-old woman with thoracic pain and newly diagnosed osteoporosis who comes to physical therapy for evaluation and treatment.

Provider-centered approach: professional as expert	*Evaluation concept*	*Patient-centered approach: professional as teacher*
Standing in treatment room with patient sitting on table. Little eye contact, reading chart as evaluation begins. Collecting data and recording on clipboard.	Establish therapeutic relationship.	Sitting face-to-face with patient. Being aware of patient's thoracic pain and providing gentle palpation of the most acute areas as patient sits on table. Engaging in personal dialogue and finding some area of common interest with the patient.
Focusing on gathering data on the joints involved, including the activities that make the symptoms worse or better. Assessing the irritability of the patient's condition (moderate), so that the therapist is able to perform a good physical assessment and localize the involved thoracic joints.	Diagnostic process of mutual inquiry.	Identifying the areas of the thoracic spine where primary symptoms occur. Discovering the patient's intense fear of fractures from the osteoporosis. Identifying that the patient's primary goal is to pick up a grandchild. Finding out that the patient walks in the mall with a group of friends 3 days a week.
Establishing that joint mobilization, grades I and II, will be the appropriate place to start. Discussing with the patient the prognosis that the manual therapy along with an exercise program should eliminate the symptoms in 2–3 weeks.	Negotiate common ground.	Identifying that patient is most likely to exercise along with her mall walking. Setting mutual short-term goals with patient to become proficient with her exercise program. Setting the long-term goal for the patient to be able to pick up her grandchild. Performing an initial assessment of self-efficacy that shows that patient's fear of fracture needs to be addressed.

Table 9-3 *continued*

Provider-centered approach: professional as expert	Evaluation concept	Patient-centered approach: professional as teacher
Proceeding with joint techniques; reassessment shows increase in movement. Giving patient a sheet of home exercises that include trunk extension and beginning mobility exercises for the trunk. Writing on the sheet for the patient to do each exercise five times twice a day.	Intervention: teaching and problem solving.	Adding an exercise log as a reminder strategy. Requesting that the patient call in with any questions about the exercise. Telling the patient that you will see her in 2 weeks, when she has achieved the short-term goal.
Noting patient complaints of difficulty in doing exercises. Reviewing the exercises, performing another session of mobilization, and adding two self-mobilization exercises. Telling the patient that you will see her in 2 weeks.	Follow-up: teaching and problem solving.	Asking the patient to demonstrate the exercises. Asking the patient how many times she did not exercise and why. Finding out that the patient has had trouble with two of the most difficult exercises. Working specifically with the patient on those exercises. Reinterpreting the patient's symptoms, because what appeared to be a barrier was the patient's fear of fracture.

with inquiring about the movement dysfunction the patient has, the therapist should begin to do an explicit assessment of the potential for patient adherence or cooperation by beginning to formulate a behavioral diagnosis.[1,8] This information is crucial for understanding potential barriers to the ideal treatment. Typical barriers include the patient not knowing how and when to do the treatment; not being confident in her or his ability to perform the treatment; having beliefs or values incompatible with the treatment; and not having the time, equipment, or support to do the treatment.

Assessing what the patient knows and believes about his or her condition and treatment is a good place to start. This assessment includes identifi-

Table 9-4 Interactional Behaviors That Facilitate or Impede the Therapist's Ability to Connect with Patients

---

Connecting behaviors
 Verbal
   Greeting the patient in a friendly manner
   Making positive comments
   Inquiring about the patient
   Reflecting on the patient's feelings
   Clarifying the patient's needs
 Nonverbal
   Facing the patient
   Making eye contact
   Leaning toward patient
   Displaying an open posture
   Using nonverbal cues to acknowledge active listening
Behaviors that impede the therapist's connection with patients
   Acting busy
   Reading notes
   Doing tasks
   Using medical jargon
   Cutting off patient's story
   Responding only to disease information
   Failing to give feedback
   Showing little empathy
   Not asking about the patient's concerns

Sources: D Meichenbaum, DC Turk. Facilitating Treatment Adherence. New York: Plenum, 1987; GM Jensen, C Lorish. Promoting patient cooperation with exercise programs: linking research, theory, and practice. Arthritis Care Res 1994;7:181; and R Carkcuff. The Art of Helping (7th ed). Amherst, MA: Human Resources Press, 1993.

cation of the patient's beliefs about the condition, the consequences of the condition, and what treatments he or she is likely to follow.[1,3,8,20] The therapist needs to identify the patient's beliefs about the positive and negative consequences of the disease or condition and how it is affecting the patient's life.

Sample questions for this assessment include

How would you describe the problem that brought you to physical therapy?
What do you think caused the problem?
Why do you think this happened to you?

The therapist must also find out about the patient's symptom experience. Some sample questions about the patient's symptom experience include

What things can you no longer do in your work or home life as a result of
your condition?

What daily activities do you need to get back to as quickly as possible?

How do others with whom you live react to your condition?

How does your body tell you that you are better or worse, and what
causes these changes?

The therapist will also want to know about the patient's treatment beliefs,
including past treatment, home treatment, and future treatment. The therapist should also identify any potential barriers that the patient may have to
treatment by asking questions like

What treatments, home remedies, or activities seem to help, and what
are you not willing to try?

What are the worst things you anticipate about treatment?

Have you ever tried exercise?

If you were to do the treatment, what difficulties would you have doing it?

Why is it so important to identify these patient beliefs? The answers to
questions like these reveal much about what the patient knows and does
not know about her or his condition, what activity the patient wants to
recover that can motivate treatment adherence, and what alternative treatments the patient may be doing in addition to the prescribed treatment.
Physical therapists are ultimately interested in facilitating patients' self-
care in terms of their movement problems. Exercise is likely to be one of the
health behaviors that is part of the treatment regimen carried out at home.
As the therapist asks the patient to reveal more about his or her understanding of the condition and what possible treatment she or he is likely to follow, the patient is also gaining information about the therapist by observing
and responding to the questions and developing or modifying beliefs about
the therapist's competence and trustworthiness.[6,20] By inquiring about the
patient's beliefs, the therapist demonstrates interest in the patient's illness
and disease process.

Finding Common Ground through Negotiation

As the therapist continues the evaluation and behavioral diagnostic process, she or he is negotiating treatment goals with the patient. The
essential question is not just what is the best treatment for this condition,
but what is the best treatment that this patient is likely to follow. To answer
this question, the therapist must continue with the behavioral diagnosis and
find out more specifically about other potential barriers (e.g., physical, sociocultural, and psychological) that were not revealed by the other questions.[1,8]

Table 9-5 Typical Positive and Negative Consequences Related to Exercise

Negative consequences
  Boring
  Takes too much time
  Too complicated
  Increases symptoms
  Takes too much energy
  Forget to do them
  Exercises have no purpose
Positive consequences
  More limber
  More energy
  Can do more valued activities
  Exercise with friends
  Feel stronger
  More independent
  Family is supportive

To discover these barriers, the therapist should begin by acknowledging that many patients find it difficult to follow an exercise program (Table 9-5). The therapist should then ask the patient

> What problems do you anticipate?
> What are your beliefs about exercise?
> What are the worst things about exercise, and what are the best things?
> What is the most important thing I can do to help you succeed?

A central aspect of the behavioral diagnosis process is the assessment of the patient's motivation to improve his or her condition. It is hoped that the patient has some important activity or symptom that will serve as a treatment goal to motivate treatment behavior. The therapist should determine what activity the patient wants most to recover, or what symptoms she or he wants most to control or eliminate.[12,19] In addition to the goal, the concept of *self-efficacy* (i.e., the state of belief in one's ability to accomplish a certain behavior) is a good predictor of motivation and behavior.[3,25] A patient also is more likely to follow the treatment if he or she believes that there is a high likelihood that the treatment will result in achieving the treatment goal. The patient's belief that the treatment will result in the desired outcome can be developed by reference to other successful patients, graded success experience with the treatment, or both. If the patient is not confident in her or his ability to perform the treatment, then practice opportunities for performing the treatment must be provided. Good questions for assessing the patient's motivation are

What is the most important activity that you wish to recover?
What symptoms do you wish to minimize first?
How confident are you in your ability to perform the exercise(s)?
Do you think these exercises will help you recover or return to your
    important activities?

The therapist should link the intervention to improving the patient's condition, so that he or she can return to valued activities and minimize the most bothersome symptoms. The therapist can then decide on reasonable short- and long-term goals with the patient and make a mutual agreement about the treatment regimen.

Teaching and Problem Solving during Intervention and Follow-Up

Instruction about the treatment regimen is critical.[3,4] Perhaps one of the most common mistakes is making the treatment regimen too complex (i.e., giving the patient too much to do with little specific instruction).[1,6] Although the therapist may believe that doing all 10 of the exercises is critical to a rapid change and that the patient can refer to the exercise handout, the likelihood of a patient's being able to successfully do all the exercises is probably quite low. If home exercise is part of the intervention, then patients should receive specific instruction in the psychomotor aspects of the exercise, clearly written instructions on what to do, specific tailoring of the exercise to the patient's lifestyle and valued activities, and, if necessary, reminder strategies to perform the exercise. The therapist should find out about social support and teach the family or significant others the exercises, if necessary. The following questions are helpful for assessing the patient's understanding of the treatment regimen:

Tell me about the home exercises you do. (Probe for exercise frequency,
    duration, and intensity.)
Can you demonstrate the exercise(s)?
What problems do you anticipate with fitting the treatment into your
    daily activities?
Do you have the necessary equipment?
Do you have a place where you can do the exercise(s)?
What should you do if the exercises are not working or are causing a negative change in symptoms?

When the patient returns for follow-up, the therapist should evaluate the patient not only for change in physical impairment measures and function, but also for treatment effect—present and future. The therapist will also

Table 9-6 Problem-Solving Skills for Practitioners

Key problem-solving steps
1. Define the problem in behavioral terms.
2. Encourage the patient to substitute general statements that he or she cannot do something with a specific application of what he or she cannot do and why.
3. Generate possible solutions for each problem or task.
4. Evaluate the positives and negatives of each solution and rank them from least practical to most practical.
5. Try out the solution. Stay flexible.
6. Reconsider the problem. Can the patient see anything different or positive about the problem?

Ideas for problem-solving methods
1. Talk to others.
2. Recall what things have worked in the past.
3. Imagine how someone else might cope.
4. Think of the future and potential barriers. Make a contingency plan.
5. Practice coping by rehearsing skills.
6. Look for a support system that provides advice and encouragement.
7. Use coping skills instead of giving up.

Source: Adapted from D Meichenbaum, DC Turk. Facilitating Treatment Adherence. New York: Plenum, 1987.

want to do some specific assessment for adherence to the regimen. Sample questions for assessment of adherence to the regimen include

Can you perform the exercise(s)?
What changes have you noticed, and what do you believe caused the changes?
Were there any negative consequences of doing the exercise(s)?
What problems did you run into in remembering to do the exercises?
What has happened with progress toward your valued activity goal?
When do you expect to notice some improvement in your condition?

Follow-up with the patient is likely to involve renegotiation and problem solving. These steps are necessary, because the patient's beliefs can change during the intervention. What was motivational or a barrier before may no longer be so because of the patient's continuing experience with the illness and treatment. The therapist will need to problem solve to eliminate any barriers to adherence. If necessary, she or he may modify the treatment, modify success indicators (if the patient has progressed), and confirm the patient's commitment to the goals. Table 9-6 provides a list of problem-solving skills that can be used when working with a variety of patients and families. These skills are general strategies and should be applied in concert with specific barriers, as described in the following section.

Removing Barriers to Treatment

Whether the patient follows the treatment regimen depends on the interaction between the therapist and the patient.[6,12,20] If the patient has a problem adhering to the intervention, the physical therapist needs to explore barriers to following the treatment. The therapist may also need to find ways to adapt or change the treatment goal and the time line to accommodate barriers that cannot be changed. Lorig and coworkers[3] outline a decision chart that can be used by the therapist for exploring with the patient how to improve adherence (Table 9-7). For example, if a patient cannot tell why he or she is not doing the exercises, the therapist may need to apply problem-solving steps as tools to access the patient's belief system. The therapist may begin by defining the problem, evaluating the positive and negative aspects of exercising, having the patient recall what has worked in the past, identifying a support system, and assisting the patient to focus on coping with the barriers instead of giving up (see Tables 9-6 and 9-7).

Role of Self-Efficacy

Several of the areas for exploration, renegotiation, and problem solving with the patient have to do with the concept of self-efficacy. Remember that *self-efficacy* is a person's belief that she or he can accomplish a behavior.[3,25]

There are four strategies therapists can focus on to enhance a patient's self-efficacy. Therapists usually begin with skills mastery, making sure the patient can perform the exercise. Often, a task can be broken into smaller tasks. The patient needs feedback about his or her performance of the exercise to increase the likelihood of mastery of the skill. See Chapter 10 for more information on effective feedback strategies. Goal setting and contracting are other methods of providing feedback.[3,25]

Modeling is another strategy for increasing self-efficacy. In one-to-one patient care, the therapist is often the model. In group education settings, the model should be most like the patient, matching as many characteristics as possible (e.g., age, sex, ethnic origin, socioeconomic status). The therapist may consider having another patient with a similar condition demonstrate. One reason why group educational intervention can be helpful is that patients are modeling to each other and, therefore, enhancing their own self-efficacy.[3,25]

Table 9-7   Suggestions for Improving Patient Adherence

Problem	Patient's response	Suggestion
Can the patient tell you why he or she is not doing the exercise?	Yes	Listen and problem solve.
Does the patient believe that adherence to the regimen will help the problem?	No	Explore the patient's belief system. Expand on the patient's current belief system.
Does the patient understand the exercise program?	No	Teach the patient why exercises are important.
Does the patient have the skills to do the exercises?	No	Teach the patient the skills. Break the regimen into smaller parts. Give the patient feedback on his or her performance.
Does adherence with the exercise program have negative consequences for the patient?	Yes	Adapt the regimen to the patient's complications. Reinterpret the patient's symptoms (if necessary).
Does non-adherence have positive consequences for the patient?	Yes	Problem solve with the patient. Provide a support structure for the patient.
Does the patient forget to do the exercises?	Yes	Design memory strategies.
Does the patient believe that he or she cannot do the exercises?	Yes	Increase the patient's self-efficacy.
What if the patient does not want to adhere to the regimen?	—	That is okay. You have tried your best.

Source: K Lorig (ed). Patient Education: A Practical Approach (2nd ed). Thousand Oaks, CA: Sage, 1996.

Two other strategies for enhancing self-efficacy include reinterpretation of physiologic signs and symptoms and persuasion. The reinterpretation of physiologic signs and symptoms can be a powerful strategy for patients. First, the therapist must find out what patients believe about their problems, or how they interpret their present symptoms (this is similar to what was discussed as part of the behavioral diagnosis). For example, if the patient believes that pain with exercise is a sign of more damage to the joint, he or she is not likely to exercise. The patient must be taught to reinterpret her or his beliefs about exercise and the symptoms. The therapist may need to teach the patient to distinguish between different types of pain. Persuasion is another common method used by therapists. For example, in verbal persuasion, the therapist urges the patient to do more by giving verbal support and encouragement during exercise. As a last resort, the therapist should emphasize to the patient the negative consequences of not doing the exercise. This strategy of emphasizing what a patient might lose should be used with care and only after some initial problem solving has been done. Although some therapists may quickly focus on sharing their knowledge with the patient by telling him or her all of the bad things that could happen, an initial focus on the positive consequences of treatment is an important aspect of patient-practitioner collaboration.[3,25]

Self-Efficacy Patient Cases

This chapter discusses the central importance of collaborating with patients in designing treatment interventions that are likely to be followed. The following three cases are grounded in the collaborative model and demonstrate specific application of concepts from self-efficacy theory. The reader should try to identify the self-efficacy concepts being used in each case.

Case 9-1

Bill is a 34-year-old man who came to physical therapy after surgical repair of his knee, which he hurt during a pickup basketball game. He currently works as a plumber. He was given a home exercise program but found the exercises hard to do, because they caused more pain. During his last visit, he said that he did not think exercise was doing him any good, and he wanted to quit and just get pain medication from the doctor.

What now? First, you attempt to understand more about Bill and explore more of his current life circumstances. When you probe more specifically about his home life, his family, and his financial status, you find that he is afraid of not being able to hold his job as a plumber because of his knee problem. He and his wife have a 2-year-old child and another baby on the way. He believes that his knee will not get better through exercise, because he associates exercise with pain. His concerns about potential unemployment and failure to fulfill his role as a husband and father and his association of exercise with pain contribute to his inability to adhere to his exercise therapy.

You identify the barriers to Bill's exercises—time, pain with exercise, and his belief that exercise doesn't matter. You work with him to set up two specific times per day to exercise that are part of his routine schedule. One of these times, he exercises at work, and the other at home. You revise the exercise program so that the pain brought on by the exercises is only temporary, and you reteach Bill the exercises by doing some joint problem solving. You also work with Bill on reinterpretation of pain as a negative consequence of exercise. You teach him about different types of pain and introduce the use of ice for pain relief.

Case 9-2

Helen has worked with physical therapists several times over her 10-year course of rheumatoid arthritis. Each time she sees a therapist, she does the exercise for a while and then quits. You are seeing her for a specific shoulder problem, but you realize in the course of treatment that Helen really needs more support for her exercise and would benefit from being involved in a regular fitness program. As you begin to discuss possibilities with her, she immediately says she could never go to a gym or health club. She says that she has arthritis and will never be fit.

At the next visit, you arrange for one of your friends who has rheumatoid arthritis and participates in the arthritis water exercise program at a local community pool to come and talk with Helen. She talks with Helen about the program, discusses her continued battle with the disease, and sets up a time to take Helen to the next class. Helen agrees. You are glad that you decided not to be a role model for Helen about the benefits of water exercise. Calling on this friend seemed to provide Helen with a powerful example of what she could do.

Case 9-3

Mr. Runningbear is an elderly Native American man who has experienced a mild stroke. He experienced a slow onset of loss of strength and increasing numbness on his right side. He has been sent to physical therapy for a home exercise program to improve his walking. In exploring with your patient his beliefs about the stroke, you find out that he is quite concerned that the stroke was some form of punishment for past events in his life.

You initiate a home program and are able to tie several of the exercises and daily functional activities to Mr. Runningbear's goal of working on his truck again. Still, you are concerned about his thoughts about deserving the stroke. You decide to contact Mr. Runningbear's daughter. After some initial discussion with her and the physician's assistant who referred Mr. Running-bear to you, you all decide to call on a Native American spiritual healer to identify some possible spiritual disturbance with your patient. In this case, you decide to enlist others to assist in persuasion and, perhaps, some reinter-pretation of your patient's physiologic symptoms.

Summary

Although little research has been done in physical therapy regarding patient-centered communication, there have been several studies in medicine investigating whether patient-centered communication makes any difference to the patient and to her or his health outcome. There is strong evidence that more patient-centered communication does lead to enhanced patient satisfaction and more positive outcomes.[26–29] In effective use of the patient-centered approach, the physician does the following:

- Asks questions about the patient's complaints, concerns, understanding of the problem, expectations, and feelings
- Shows support and empathy
- Allows the patient to express himself or herself completely
- Allows the patient to perceive that a full discussion of the problem has taken place
- Allows the patient to ask more questions
- Uses information and educational materials for patients
- Is willing to share decision making with patients

We have presented a model for patient-practitioner collaboration that, we hope, can be useful in clinical practice. This chapter provides the reader with many examples of how to use this patient-practitioner collaboration model in designing specific educational interventions for patients and families. Chapter 10 continues the discussion on successful educational interventions by focusing on facilitating patient adherence to healthy life styles. We firmly believe that atten-tion to and integration of adherence procedures should be part of every physical therapist's and physical therapist assistant's therapeutic interactions with all patients. The following treatment adherence guidelines, suggested by Meichen-baum and Turk,[6] provide a good summary of the key ideas in this chapter:

Guideline 1   Anticipate non-adherence.
Guideline 2   Consider the prescribed self-care regimen from the
              patient's perspective.
Guideline 3   Foster a collaborative relationship based on negotiation.

Guideline 4   Be patient-oriented.
Guideline 5   Customize treatment.
Guideline 6   Enlist family support.
Guideline 7   Provide a system of continuity and accessibility.
Guideline 8   Make use of other health care providers as well as
               community resources.
Guideline 9   Repeat everything.
Guideline 10   Do not give up.

References

1. Bartlett EE. Behavioral diagnosis: a practical approach to patient education. Patient Couns Health Educ 1982;4:29.
2. American Physical Therapy Association. Guide to physical therapist practice. Phys Ther 2001;81.
3. Lorig K (ed). Patient Education: A Practical Approach (3rd ed). Thousand Oaks, CA: Sage, 2000.
4. Redman BK. The Process of Patient Education (5th ed). St. Louis: Mosby, 1984;21.
5. Haynes R. Ten-year update on patient compliance research. Patient Educ Couns 1987;10:107.
6. Meichenbaum D, Turk DC. Facilitating Treatment Adherence. New York: Plenum, 1987.
7. Slujis EM, Knibbe J. Patient compliance with exercise: different theoretical approaches to short-term and long-term compliance. Patient Educ Couns 1991;17:191.
8. Jensen GM, Lorish C. Promoting patient cooperation with exercise programs: linking research, theory and practice. Arthritis Care Res 1994;7:181.
9. Slujis EM, Kok GJ, van der Zee J. Correlates of exercise compliance in physical therapy. Phys Ther 1993;73:771.
10. Jette AM. Improving patient cooperation with arthritis treatment regimens. Arthritis Rheum 1982;25:447.
11. Turk D. Correlates of exercise compliance in physical therapy [commentary]. Phys Ther 1993;73:783.
12. Glanz K, Lewis FM, Rimer B. Health Behavior and Health Education. San Francisco: Jossey-Bass, 1997;33.
13. Eddy D. Principles for making difficult decisions in difficult times. JAMA 1994;271:1792.
14. National Health Promotion and Disease Prevention Objectives. Healthy People 2000. DHHS Publication No. (PHS) 90-50212. Wash-

ington, DC: U.S. Department of Health and Human Services, GPO, 1990.

15. Commission on Accreditation in Physical Therapy Education, American Physical Therapy Association. Evaluative Criteria for Accreditation of Education Programs for the Preparation of Physical Therapists. Alexandria, VA: American Physical Therapy Association, 1998.

16. Commission on Accreditation in Physical Therapy Education, American Physical Therapy Association. Evaluative Criteria for Accreditation of Education Programs for the Preparation of Physical Therapist Assistants. Alexandria, VA: American Physical Therapy Association, 1998.

17. American Physical Therapy Association, Education Division. Coalitions for Consensus: A Normative Model of Professional Education. Alexandria, VA: American Physical Therapy Association, 2000.

18. Kleinman A. The Illness Narratives: Suffering, Healing, and the Human Condition. New York: Basic Books, 1987.

19. Levanthal H. The role of theory in the study of adherence to treatment and doctor-patient interactions. Med Care 1985;23:556.

20. Stewart M, Brown J, Weston W, et al. Patient-Centered Medicine: Transforming the Clinical Method. Thousand Oaks, CA: Sage, 1995.

21. Jette A. Physical disablement concepts for physical therapy research and practice. Phys Ther 1994;74:380.

22. Jette A. Outcomes research: shifting the dominant research paradigm in physical therapy. Phys Ther 1995;75:965.

23. Miller WL, Crabtree BF. Clinical Research: Conversing the Wall. In: Denzin NK, Lincoln YS (eds). Handbook of Qualitative Research (2nd ed). Thousand Oaks, CA: Sage, 2000;618.

24. Carkcuff R. The Art of Helping (7th ed). Amherst, MA: Human Resources Press, 1993.

25. Bandura A. Social Foundations of Thought and Action: A Social Cognitive Theory. Englewood Cliffs, NJ: Prentice-Hall, 1986.

26. Evans B, Kiellerup F, Stanley R, et al. A communication skills programme for increasing patient satisfaction with general practice consultations. Br J Med Psychol 1987;60:373.

27. Kaplan S, Greenfield S, Ware J. Assessing the effects of physician-patient interactions on the outcomes of chronic disease. Med Care 1989;275:5110.

28. Roter D, Hall J. Doctors Talking with Patients, Patients Talking with Doctors. Dover, MA: Auburn House, 1992.

29. Levinson W. Physician-Patient Communication [editorial]. JAMA 1994; 272:1619.

Annotated Bibliography

Bandura A. Self-Efficacy: The Exercise of Control. New York: WH Freeman, 1997. Bandura describes each of the core components of his self-efficacy work in great detail in the initial theory-based chapters. The second section of the book contains an excellent discussion of research that applies theory to practice across the broad areas of cognitive functions, health functions, clinical function, and organizational function. The chapter on perceived self-efficacy in health promoting behavior is of particular interest to physical therapists.

Green LS, Dreuter MW. Health Promotion Planning: An Ecological and Educational Approach (3rd ed). Mountain View, CA: Mayfield Press, 1999. An excellent resource for any physical therapist involved in health-promotion planning, implementation, and evaluation. The book provides detailed guidance for implementation of the PRECEDE (for identifying *p*redisposing, *r*einforcing, and *e*nabling factors in educational interventions)–PROCEED (for *p*olicy, *r*egulatory and *o*rganizational factors that need to be considered) model. The book also includes several case examples of how the model has been used in various community and institutional settings.

Klcinman A. The Illness Narratives: Suffering, Healing, and the Human Condition. New York: Basic Books, 1987. Dr. Klcinman is a psychiatrist and anthropologist who has written extensively in the area of medical anthropology. He is a strong advocate for bridging the gap between the patient and the practitioner. His work on explanatory models is used by many.

Lorig K (ed). Patient Education: A Practical Approach (3rd ed). Thousand Oaks, CA: Sage, 2000. This is a great book for clinicians. It is very readable, with lots of examples. The book takes the reader through a process of conceptualization, design, implementation and evaluation of patient education programs. The chapters on application of self-efficacy theory and other simple behavioral theories are exceedingly well done. The book contains a number of examples of how to create health education programs for groups.

Meichenbaum D, Turk DC. Facilitating Treatment Adherence: A Practitioner's Guidebook. New York: Plenum, 1987. This book is another classic. The book is the most well-known text on what to do about enhancing patient adherence. There are several chapters on clinical guidelines and techniques for health care professionals dealing with issues of non-adherence. The book is written for broad application across the health professions.

Ozar MN, Payton OD, Nelson C. Treatment Planning for Rehabilitation: A Patient-Centered Approach. New York: McGraw-Hill, 2000. This book provides useful techniques for involving patients, families, and other caregivers in maximizing patient participation. Case studies include teaching points as well as insights for application in clinical practice.

Stewart M, Brown J, Weston W, et al. Patient-Centered Medicine: Transforming the Clinical Method. Thousand Oaks, CA: Sage, 1995. This text, although written from work in medicine, has a number of examples that can be applied across the health professions. The authors make a strong case for a patient-centered model and then describe, in detail, all elements of this model, as well as several case examples. In addition, the authors discuss how to go about teaching a more patient-centered clinical method in medical education. The book provides a good overview of research on patient-centered communication.

10

Facilitating Adherence to Healthy Lifestyle Behavior Changes in Patients

Christopher D. Lorish and Judith R. Gale

Experienced therapists know that many patients present with musculoskeletal problems that are the result of lifestyle choices that also put them at risk for other serious diseases and premature death. Even more frustrating is the patient who does not follow the home program, resulting in no or delayed improvement. Perhaps you have encountered a patient like Mr. Smith.

> Mr. Smith, a 42-year-old white man, comes to your clinic complaining of knee pain, the result of a football injury sustained in high school. He has a body mass index of 32, which classifies him as obese; smokes two packs of cigarettes a day; except for weekly bowling, works at a sedentary job; and watches 4 hours of television at night. On weekends, he watches sports on television. After examining his knee, your diagnosis is that he likely has osteoarthritis and an altered gait pattern because of his knee pain. You teach him appropriate strengthening and stretching exercises, after setting strength and range-of-motion goals. The patient returns in 2 weeks to assess progress. He tells you that the exercises were boring, and, as result, he did them "off and on." In addition, he has gained a pound, still smokes two packs a

day, and is watching even more television, because it is the start of the new football season. What should you do? Explain the treatment again? Change the exercises? Try to scare him into doing the program with a threat of surgery? Label him as non-compliant and wish him good luck? Or none of the above?

Before discussing this dilemma, you are challenged by the following assertion: If a physical therapist wants to be an effective practitioner, the therapist must become an influential person in each patient's life. Technical competence in assessment and intervention planning, although very important, means little if the patient goes home and does not follow the home program, or continues the unhealthy habits contributing to the musculoskeletal problem. Although a physical therapist cannot control what a patient does at home, she or he can influence the patient so that there is a greater likelihood that what is prescribed is followed at home. The therapist can also work at helping the patient modify unhealthy habits (e.g., inactivity, smoking, poor diet, obesity) to prevent premature illness and death. The challenge is to negotiate the most efficacious intervention or prevention plan that the patient will be motivated to follow. Now, back to the dilemma posed in the patient scenario.

This chapter is about the "none of the above" option. This option does not imply that the situation is hopeless because there is no other option. Rather, it implies that there are ways that therapists can use themselves as agents to promote the patient's intervention adherence, or the initiation of healthier lifestyle habits (e.g., regular exercise, weight loss, quitting tobacco), or both. After developing the justification for negotiated programs, a detailed behavioral intervention protocol is described to help the reader know how to address patients' adherence problems or lifestyle risks. Variations of this protocol are developed to illustrate the slight differences between adherence and lifestyle negotiation.

Chapter Objectives

After completing this chapter, the reader will be able to

1. Discuss the role of the therapist-patient relationship in promoting adherence.
2. Identify the major behavioral theories for promoting adherence and behavioral changes.
3. Compare and contrast the Health Belief Model, the Transtheoretical Model of Change, and the Five A's Behavioral Intervention Protocol.
4. Apply the Five A's Protocol to clinical cases encountered in physical therapy practice.

Justification for Physical Therapists to Counsel Patients on Lifestyle Changes

Adherence versus Non-Adherence

Physical therapists should integrate adherence and lifestyle counseling into their practices for a variety of reasons. Although good studies on non-adherence with physical therapy interventions are few, the data suggest that non-adherence exists. Reports of adherence rates to supervised exercise, the kind typically associated with cardiac rehabilitation or other hospital- or clinic-based programs, range from 70% to 94%,[1,2] whereas adherence to unsupervised exercise and home programs ranges from 18% to 57%.[3-7] We might infer, then, that adherence rates in supervised programs are considerably better than adherence rates in unsupervised programs.

Non-adherence can take the form of the patient doing less or more of the prescribed intervention, never starting, temporarily stopping, adding other components, or quitting before the full benefit is experienced. These variations of non-adherence represent a potential threat to a patient's recovery and level of function. Evaluation of the patient's non-adherence by the therapist at each follow-up visit is necessary to determine the degree of risk to the patient's continued progress or well-being. For example, it would likely be a serious risk to a patient's recovery after a rotator cuff repair if the patient were to substitute or add several shoulder exercises with weights to "hurry things up." Thus, it is in the best interest of both the patient and the physical therapist to negotiate the most efficacious treatment program that the patient is willing to follow.

Even if a patient is doing well at a follow-up visit, it is useful to know whether the patient is doing more, less, or something different than prescribed. The effects of the modifications on the patient's condition and function may be both large and negative and may not become apparent until after the visit. Whether the therapist should do anything about the patient's non-adherence, once it is recognized, depends on the effects of non-adherence on the patient's long- and short-term functioning, as well as its potential harmful effects. Thus, it is quite possible that some non-adherence can be tolerated, as when a patient consistently does less of the program, affecting only the rate of progress toward the desired functional goals.

Changes in Health Care Delivery and Reimbursement

Some physical therapists may object to the view that part of their responsibility is to work with the patient's non-adherence or lifestyle risks, believing that the patient is responsible for intervention implementation and that the therapist's responsibility ends with providing the best advice possible regarding intervention or healthy habits. However, structural changes in the way health care is delivered and reimbursed have affected, and will continue to affect, how physical therapists work with patients.

One stimulus for more attention to lifestyle modification during the clinical encounter is the development and increasing use of the Health Plan Employer Data and Information Set (HEDIS), a set of common data indicators for the examination of managed care organization performance developed by the National Committee on Quality Assurance. The latest version of HEDIS requires managed care organizations to report on more than 50 prevention-oriented indicators.[8] Because of the marketing importance of HEDIS data in recruiting businesses and patients to purchase managed care organizations' plans, it is quite likely that these organizations will be under increasing competitive pressure to provide more health promotion programs to address HEDIS-related issues.[9]

Although HEDIS is a stimulus for promoting more prevention activity, the growth of managed care organizations is likely the most significant structural change affecting how physical therapists work with patients. In 1989, 18% of the population reported that they were covered by some form of managed care. As of June 30, 1998, more than 16 million people—54% of Medicaid beneficiaries—were enrolled in managed care programs.[10]

One consequence of these structural changes is that health care practice is being altered.[11,12] Cost control mechanisms, such as case managers, utilization reviews, and managed care policies, as well as competition with other clinics for patients, appear to be causing a decline in the number of clinic visits approved. Under this scenario, the burden of therapeutic work has shifted from therapist-supervised clinic visits to independent, unobserved home exercise programs that patients are expected to follow. When the patient does come to the clinic for the allotted visits, the therapist may have less time to spend, because therapists' patient loads have increased to compensate for declining or static reimbursement for services. Although no study has documented the amount and effects of patient non-adherence to home therapeutic programs, it is quite possible that non-adherence will increase as physical therapists rely more on home exercise programs, resulting in decreased intervention efficacy and, subsequently, a less-than-optimal patient outcome.

Role of Lifestyle in Morbidity and Mortality

Because physical therapists often see patients with musculoskeletal problems partially caused or worsened by chronic inactivity, obesity, and tobacco or alcohol abuse, the statistics surrounding these risk behaviors are highlighted in this chapter. Patients who present with one or more of these lifestyle risk factors are likely to benefit from attempts to modify their health risks. Physical therapists can play an important role in supporting their patients' efforts to change.

There is significant evidence that these lifestyle risks contribute to premature morbidity and mortality. Healthy People 2010 targets several indicators of health, the top three being physical activity, obesity, and tobacco use (information is available online at http://www.health.gov/healthypeople/). Because more than 875,000 deaths in the United States in 1990 were considered attributable to lifestyle-related behaviors,[13] the U.S. Preventive Services Task Force report (available online at http://www.ahrq.gov/clinic/cpsix.htm) recommended universal risk assessment of patients' cigarette and alcohol consumption, seat belt use, diet, stress, safe sex practices, voluntary exercise, and discussion of these health risks with patients when indicated.[14] To assist clinicians with counseling patients about unhealthy lifestyle habits, the U.S. Preventive Health Services Task Force also produced *Clinician's Handbook of Preventive Services: Put Prevention Into Practice* (available online at http://www.ahrq.gov/clinic/ppiphand.htm). This handbook is intended to be a practical guide written for clinicians, to assist their prevention efforts in the clinical setting.

Physical therapists are likely to discuss inactivity, obesity, and smoking with patients, because exercise can be part of the solution for all three of these risk behaviors, as well as for the patient's musculoskeletal problem. However, the musculoskeletal problem or the risk behaviors, or both, may affect the patient's ability to exercise. A brief review of the scope of obesity, physical inactivity, and tobacco use will help the reader realize how widespread these problems are, even if they are not directly implicated in a patient's musculoskeletal problem. In 1997, 64% of adolescents engaged in the recommended amount of physical activity. In the same year, only 15% of adults performed the recommended 30 minutes of daily physical activity, and 40% of adults engaged in no leisure-time physical activity. Women are less active than men at all ages. People with lower incomes and less education typically are not as physically active as those with higher incomes and more education. African-Americans and Hispanics are generally less physically active than Caucasians. Adults in northeastern and southern states tend to be less active than adults in north-central and western states. People with disabilities are less physically active than people without disabilities. By age 75 years, one in three men and one in two women engage in *no* regular physical activity. Inactivity is a major risk factor for obesity.[15]

Research has demonstrated that intervening with inactive patients is likely to be helpful, because virtually all individuals benefit from regular physical activity. *The Surgeon General's Report on Physical Activity and*

Health concluded that moderate physical activity can substantially reduce the risk of developing or dying from heart disease, diabetes, colon cancer, or high blood pressure.[15] Physical activity may be effective in the prevention of low back pain and may afford protection against some forms of cancer (e.g., breast cancer), but the evidence is not yet conclusive.[16,17]

Poor nutritional habits and obesity contribute substantially to the burden of preventable illnesses and premature deaths in the United States.[18] The number of overweight children, adolescents, and adults has risen over the past four decades. Total costs (direct medical costs and lost productivity) attributable to obesity alone amounted to an estimated $99 billion in 1995. Between 1988 and 1994, 11% of children and adolescents aged 6 to 19 years were overweight or obese. During the same years, 23% of adults aged 20 and older were considered obese. Indeed, dietary factors and obesity are associated with 4 of the 10 leading causes of death: coronary heart disease, some types of cancer, stroke, and type II diabetes.[19,20] These health conditions are estimated to cost society more than $200 billion each year in medical expenses and lost productivity.[21] Dietary factors also are associated with osteoporosis, which affects more than 25 million people in the United States and is the major underlying cause of bone fractures in postmenopausal women and in the elderly.[22]

Finally, despite what smokers and nonsmokers know of the health risks of tobacco use, more than 430,000 smoking-related deaths occur each year among adults in the United States. This represents more than 5 million years of potential life lost.[23] Cigarette smoking causes heart disease, several kinds of cancer (lung, larynx, esophagus, pharynx, mouth, and bladder), and chronic lung diseases such as emphysema. Cigarette smoking also contributes to cancer of the pancreas, kidney, and cervix. Smoking during pregnancy causes spontaneous abortion and low birth weight, and it may lead to sudden infant death syndrome.[24] Other forms of tobacco are not safe alternatives to smoking cigarettes. Use of smokeless tobacco causes a number of serious oral health problems, including cancer of the mouth and gum, periodontitis, and tooth loss.[25,26] Cigar use causes cancer of the larynx, mouth, esophagus, and lung.[25]

More information on how to assist patients to stop smoking is available online at http://www.surgeongeneral.gov/tobacco/default.htm. This information might be useful to the physical therapist in assisting and supporting patients' efforts to change.

Therapeutic Context to Promoting Prevention

Unlike the physicians and nurses with whom patients come in contact, physical therapists can exploit the fact that they probably will be recommending, teaching, and monitoring the effects of therapeutic exercise.

In this therapeutic role, physical therapists can include recommendations for a safe voluntary exercise program using the American College of Sports Medicine's guidelines for exercise testing and prescription.[27] Because physical therapists are likely viewed by their patients as credible sources regarding exercise, diet, and smoking, and since therapists likely see patients for multiple visits during which voluntary exercise can be discussed, the potential for influencing patients' choices to change unhealthy habits is enhanced. In addition, because patients are increasingly expected to adhere to home exercise programs, the same behavioral strategies used to enhance patients' adherence can be applied to the initiation or maintenance of voluntary exercise (see Chapter 9). The commonality between adherence to therapeutic exercise and initiation of voluntary exercise is that, in both cases, the patient makes the daily choice to exercise, a choice that can be influenced by physical therapists. To more effectively influence patients' choices, some behavior theory concepts need to be understood.

Behavior Theory

In today's managed care environment, in which time to work directly with the patient during a clinic visit is less likely, it is important that the efforts to promote treatment adherence, lifestyle modification, or both be time efficient and effective. Recent work in behavior theory has provided important concepts and insights that can guide physical therapists' work with patients. Three models of behavior theory are presented in this chapter: the Health Belief Model, the Transtheoretical Model of Change, and the Five A's Behavioral Intervention Protocol. All of these theories posit key beliefs of patients as causal determinants of their behavior. To maximize adherence or to help the patient alter unhealthy habits, the basic strategy is to use written or oral questions to help the patient identify the reasons that will motivate him or her to adhere to or to change a habit. Sometimes, patients just need help with verbalizing why it is in their best interest to follow the intervention or to change a habit. Sometimes, additional reasons must be suggested by the physical therapist if the patient is not verbal, insightful, or knowledgeable about the consequences of poor adherence or unhealthy habits. Present information from a credible source—you, a former patient, the physician, a significant other, or someone else whose word the patient trusts—challenging the basis of the patient's beliefs or supporting the desired behavior. One way to challenge the patient's belief, for example, that "a pill taken before sleep is sufficient to lose weight" is by involving the patient in an informal, single-subject "study" to disprove the patient's belief in the efficacy of a home remedy or to prove the efficacy of a prescribed treatment. Key concepts from three of the most cited cognitive behavior theories can guide therapists' inquiries into the beliefs that motivate patients' behavior.

Health Belief Model

The Health Belief Model asserts that, to make a behavioral change, an individual must believe that she or he is susceptible to a disease or condition, that the disease has serious consequences, that making a change such as increasing activity can reduce the threat, that the costs or barriers of changing are less than the benefits, and that she or he is able to successfully make the change.[28] Application of these concepts suggests the importance of asking what the patient sees as the worst consequence of poor adherence or continued inactivity (e.g., loss of meaningful activities, onset of serious disease). Asking whether the patient believes that the intervention or increased activity is likely to help prevent this consequence and asking what the patient believes are the costs and benefits of the intervention or increased activity yield important information for the therapist. If the patient does not believe that the personal consequence of the presenting condition or a life of continued inactivity is serious, does not believe that the intervention is likely to help, or believes that there are too many barriers and "costs" to the intervention, then attempts to modify any and all of those beliefs should be initiated. Giving information from credible sources and asking the patient to discuss these issues at the next visit are reasonable first steps. It is important to realize that this conversation may only start the patient thinking about changing, with attempts at making a change coming later, even after this episode of care with the physical therapist is completed.

Transtheoretical Model of Change

As Figure 10-1 shows, the Transtheoretical Model of Change suggests that making a behavior change, such as following a home exercise program, follows a non-linear progression of five stages: not thinking about changing (*precontemplation stage*), thinking about making a change (*contemplation stage*), making preparations to change (*preparation stage*), implementing the change (*action stage*), and maintaining the change (*maintenance stage*).[29] Relapse to a previous stage is common, may occur at any time and to any prior stage, and is an integral part of the change process. An important insight from this theory is that different educational strategies are successful, depending on the patient's stage. The application of this stage-process model of change implies that therapists first assess a patient's stage and then use education and persuasion to try to move the patient closer to the action stage. For

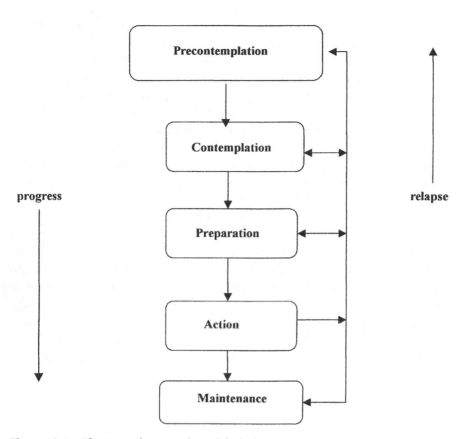

Figure 10-1 The Transtheoretical Model of Change. Relapse can occur at any stage. Strategies for facilitating change are stage dependent. (Adapted from S Rollnick, P Mason, C Butler. Health Behavior Change: A Guide for Practitioners. Philadelphia: Churchill Livingstone, 1999.)

example, if a patient indicates that she or he has not thought of increasing her or his activity level (*precontemplation*), then discussion of the reasons that it is in the patient's best interest to adhere to an exercise program or modify an unhealthy habit would be appropriate. During a subsequent visit, if the patient indicates that she or he has been thinking about exercise (*contemplation*), then asking about and helping to problem solve the barriers to starting is appropriate. If the patient reaches the implementation (*action*) stage during the sequence of visits to the therapist, strategies to help the patient maintain that stage or to prevent relapse can be discussed. Such discussion can be accomplished by problem solving potential new barriers, identifying rewards for adherence or increased activity, or reminding the patient of the risks of non-adherence and inactivity and of the benefits of adherence and activity.[30,31]

Patients who come to a therapist are likely in the preparatory or implementation (action) stages regarding their musculoskeletal problems, because they have come to the therapist seeking help regarding their symptoms. They may have already tried home remedies or prescribed medications to reduce their symptoms. The task is to encourage and maintain adherence to the intervention by reviewing the reasons that the patient believes it is important to continue the intervention and the problem solving of any barriers to adherence. However, starting a voluntary exercise program may be a change that the patient has never considered (*precontemplation*). A precontemplative, sedentary patient first needs to reflect on and verbalize the positive consequences for changing his or her behavior, and the negative consequences of not changing, through discussion with the physical therapist. The consequences must be personally important to the patient, typically centering on losses in valued work, family, and leisure activities, and on other valued relationships. Verbalizing consequences helps the patient move from the precontemplative to the contemplative and action stages. When a patient reaches the latter two stages, it is appropriate to negotiate a voluntary exercise program or some other health-risk modification. Although this initial program may not reflect the plan that the physical therapist believes is ideal for the patient, it reflects one that the patient is more likely to follow, and it leaves open the possibility that the plan can be renegotiated more (toward the ideal) at future visits.

Social Learning Theory

The Social Learning Theory posits that behavior is the product of the continuous, reciprocal interplay between social or physical environmental factors and psychological factors such as emotions, self-appraisals, beliefs about behavioral consequences, and confidence in the ability to execute the desired behavior (*self-efficacy*).[31,32] The application of these concepts stresses confidence-building practice in the performance of the exercise, goal setting, identifying of immediate and future rewards for adherence or voluntary exercise, and implementing self-monitoring strategies. A more complete elaboration of these theories, as well as practical suggestions for working with patients' motivation to change, is found in Chapter 9.

Reading these brief accounts of the key behavior theories may make it seem impossible to apply them in any coherent and time-efficient way. Fortunately, a brief behavioral intervention has been developed for clinicians to use in assisting patients to stop smoking.[33] This behavioral intervention process can be generalized to apply to issues of adherence to home programs, the initiation of a voluntary exercise program, or dietary modifications to promote weight loss. The full process is described first, followed by a brief variation that is useful when you only have a minute of time to address these issues.

The Five A's Behavioral Intervention Protocol

Preliminaries

Once a patient leaves the clinic, you have no control over whether the treatment is followed as prescribed or whether your advice to start a regular exercise program, lose weight, or quit smoking is followed. The challenge is to find ways to work effectively and quickly with patients, so that they are more likely to do what they need to do to maintain function, minimize morbidity, or delay mortality. The usual method—giving advice and information—may not be the best approach, especially if the patient is not motivated to change. The advice- and information-giving approach usually fails to address the patient's motivation to follow a treatment program or to change an unhealthy habit, as well as the barriers the patient likely encounters in attempting to follow the program. The Five A's Behavioral Intervention Protocol reflects a systematic process for working with patients to maximize the physical therapist's influence and for addressing the shortcomings of the advice- and information-giving approach. The Five A's protocol uses the theoretical concepts discussed previously and has been empirically tested by physicians in counseling patients to quit smoking.[33] It consists of five steps: address the issue, assess the patient, advise the patient, assist the patient, and arrange follow-up. When these five steps are applied consistently and with some skill, they are likely to be more effective than information- and advice-giving for influencing patients' choices about following their home programs, starting prevention programs, or both, once they leave your office. Skilled use of the Five A's protocol requires understanding the sequence of the steps and their purposes. It also requires efficient phrasings—like the ones suggested in the section Implementing the Five A's Behavioral Intervention Protocol—to minimize the time spent asking the patient a question or getting diverted by a side issue. A skilled clinician would take 3–10 additional minutes to complete the protocol.

Necessary Conditions

Let us return to Mr. Smith, the man we met at the beginning of this chapter, with a bad knee and a history of obesity, inactivity, and tobacco use. If Mr. Smith were told by a stranger on the street to go home and do 50 straight leg raises three times a day, or to go on daily walks and cut out junk food to lose weight, it is likely that the patient would look at the stranger as if she or he were crazy, and walk away. However, if a physical therapist told Mr. Smith the same thing at the first visit, Mr. Smith would be more likely to listen and be inclined to do something. The difference is that the physical therapist's influence is derived from the expertise and authority symbolized by the "white coat" and by his or her respectful, caring, and empathetic behavior, which allows the patient to be open to the therapist's influence as intervention plans are negotiated or unhealthy habits are discussed. Negotiating the most efficacious plan of care that Mr. Smith is willing to follow at home implies establishing a partnership in which Mr. Smith views the physical therapist as an ally in solving his problem or modifying his unhealthy habits. Such negotiation implies that the agreed-on intervention may not be the most efficacious one, but it should be effective enough to allow Mr. Smith to make some progress. Follow-up visits are used to problem solve difficulties that the patient had following the program, as well as to negotiate a more ideal plan. Negotiating a plan also implies that the physical therapist strives to understand how the condition affects activities important to Mr. Smith, what his goals and motivations are, and the potential barriers to following whatever intervention or prevention plan is agreed on.

General Strategy

Initiating and maintaining a behavior change, like a home exercise or voluntary exercise program, usually involves addressing three conditions: knowledge, motivation, and resources. Compared to the more typical advice-giving or telling approach that is often used, the Five A's protocol is a better strategy to promote the patient's adherence or behavior change, because it systematically addresses all three conditions. In addition, the Five A's process is one in which the intervention or prevention program develops through a shared perspective and negotiation, which should reduce patient resistance.

The first condition for initiating a behavior change is *provision of information*. A patient like Mr. Smith needs knowledge and understanding of the condition and of the intervention or prevention program—what the problem or condition is, what may have caused the problem, how and when to do the treatment program, when not to do the treatment, its possible side effects, the length of time before positive effects of the program will be noticed, and how the treatment will positively impact present and future health and functioning in ways important to the patient. Mistaken beliefs that the patient reveals during the Assess step may need to be addressed as potential barriers. Patients may also need to be informed about the possible negative consequences important to them regarding present and future health and functioning that might occur if they do not follow the intervention or do not change an unhealthy habit. Educating patients about how the health risks associated with poor treatment adherence or their lifestyle habits jeopardize valued activities and relationships helps to develop or strengthen the motivation to adhere to a program or change a habit. In addition, because most home programs involve performing a sequence of exercises or movements, patients need to develop confidence, through supervised practice, that they can correctly perform the behavior at home. Because studies suggest that patients misinterpret or do not remember up to one-third of what a physician tells them immediately after a visit,[34–36] a better strategy is to inform the patient as an issue arises during the visit and provide a take-home handout summarizing the program like the one shown in Figure 10-2, or do both.

The second condition for initiating a behavior change is *motivation* to follow a home program or to start a regular exercise, diet, or tobacco-cessation program. This motivation involves the therapist asking a patient like Mr. Smith to identify and state all the reasons important to him for following the treatment or for changing an unhealthy habit. These reasons function as incentives to follow the program. Put another way, a patient is motivated when she or he believes that more is to be gained from following the program than from not following it. The physical therapist helps the patient realize that there is more to be gained than lost through questions that encourage the patient to reflect on all of the positive consequences of following the home program and all of the negative consequences of not doing so. Although it may be necessary to suggest some of these reasons to a patient who is not very knowledgeable, reflective, or verbal, the better strategy is to use questions that allow the patient to verbalize the consequences that are personally important. Doing so may take more than one visit to accomplish. The process of helping the patient to reflect and verbalize important consequences helps to minimize resistance, facilitate movement from the precontemplative to the action stage, and maintain the patient's behavior once the program is started.

The third condition for initiating a behavior change is *resources*. Carrying out a home intervention, diet, exercise, or smoking-cessation program often requires time, money, equipment, space, and assistance from others. The absence of these resources can undermine the patient's willingness to initiate or maintain a program.

Although many patients are ready to try a home program that promises relief of their symptoms, many will not be ready to change an unhealthy habit. Time should be spent efficiently exploring the patient's motivation and helping the patient verbalize and understand all the personal reasons why quitting smoking or exercising is in her or his best interest. The patient's decision to change may not occur during the first, second, or even third visit, but may occur later, perhaps while he is having difficulty keeping up with his friends while hunting, or when she realizes that she can only work in the garden for 10 minutes before becoming short of breath. Without the prior conversations with the physical therapist, that decision to change may never occur. Some patients come to the clinic contemplating making a

Home Program Record

Name:_____   Date:_____

(The Home Program Record and Treatment Log should be back to back.)

1. My diagnosis is: (Should be term[s] that you and the patient both understand as an initial part of creating the common ground of understanding that promotes collaborative treatments.)

2. My treatment goals are: (This section should reflect the goals important to the patient and revealed by the patient that will help motivate her or him to follow the treatment. The idea is to make the patient believe that there is more to be gained by following the treatment than by not doing it.)

Activity: (This should reflect the work, leisure, social, family activities, and relationships the patient wishes to recover or maintain that serve as her or his incentive to follow the treatment.)

Symptom: (This should reflect the symptom[s] most bothersome to the patient that she or he would like to eliminate or reduce through the treatment.)

3. My treatment options are: (This section lays out the plan collaboratively negotiated.)

a. **If I do nothing, the likely result is:** (This helps ensure the patient understands the consequences of not following treatment on her or his Activity and Symptom goals. Could also specify other likely negative consequences. The idea is to try to make the patient believe that it is not in her or his best interest to do nothing.)

b. **My home exercise program is:** (List the details: what, when, how many, how often, intensity, etc.)

Likely positive consequences are: (List the more immediate outcomes [if any] that are related to the desired goals above, and explain how achieving these outcomes moves the patient toward the goals. Include any rewards that are negotiated for following the treatment program.)

Likely negative consequences are: (List any negative consequences or side effects–time, money, temporary pain that might result from the program. If necessary, problem solve to try to reduce the negatives. The idea is for the patient to believe that there are more positive than negative consequences.)

Time to notice improvement: (Tell the patient how long it will take for results to be noticed and what changes the patient will notice to indicate that improvement is being made. This will prevent the patient from prematurely stopping the program, thinking that it is not working.)

c. **My group land or water exercise program is:** (If you are able to negotiate a group or community program, then list its details. Group programs can help support the patient's motivation to continue the programs once the patient feels an affiliation with group.)

4. Special instructions

Figure 10-2 The Home Program Record summarizes the negotiated program for the patient. Its purpose is to assist the patient in gaining confidence that she or he is able to correctly perform the program.

lifestyle change. For them, the physical therapist will likely be able to negotiate a plan and problem solve any anticipated barriers during the first visit.

Studies of the Transtheoretical Model of Change document that people go through different stages during the process of change.[37,38] These include not thinking about making a change, making a change, and relapsing to not following the home program or to an unhealthy habit. It is helpful, then, if each physical therapist views intervention, adherence, and prevention as an ongoing conversation that occurs with each patient at each visit. In addition to writing a chart note so that the conversation can be resumed with the patient at the next visit, having the patient keep a treatment log, like the one shown in Figure 10-3, will also help to keep the conversation going and promote the patient's belief that you will not forget.

Implementing the Five A's Behavioral Intervention Protocol

The Five A's process is presented as a sequenced, scripted protocol that is applied during the initial visit and at subsequent visits (Figure 10-4). Each step has a purpose, and, if performed well, is likely to achieve its intended effect. Skipping a step because of time constraints may be necessary but may diminish the overall effectiveness of the process. The suggested phrasings for each step are focused and time efficient. Separate questions for addressing the adherence and prevention issues are given in each step.

The Five A's protocol builds on the behavioral theories introduced earlier in this chapter. The three models—the Health Belief Model, the Transtheoretical Model, and the Five A's Behavioral Intervention Protocol—are actually very similar in their processes of behavior change. Table 10-1 highlights how the behavior theories are incorporated into the Five A's protocol.

Step One: Address the Issue

Rationale: Patients like Mr. Smith come to the physical therapist with agendas, typically seeking symptom relief. This means that patients are willing to discuss the problems that brought them but probably did not come thinking that they would talk about their weight, activity level, or smoking. After the physical therapist has obtained Mr. Smith's focused history, completed an examination, formulated a physical therapy diagnosis, developed a plan of care for the presenting problem, and identified one or more prevention concerns, the adherence issue must be addressed as part of negotiating the most efficacious intervention that Mr. Smith is willing to follow. After the plan of care is negotiated, a prevention issue may be addressed or put off to the follow-up visit.

My Treatment Log

Prescribed activity	Day 1	Day 2	Day 3	Day 4	Day 5	Day 6	Day 7
1.	——	——	——	——	——	——	——
2.	——	——	——	——	——	——	——
3.	——	——	——	——	——	——	——
4.	——	——	——	——	——	——	——
5.	——	——	——	——	——	——	——
Activity rating Symptom rating	W/S/B W/S/B	W/S/B W/S/B	W/S/B W/S/B	W/S/B W/S/B	W/S/B W/S/B	W/S/B W/S/B	W/S/B W/S/B
Problems with doing any of the exercises? Please bring this Log to your next visit. We will talk about it.							

Figure 10-3 Keeping a treatment log stimulates conversation about the home program and can help to identify problems with its successful completion. The log is used effectively in combination with the Home Program Record (see Figure 10-2). Stress that any problems will be discussed at the follow-up visit or over the telephone if the patient thinks she or he cannot tolerate the program and wants to quit. (B = better than yesterday; S = same as yesterday; W = worse than yesterday.)

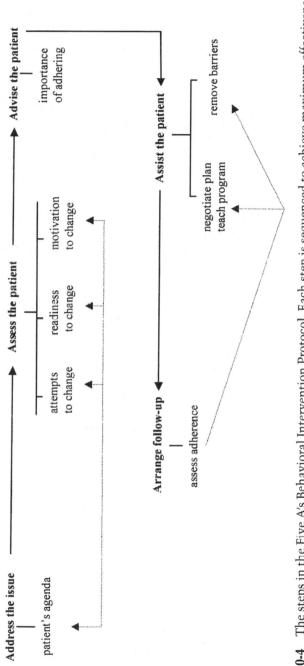

Figure 10-4   The steps in the Five A's Behavioral Intervention Protocol. Each step is sequenced to achieve maximum effectiveness as the patient moves through the stages.

Table 10-1 The Five A's Protocol and Behavior Theory

Five A's Protocol	Social Learning Theory	Health Belief Model	Transtheoretical Model of Change
Step One: Address the issue			
Step Two: Assess			
Task 1: Prior attempts	Reveals patient self-efficacy about prior programs		Reveals if patient is in action stage
Task 2: Readiness to change			Reveals if patient is in precontemplative or contemplative stage
Task 3: Motivational reflection	Personal positive and negative consequences		Facilitates movement to next stage
Step Three: Advise	Establish social performance expectation	Provide cue to action	
Step Four: Assist			
Task 1: Negotiate	Identify goal, steps, and rewards		Establish stage-appropriate plan
Task 2: Educate	Develop program self-efficacy	Address patient's problem susceptibility, severity, program effectiveness	Facilitates movement to next stage
Task 3: Address barriers		Problem solve program costs and positive consequences of not changing	Facilitates movement to next stage
Step Five: Arrange follow-up	Establishes monitoring expectation		

- Addressing adherence to the home program

  "Mr. Smith, I think the best intervention for your problem is (briefly state the intervention), but before we agree that that is what you will do, I would like for us to talk about what you are *willing* to do at home to get better."

- Addressing a prevention issue

  "Now that we have agreed to a home program for your knee problem, I am wondering whether we could talk about your [smoking, weight, inactivity]? I think it is important to your problem and to your long term health."

  Application: To have maximum impact on getting the patient's attention and cueing her or him to think that an important issue is about to be discussed, one or more of the following nonverbal behaviors can help: moving in front of the patient and looking the patient in the eye; leaning toward the patient; and lowering or raising your voice. These nonverbal cues signal a change in topic, the importance of what is to come, and concern of the physical therapist.

  Step Two: Assess the Patient
  At least three areas should be assessed: recent attempts to follow a home program or change an unhealthy habit, the patient's readiness to change an unhealthy habit, and the patient's motivation to follow a home program or change an unhealthy habit. Information about a patient's dietary, smoking, and exercise habits can be obtained by a waiting room survey or while taking the patient's history.

Recent Attempts

  Rationale: Probing the patient's recent attempts to follow a medication regimen or a prescribed exercise program or to change an unhealthy habit provides important information that will be helpful when negotiating a home program or a behavioral plan to modify an unhealthy habit. The patient will likely reveal what has worked and what has not worked, mistaken beliefs, barriers that caused the patient to quit or to not start, and how confident the patient feels about making a change to an unhealthy habit.

- Addressing adherence to the home program

  "Following an intervention program at home or taking medicines according to directions is difficult. I know I sometimes have difficulty doing my exercise program daily. Can you think of any problems you had the last time you were prescribed an exercise program or medicines, like forgetting to do your program or deciding to quit it? Can you think of what helped you to do the program every day?" (Note the problems to address later in the Assist phase.)

- Addressing previous prevention attempts

  "Mr. Smith, have you tried to [lose weight, exercise regularly, stop smoking] in the last 3 months?" If yes, ask, "What did you do? How successful were you? What problems did you have, and why did you stop?"

  Application: When addressing prior adherence, it is useful to reveal to the patient your own problems with following an exercise program or taking medicine as prescribed. Your acknowledgment of your imperfections allows the patient to more easily admit his or her own. The last 3 months is a reasonable time frame for assessing recent attempts. Be sure to note areas of ignorance, confusion, or mistaken beliefs, because the patient will need to be informed later in the Assist step. The question about whether the patient has tried to lose weight, exercise, or stop smoking may also reveal barriers or problems that caused the patient to quit. Any new treatment or prevention program would have to avoid this barrier, or, if not, a solution would have to be found.

READINESS TO CHANGE AN UNHEALTHY HABIT

  Rationale: Because most patients come to a physical therapist ready to do something to obtain relief from the symptoms that brought them, the question about the patient's recent efforts toward modifying health habits is typically only used when addressing a prevention issue and when the patient is not doing something about her or his weight, smoking, or inactivity at the time of the visit. If the patient is doing something, she or he is in the action stage already, but you may want to negotiate a more effective plan to replace one that is often based on misinformation and of dubious value. Derived from Prochaska's and DiClemente's Stages of Change theory, this question determines whether the patient is at the precontemplative stage and determines what the physical therapist does with the patient during the rest of the visit. If the patient says "No" to the question about recent efforts, she or he is in the precontemplative stage. The physical therapist needs to spend the rest of the visit helping the patient explore the reasons for changing an unhealthy habit, and educating him or her about health risks to try to help the patient decide to adhere to the treatment or to change an unhealthy habit. Doing so is analogous to moving the patient from the precontemplative stage to the contemplative and preparatory stages in the Transtheoretical Model. If the patient says "Yes," she or he is at least in the contemplative stage. There is likely enough motivation to negotiate an initial plan that can be modified at subsequent visits, as the patient experiences some success.

- Addressing prevention readiness

    "Mr. Smith, have you thought about trying to [lose weight, start an exercise program, stop smoking] *in the last month?*"

    Application: If Mr. Smith says "No," the physical therapist can use the remaining time in the visit to help him explore the reasons why it is in his best interest to change. After this exploration, the physical therapist gives an Advise statement (step three in the Five A's protocol) (e.g., informs the patient about health risks related to poor adherence or unhealthy habits and about how she or he may jeopardize valued activities and relationships). Finally, a follow-up visit is scheduled if possible, with the expectation communicated to the patient that she or he will discuss the issue again at the next visit. The physical therapist can also assure the patient that he or she is there to help the patient with the behavioral change, when the patient decides to make it. It is important for the patient to view the therapist as an ally and not as a nag; which often causes the patient to resist longer.

    If Mr. Smith says "Yes," then the physical therapist can use motivational reflection to help the patient expand the reasons for making a change. After a brief Advise statement, an initial goal and plan are negotiated, health risks and areas of misinformation are discussed, solutions to any barriers are discussed, and a follow-up visit is scheduled to address progress and problems encountered while following the plan.

- Motivation to change an unhealthy behavior or follow a home exercise program

    Rationale: People initiate change because they want to avoid personally important negative consequences, or experience positive consequences in the near and distant future, or both. Although consequences can be things, money, relationships, and activities, the specific ones of those that motivate a patient to act have to be identified by engaging the patient in motivational reflection. Although a therapist can tell patients about all the medically bad things that can happen if they do not follow their home programs or change unhealthy habits, such warnings are likely not as motivationally powerful as patients' understanding the positive and negative consequences that are personally important to them, now and in the future. Through some simple questions, the physical therapist can ask the patient to reflect on and verbalize the positive and negative consequences that are meaningful to the patient and are at risk because of poor adherence or unhealthy habits. The more of these consequences that the physical therapist can help the patient identify, the more powerful the incentive to change. Even if the patient is contemplative about making a change or expresses a willingness to follow a home program, it is still important to explore her or his motivation; doing so will likely help the patient realize even more incentives.

- Eliciting adherence motivation

    "Mr. Smith, if your problem did not improve, what important activities would this cause you to quit or do less of now and in the future?" Follow up each item with "What is the worst thing about that?" Then ask, "With all that at stake, what do you think would happen if you did not do your home program?"

- Eliciting prevention motivation

    "Mr. Smith, what activity, now or in the future, would you most hate to give up or do less of?" If necessary, cue the patient with "What about [work, leisure, home, social activities, relationships]?" For each answer the patient gives, follow up with, "What is the worst thing about that?" Then, go back to the beginning and ask, "What other activities, now or in the future, would you most hate to give up or do less of?" using the same follow-up question. Then ask, "Given all that is at stake, how do you think your [smoking, weight, inactivity] affects those activities, now and in the future?"

Application: These questions are designed to help the patient to more fully understand what may be at risk or lost if he or she does not follow the home program or change an unhealthy habit. In the adherence question, Mr. Smith must realize what is at stake and how not doing his home program may put his recovery and those activities at risk. The prevention question helps Mr. Smith understand how his unhealthy habit puts current and future valued activities at risk. Asking the follow-up question, "What is the worst thing about . . . " helps Mr. Smith understand the chain of consequences of his behavior that he probably did not understand before. The incentive to change is made more powerful as the patient verbalizes more consequences and better understands the connections between one consequence and another. If time permits, you can also ask, "What good things might happen in your life if you [lost weight, quit smoking, started exercising, took your medicine]?" and "What would be the best thing about that?" It may take several visits to explore the personalized, positive consequences of new, healthy behaviors and the negative consequences of current unhealthy habits. Reviewing these personalized consequences at subsequent visits is also useful, because patients may decide to value an activity differently after the initial visit.

Step Three: Advise the Patient

Rationale: In this step, the physical therapist is exerting whatever influence exists (owing to the symbolism of the "white coat" and the relationship based on respect and caring) to advise the patient of the importance of adhering to the home program or initiating a lifestyle change. The physical therapist conveys this advice to the patient, not only by what is said, but also by how it is said. Social pressure, especially if exerted by persons viewed as important in the patient's life, can be an important influence.

- Addressing adherence

  "Completing a home program regularly and correctly is important to your getting well and for getting back to the activities that are meaningful to you. Because it is important that you perform the program as prescribed, we need to agree on the most effective treatment that you are willing to do regularly and correctly." This statement reinforces the expectation in the patient that the therapist is an ally, willing to negotiate.

- Addressing prevention

  "Mr. Smith, as your physical therapist, I believe it is important that you [start a diet, start an exercise program, quit smoking] for health reasons, but more importantly, for all of the reasons in your life that you mentioned earlier."

  Application: If the patient answered "No" to the previous readiness-to-change questions, you can say, "I know you are not ready to start with a diet, exercise, or quit-smoking program today, but when you do decide, I will assist you with your efforts." Then, inform the patient about likely health risks that may jeopardize valued activities or relationships. If the patient answered "Yes" to the readiness question, you can go directly to the Assist step by asking what food the patient is willing to give up, what activity or exercise the patient is willing to start or do more of, or on what day the patient would like to quit smoking. Focus the patient's attention on your message, using one or more of the same techniques as in Step One: Address the Issue—face the front of the patient and look her or him in the eye, lean forward, change the level of your voice, or slow the rate of your speech.

  Step Four: Assist the Patient

  Rationale: During this step, the physical therapist tries to accomplish three things: negotiate a plan, educate the patient about the home program and about any other mistaken beliefs or areas of ignorance, and problem solve any barriers to following the home program or behavior change plan.

- Negotiating the home treatment program

  To negotiate the most efficacious program that the patient is willing to follow, ask, "Mr. Smith, how much of the plan (the one you described in Step One: Address the Issue) would you be willing to do regularly and correctly at home?"

- Negotiating the health risk modification program

  "What activity or exercise, like brisk walking, would you be willing to start or do more of tomorrow?" or "What junk food or other high-fat food that you regularly eat would you be willing to give up or eat less of starting tomorrow?" or "When would you like to set a quit date to stop smoking?"

- Negotiating more

  "To achieve your goal, what else would you be willing to do?" or "Would you be willing to supplement your bike riding with 10 minutes of walking on the days you don't bike?" Note that the second question involves your making a modest suggestion that may not be ideal, but moves the patient closer to the ideal program. How much you push the patient may depend on what you sense the patient's current motivation is, how frustrated the patient was with prior change attempts, or both.

  Application: If the patient responds that she or he is willing to do something less than the full program, it would be appropriate to inform the patient, without being judgmental, of the likely consequences of doing less, and to ask the patient if such consequences are acceptable. Informing the patient of the consequences of not treating or inadequately treating the medical problem can be an important boost to the patient's motivation, because those consequences are likely something the patient would want to avoid. Review the positive consequences of following the home program as prescribed relative to both the musculoskeletal dysfunction and the patient's ability to maintain, recover, or increase valued activities. If appropriate, ask again what the patient is willing to do, and either accept his or her choice or come up with a different intervention. Asking the patient what barriers there might be to doing the program at home correctly and regularly can lead to finding solutions to the barriers or changing the program to avoid the barriers.

Once a home program has been agreed on, educate the patient on how to do it, when to do it, what side effects to expect and what to do if they occur, the time frame in which the patient should notice improvement, and what the patient will notice as evidence of the improvement. Give the patient enough practice in doing the program in the clinic so that she or he has sufficient confidence that she or he can do it correctly at home. Complete the Home Program Record (see Figure 10-2) and instruct the patient on how to complete the treatment log (see Figure 10-3), indicating that you will use the log as an important source of information to help solve any problems with the program and to aid in renegotiation of the plan at the next visit. As a record of the patient's behavior away from the clinic, the log communicates to the patient that you are interested in what he or she does.

To negotiate a change to an unhealthy habit, recall that Step Four (Assist step) occurs only if Mr. Smith answers "Yes" to the readiness-to-change question in Step Two or indicates in a subsequent visit that he is ready to start a program. Because commitment to changing an unhealthy habit is likely tenuous, the strategy is to ask what the patient is willing to do tomorrow, and then try to negotiate a bit more. For example, the physical therapist might ask Mr. Smith how often he is willing to perform aerobic exercise; the therapist should acknowledge his response as a good start, however modest it might be. Start with what the patient gives, and then try to negotiate a better program, realizing that, at subsequent visits, the program can be renegotiated to something more efficacious if needed. If Mr. Smith says that he is willing to ride the stationary bike every other day for 7 minutes, acknowledge that doing so is an important start, even though its effect on endurance will only be minimal. The point is to try to negotiate an initial program through which the patient will experience success to help maintain her or his motivation to continue.

To negotiate a better program from what the patient initially says that he or she is willing to do, the physical therapist can probe further into the patient's goals of how much activity she or he would like to do before becoming tired or breathless, and in what time frame, and tie the patient's response to maintaining or improving a valued activity. Because a patient may have an unrealistic goal or time frame for achieving his or her goals, it is helpful to educate the patient about strength and aerobic fitness to allow her or him to set more realistic goals. For example, Mr. Smith may want to be able to walk 10 miles while hunting, without getting short of breath, within the next 2 weeks. Telling the patient about strength and aerobic fitness programs, the weight loss process, healthy diets, or the smoking cessation process, or providing the patient with appropriate, understandable handouts on such topics, can assist the patient in making informed decisions and setting realistic goals. Handouts, if presented in a format that the patient can understand, have the great advantage of being re-read at a later time, when the patient may have forgotten what the physical therapist said. Referrals to community programs may be appropriate at this time or, more likely, at a follow-up visit, after the patient has experienced some initial success. Community programs can be very helpful in bolstering patients' resolve to change, and their success in doing so, because of the social bonding with others in the program that often occurs.

Once an initial goal and a program of action have been decided, ask the patient to keep a daily treatment log, as in Figure 10-4, of what she or he did and the problems encountered in carrying out the program. By acknowledging that there may be some problems following the plan and that possible solutions will be discussed at the next visit, the patient is, in effect, absolved of guilt about not adhering completely to the plan, making it easier to admit any non-adherence and to address the problems. The treatment log also lets the patient know that you are monitoring her or him for discussion of progress at future visits.

- Assessing barriers

  "Can you think of anything—for example, time, equipment, or space—that would prevent you from starting this program and being successful?" Note that "not enough time" often means that the activity is not important enough to the patient to put it in his or her daily routine. Work at the motivation component.

Application: As with the adherence-to-the-program issue, the last step includes anticipatory problem solving of barriers, or addressing beliefs the patient has about the seriousness and severity of her or his problem or the effectiveness of the program, or both. Ask Mr. Smith whether he can think of anything that might prevent him from carrying out the plan, starting the next day. For example, although he has agreed to start riding the stationary bike for 7 minutes every other day, he may realize that he only has access to the bike during his lunch hour at work, and he often has meetings over lunch. Usually, the patient can think of nothing, but if he or she does, then you ask how she or he might solve the problem, making suggestions only if the patient cannot think of a solution. The point is to encourage the patient's independent problem solving—not dependence on you.

Developing an initial program based on what the patient gives you and trying to negotiate more, rather than simply informing the patient of the program you want her or him to do, increases the likelihood that the patient will return having been more adherent and successful. Such success would be due, in part, to the fact the patient decided what to do for himself or herself. At a follow-up visit, reviewing Mr. Smith's reasons to adhere to or follow a prevention program; assessing his progress; and problem-solving difficulties that he had or renegotiating the program, or both, are important tasks.

Step Five: Arrange for Follow-Up

Rationale: In addition to the legitimate desire to follow up with Mr. Smith's medical problem, as well as with his progress with any prevention program, the other important function of the Follow-Up step is to communicate to the patient that you expect to discuss the adherence issue, the prevention issue, or both, at the next visit. Mr. Smith was told, in the Advise statement, what the physical therapist's position is. Arranging follow-up conveys to the patient that she or he is accountable.

- Addressing treatment adherence follow-up

"When you come back in ____ weeks, we'll talk about how you are doing and what problems you had following your home program."

- Addressing prevention program follow-up

  If you discussed only the reasons why making a lifestyle change would be in the patient's interest, say, "I will see you in ____ weeks to see how your medical problem is doing, and to see whether you have thought of any more reasons why starting a [diet, exercise, smoking cessation] program would be good for you."

  If you negotiated a prevention program, say, "I will see you in ____ weeks to see how your medical problem is doing, check how much progress you have made on your [weight loss, exercise, smoking cessation] goal, and, most important, discuss any problems you had with following the plan."

  Application: If a prevention program is negotiated at this visit, write a chart note that includes the behavioral issue, the negotiated goal, the actions that the patient agreed to take toward achieving the goal, and the patient's motivation, so that you can continue the discussion appropriately at the next visit.

  Five A's Behavioral Intervention Protocol Variation: Brief Behavioral Intervention Protocol
  Because of the reality of increasingly busy clinics, it is likely that the physical therapist will have limited time to devote to applying the full Five A's protocol to every patient. However, a shorter version of the intervention may be possible and can serve to start a conversation with the patient about adherence or changing an unhealthy habit. The therapist may connect with the patient at just the right time and be able to quickly negotiate an initial program.

- Addressing adherence

  "Mr. Smith, the program I have developed for you is your best bet for being able to return to the activities that are important to you and that you need to do. I am wondering what problems you anticipate in doing your program at home every day as you have done it here."

- Addressing prevention

> "Mr. Smith, I am wondering what would stop you from [starting a modest diet, starting an exercise program, quitting smoking] tomorrow to maintain or improve your health, or to allow you to continue doing the activities that are important to you, now and in the future. I would be glad to assist you in your efforts."

> **Application:** If Mr. Smith recoils and utters several excuses, the physical therapist can indicate that he does not seem ready to start and can give some reasons why it might be in his interest to change. Finish by indicating that you would like to discuss this matter at the next visit, and that you are ready to help him when he decides that he is ready to start. If the patient appears receptive, then perform the Assist step, attempting to negotiate the best plan that you can. If you have enough time, precede the question about what would stop the patient from initiating changes with a motivational question such as, "Mr. Smith, can you think of how the activities important to you, such as work, leisure, family, household chores, or hobbies, might be better now or in the future if you [lost weight, ate healthier foods, quit smoking, exercised regularly]?" Or you might ask, "How are those activities being affected negatively because of your [weight, smoking, inactivity]?" If nothing is elicited, you can suggest some positives and negatives. Then, ask the question about what would keep the patient from starting a program tomorrow.

Final Comments

Although physical therapists are powerless to force Mr. Smith, or patients like him, to do anything once he leaves the clinic, it does not follow that the therapist is absolved of all responsibility if Mr. Smith does not perform the home program. The Five A's protocol is a process that helps the therapist become more influential in Mr. Smith's life. Through engaging Mr. Smith in a discussion of what is at stake for him personally, negotiating the most efficacious treatment or behavioral plan he is willing to follow, and problem-solving barriers that might undermine the patient's good intentions, the physical therapist and Mr. Smith are creating a therapeutic alliance. This partnership is based on genuine caring and respect. The Five A's protocol provides a system for maximizing the physical therapist's ability to

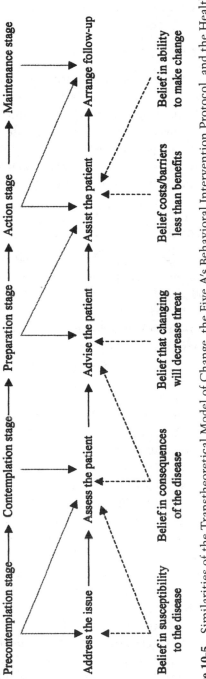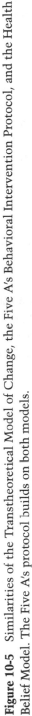

Figure 10-5 Similarities of the Transtheoretical Model of Change, the Five A's Behavioral Intervention Protocol, and the Health Belief Model. The Five A's protocol builds on both models.

influence the patient's personal choices and behavior outside the clinic. This protocol can be applied, entirely or in part, in any clinical setting.

Summary

This chapter has presented ways to promote adherence to healthy lifestyle behavior changes. Figure 10-5 shows the relationship among the models discussed in this chapter for what patients believe, how patients think and act relative to lifestyle behavior changes, and what physical therapists can do to provide supportive and successful interventions. Reading Chapters 9 and 10 together should provide the reader with the knowledge, insight, and understanding to provide outstanding patient education.

References

1. Pollock M, Carroll J, Graves J, et al. Injuries and adherence to walk/jog and resistance training programs in the elderly. Med Sci Sports Exerc 1991;23:1194–1200.
2. Malounin F, Potvin M, Prevost J, et al. Use of an intensive task-oriented gait training program in a series of patients with acute cerebrovascular accidents. Phys Ther 1992;72:781–789.
3. Parker L, Bender L. Problem of home treatment in arthritis. Arch Phys Med Rehabil 1957;38:392–394.
4. Moon M, Moon B, Black W. Compliance in splint-wearing behaviour of patients with rheumatoid arthritis. N Z Med J 1976;83:360–365.
5. Feinberg J, Brandt K. Use of resting splints by patients with rheumatoid arthritis. Am J Occup Ther 1981;35:173–178.
6. Sluijs E, Kok G, van der Zee J. Correlates of exercise compliance in physical therapy. Phys Ther 1993;73:771–786.
7. Taal E, Rasker JJ, Seydel ER, Wiegman O. Health status, adherence with health recommendations, self-efficacy, and social support in patients with rheumatoid arthritis. Patient Educ Couns 1993;20:63–76.
8. HEDIS 2001: Health plan employer data and information set. Vol 2. Washington, DC: National Committee for Quality Assurance, 2000.
9. Chapman, LS. Worksite health promotion in the managed care era. Am J Health Prom 1998;1:1–7.
10. U.S. Department of Health and Human Services. Health, United States, 1998. With health and aging chartbook. Hyattsville, MD: Centers for Disease Control and Prevention, National Center for Health Statistics, 1998.
11. Brown G. Changing health care environments—implications for physical therapy research, education and practice. Phys Ther 1986;66:1242–1245.

12. Monahan B. A look overseas: the United States is not the only nation in which the health care system is being restructured. Phys Ther 1995;3:29–31.

13. McGinnis J, Foege W. Actual causes of death in the United States. JAMA 1993;270:2207–2212.

14. U.S. Preventive Health Services Task Force. Guide to Clinical Preventive Services (2nd ed). Baltimore: Williams & Wilkins, 1996.

15. U.S. Department of Health and Human Services. Physical activity and health: a report of the surgeon general. Atlanta: Centers for Disease Control and Prevention, National Center for Chronic Disease Prevention and Health Promotion, 1996.

16. Frost H, Klaber Moffett JA, Moser JS, Fairbank JC. Randomised controlled trial for evaluation of fitness programme for patients with chronic low back pain. BMJ 1995;310:151–154.

17. McTiernan A, Stanford JL, Weiss NS, et al. Occurrence of breast cancer in relation to recreational exercise in women age 50–64 years. Epidemiology 1996;7:598–604.

18. Frazao E. The High Costs of Poor Eating Patterns in the United States. In E Frazao (ed), America's Eating Habits: Changes and Consequences. Washington, DC: U.S. Department of Agriculture, Economic Research Service, Food and Rural Economics Division, 1999.

19. U.S. Department of Health and Human Services. National Center for Health Statistics. Report of final mortality statistics, 1995. Monthly Vital Stat Rep 1995;45(11 suppl 2).

20. Anderson R, Kochanek M, Murphy S. Report of final mortality statistics. Monthly Vital Stat Rep 1997;45:1–80.

21. Frazao E. The american diet: a costly problem. Food Rev 1996;19:2–6.

22. National Institutes of Health Consensus Development Conference. Optimal calcium intake. JAMA 1994;272:1942–1948.

23. Centers for Disease Control and Prevention. Cigarette smoking–attributable mortality and years of potential life lost—United States, 1984. MMWR Morb Mortal Wkly Rep 1997;46:444–451.

24. DiFranza JR, Lew RA. Effect of maternal cigarette smoking on pregnancy complications and sudden infant death syndrome. J Fam Pract 1995;40: 385–394.

25. U.S. Department of Health and Human Services. The Health Consequences of Using Smokeless Tobacco. A report of the advisory committee to the surgeon general. NIH Publication No. 86-2874. Bethesda, MD: HHS, Public Health Service, Centers for Disease Control, Center for Health Promotion and Education, Office on Smoking and Health, 1986.

26. U.S. Department of Health and Human Services. Reducing the health consequences of smoking: 25 years of progress. A report of the surgeon gen-

eral. HHS Pub. No. (CDC) 89-8411. Atlanta: HHS, Public Health Service, Centers for Disease Control and Prevention, National Center for Chronic Disease Prevention and Health Promotion, Office on Smoking and Health, 1989.

27. American College of Sports Medicine. Guidelines for Exercise Testing and Prescription. Philadelphia: Lippincott Williams & Wilkins, 2000.

28. Maiman LA, Becker MH. The health belief model: origins and correlates in psychological theory. Health Educ Monogr 1974;2:336–353.

29. Prochaska JO, Norcross JC, DiClemente CC. Changing for Good. New York: W. Morrow, 1994.

30. Marcus BH, Simkin LR. The transtheoretical model: applications to exercise behavior. Med Sci Sports Exerc 1994;26:1400–1464.

31. Bandura A. Social Foundations of Thought and Action: A Social Cognitive Theory. Englewood Cliffs, NJ: Prentice-Hall, 1986.

32. Bandura A. Self-Efficacy: The Exercise of Control. New York: W. H. Freeman, 1997.

33. The Tobacco Use and Dependence Clinical Practice Guideline Panel, Staff, and Consortium Representatives. A clinical practice guideline for treating tobacco use and dependence. JAMA 2000;283:3244–3254.

34. Ley P, Spelman MS. Communication in an outpatient setting. Br J Soc Clin Psychol 1965;4:114–116.

35. Ley P. Psychological Studies of Doctor-Patient Communication. In S Richman (ed), Contributions to Medical Psychology. Vol 1. Oxford, UK: Pergamon Press, 1977.

36. Mazullo JM, Lasagna L, Griner PF. Variations in interpretation of prescription instructions. JAMA 1974;227:929–930.

37. DiClemente C, Prochaska J, Fairhurst S, et al. The process of smoking cessation: an analysis of precontemplation, contemplation and preparation stages of change. J Consult Clin Psychol 1991;59:295–304.

38. Prochaska J, DiClemente C, Norcross J. In search of how people change: applications to addictive behaviors. Am Psychol 1992;47:1102–1114.

Annotated Bibliography

Huff RM, Kline MV. Promoting Health in Multicultural Populations: A Handbook for Practitioners. Thousand Oaks, CA: Sage, 1999. An excellent reference text for any health professional involved in facilitating behavior change and promoting healthy behaviors in multicultural populations. The Foundations section of the book provides a sound overview of health promotion in the context of culture. The remainder of the book describes actual case examples across several ethnic groups.

Prochaska JO, Norcross JC, DiClemente CC. Changing for Good. New York: W. Morrow, 1994. This inexpensive text is a comprehensive, easily understood explanation of the Stages of Change theory by its developers. The book is full of examples and practical suggestions for people trying to make a change or those trying to help. If you only read one other reference related to this chapter, this book would be a place to start for those who have not studied behavior change theory.

Rollnick S, Mason P, Butler C. Health Behavior Change: A Guide for Practitioners. Philadelphia: Churchill Livingstone, 1999. This book provides health professionals with an efficient, simple method for helping patients make decisions about health behavior change in clinical and community settings. The introductory section on theory and practice is exceedingly clear and contains several visual models of application of theoretical concepts to practice. Examples from clinical practice include a focus on multiple health behaviors (e.g., overeating, physical inactivity, and smoking), as well as health promotion consultation. The authors maintain a strong philosophic commitment to patient-practitioner collaboration, rather than the professional-as-expert perspective.

11

Teaching Psychomotor Skills

Diane E. Nicholson

Recently, I worked with a 5-year-old child named David who had a left hemiparesis secondary to cerebral palsy. David was independent in most of his age-appropriate functional skills, including gait, transfers, dressing, and feeding; however, he performed these activities with minimal, if any, contribution from his left arm and hand. For example, after toileting he would pull up, snap, and zip his jeans using solely his right arm and hand. David's mother was thrilled that David was independent with his functional skills; however, she wanted him to use his left arm and hand during functional tasks—specifically, she wanted David to learn bilateral strategies for performing upper-extremity tasks.

A physical therapy examination was performed to determine David's potential to learn bilateral upper extremity tasks. The examination revealed that physically, David could perfom active movements with his left arm and hand, but his movements were slow, uncoordinated, and required moderate to maximal effort. Emotionally, David and his family were motivated and willing to work hard to achieve his physical therapy goals. The results of his evaluation suggested that David had a favorable prognosis for learning bilateral strategies for upper extremity tasks.

Physical therapy interventions were initiated and continued for 2 months. As his physical therapist, one of my primary roles with David was to be an educator. I provided knowledge about the effects of practice, I prescribed an exercise program that (1) focused on speed and accuracy during functional tasks, and that (2) was challenging, yet achievable. I used a learning contract, and provided motivation. In essence, I provided David with a "map" for success. David's focus was on practice and hard work. He worked diligently in therapy and in home exercise programs (HEPs)—he worked, and worked, and worked. The result is that today David performs upper extremity tasks using bilateral strategies (Figure 11-1). For example, he uses two hands to pull up, snap, and zip his jeans, he uses active finger movements in both hands to button a shirt, and he uses a fork and knife in the typical manner of an elementary school child without a disability.

The primary goals for David's physical therapy program were to learn and to use novel strategies to perform functional tasks. To develop novel strategies, David learned new sensory-motor relationships and processes; then he retained the new relationships and processes in his memory for use at a later time; and then he problem solved methods to generalize the novel strategies to unpracticed tasks and environments. Thus, although strength and endurance training were a part of David's physical therapy program, these training techniques were not the focus of David's program. The focus was on learning to optimize motor performance—that is, the enhancement of daily functional activities. Motor learning focuses on the processes to develop new strategies, to retain strategies, and to generalize strategies. An understanding of motor learning principles (content knowledge) is as important to the practitioner in physical therapy as are the elements of didactic teaching (pedagogic knowledge) presented in Chapters 2, 3, 9, and 10. The primary purpose of this chapter is to present variables related to motor learning that therapists can manipulate to facilitate client acquisition of psychomotor skills.

Chapter Objectives

After completing this chapter, the reader will be able to

1. Differentiate between motor performance and motor learning.
2. Describe the following processes that influence motor performance and motor learning: attention and automaticity, error detection, motor memories, exemplar and generalized memories, forgetting, retrieval of memories, learning actions, and learning to optimize peripheral constraints.

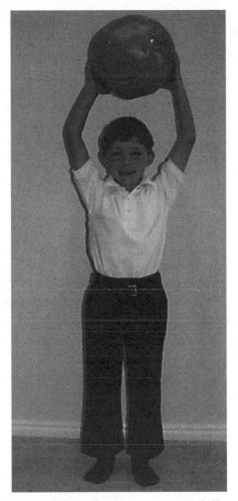

Figure 11-1   Child learning bilateral upper-extremity skills.

3. Describe Adams', Schmidt's, and Newell's motor learning theories.
4. Discuss Fitts' and Posner's stages of motor learning, and Gentile's motor tasks taxonomy.
5. Describe person, task, and environment influences on motor performance and motor learning.
6. Manipulate the following practice variables to optimize motor learning: prepractice variables; amount of practice; frequency, scheduling, and timing of augmented feedback; videotape feedback; discovery learning and guidance; practice variability; contextual interference; part- and whole-task practice; speed-accuracy trade-off; and audience effects.
7. Adapt motor learning principles for pediatric and older adult populations.

Table 11-1 Variables That Produce Temporary or Permanent Effects on Motor Performance and Measurement Methods

Primarily temporary effects	Primarily permanent effects	To measure primarily temporary effects	To measure primarily permanent effects
Motivation	Maturation and aging	Evaluate performance during practice	Evaluate performance during retention or transfer
Guidance			
Fatigue	Practice and learning		
Stress			
Boredom			
Pharmacologic agents			

Distinction between Motor Learning and Motor Performance

Motor *learning* is a process associated with practice or experience that results in a relatively permanent change in a patient's capability of performing skilled actions (motor performance).[1] Because it is a process, motor learning cannot be evaluated directly, but rather, it is evaluated indirectly most often by measuring *performance* on a motor task. For example, in physical therapy, motor learning can be evaluated by measuring change in a client's performance on a functional task, such as the "get-up-and-go" test.

At any point, however, motor performance is influenced by variables other than motor learning. Table 11-1 lists variables that may yield temporary or permanent effects on performance. Note that maturation and practice result in relatively permanent changes in performance. A common method of separating the permanent effects of maturation and practice is to measure changes across days or weeks instead of years. However, this method is ineffective when one is attempting to measure learning in pediatric and elderly populations, because maturation can result in physical changes over days or weeks in children and older adults. To separate maturation and practice influences on performance in these populations, comparisons of practice and nonpractice groups are usually necessary. For example, several studies have used two group experimental designs to separate performance changes due to maturation and participation in early intervention programs.[2,3]

Temporary factors, such as motivation, physical or verbal guidance, fatigue, stress, and boredom from long therapy sessions, also influence performance. During my initial years as a therapist, I essentially ignored these temporary effects. I now recognize, however, that temporary and permanent effects of these variables can have remarkably different effects on performance.

To measure motor learning, the effects of temporary factors on performance should be minimized. The most common method used to reduce the temporary effects of variables on performance is to allow a rest interval between the practice and the evaluation session. In physical therapy settings, the effects of temporary factors can be minimized by evaluating a client's performance after he or she rests, or by evaluating performance at the beginning of a subsequent therapy session.

Separating the effects of temporary and permanent factors on performance is critical for documentation. During the first 10 years of my clinical practice, I mistakenly documented client function using the best performance I observed in therapy. These performances could easily have been influenced by the temporary effects of therapy (e.g., hands-on guiding facilitation techniques). Now, I instead attempt to document temporary and permanent effects of variables. I document the permanent effects of practice by evaluating performance at the beginning of a therapy session. Then, I document client performance during therapy, which represents temporary and permanent effects of practice.

Goals of practice include capability to perform a practiced task at a later time and capability to modify a practiced task so that it can be performed in a different environment, at a different speed, or both. For example, goals for gait training might include the ability to walk at slow, medium, and fast velocities; on tile, carpet, grass, or snow; or in a crowded or dimly lit hallway. Often, the physical therapy environment does not include all environments that clients will encounter at a later time.

The field of motor learning distinguishes between evaluations in practiced and new environments. Evaluation in the same environment used during a practice or therapy session is termed a *retention test*, whereas evaluation in a different environment than that used during a practice session is termed a *transfer test*. For example, if a client practices walking on tile during therapy, he or she would undergo a retention test when evaluated on tile, and a transfer test when evaluated on carpet. Retention and transfer tests are used for measures of learning. Retention tests measure how well performers learn practiced tasks. Transfer tests measure how well performers learn to generalize learning and to perform the task unpracticed in a different environment.

Overview of Processes of Motor Learning

At least two major themes emerge from studying the processes of motor learning. First, learning is process specific: Performers remember processes, not specific movement patterns. Therefore, to optimize learning, therapists should understand the processes that clients practice in therapy. Second, practice conditions that encourage (or possibly force) performers to problem solve (i.e., process information and engage in sensory encoding and memory retrieval processes) are more effective for learning than practice conditions in which solutions are provided for performers. This theme suggests that clients in physical therapy should be active participants in not only the production of their movements, but also in the planning of their movements. Instead of performing therapy on patients for whom therapists provide all the solutions, therapists should act as educators by encouraging clients to solve problems. The processes of motor learning are listed in Table 11-2.

Stages of Learning

In 1967, Fitts and Posner proposed three sequential stages of motor learning: (1) cognitive stage, (2) associative stage, and (3) autonomous stage.[4] During the cognitive stage, performers focus on understanding a task goal and developing strategies to most efficiently achieve a goal. Because this stage is characterized by rapidly improving and variable performance, it is

Table 11-2　Summary of Processes of Motor Learning

1. Performers remember processes, not specific movement patterns.
2. Relative to guidance, problem solving enhances learning.
3. The three sequential stages of learning are cognitive, associative, and autonomous.
4. Automaticity develops by learning to focus on a critical subset of perceptual cues and motor strategies, and by reorganizing information in units (termed *chunking*).
5. The capability to detect and correct errors enhances learning. Error detection and correction occur on-line, or during slow, positioning movements. They occur after the movement in fast, timing tasks.
6. Exemplar and generalized sensory and motor memories are thought to be stored in memory.
7. Retrieval practice enhances learning more than repetitive drills.
8. Instead of focusing on individual elements of a functional task, performers should focus on the goals of a task.
9. Actions become more efficient when performers learn to exploit the biomechanics of a task.
10. Categorizing tasks based on task goals and environmental and performer contexts can enhance understanding of task requirements.

thought to require cognitive processes, such as attention. Teaching techniques and strategies are probably most useful in this stage of learning.

A classic example of the cognitive stage is the first few months of learning to drive a car. My personal performance at this stage consisted of gripping the steering wheel, being unable (or at least, unwilling) to remove my visual focus from the road, and having difficulty engaging in a conversation with another passenger or resetting the radio station. All of my attention was directed at trying to understand the relationships between the steering wheel, the gas pedal and the brake pedal, and keeping the car on the right side of the road and not in a ditch. In essence, driving demanded all my attention.

Each time I attempt a new motor task (e.g., juggling, in-line skating, or snowboarding), and often when I perform a well-learned task in an infrequently practiced environment (e.g., driving a car on icy, snowy roads, or skiing down a steeper hill than I am used to), I use this cognitive stage of learning. I often observe clients going through similar processes when they are in therapy. After a total knee replacement, clients often have difficulty performing a straight-leg raise. Yet, after they perform one straight-leg raise, they can often perform three or four in a row. Clients have reported that the limiting factor for their first straight-leg raise was not strength, but rather that their muscles were not performing the desired action. This suggests that clients need to think about and relearn the relationship between the action goal ("raise my leg") and the neuronal commands that achieve that goal.

After the cognitive stage of learning, performers enter the associative stage of learning. Here, the goal is to fine tune a skill. During this stage, the focus is on how to produce the most efficient action. Relative to the cognitive stage, this stage is characterized by slower gains in performance and reduced variability. Most motor learning studies have focused on this stage of learning.

To continue the previous example, the first few years after learning to drive an automobile represent the associative stage of learning. After time, I learned to smoothly accelerate and decelerate the car at intersections, and to smoothly change gears using the gearshift, clutch, and gas pedals. The associative stage is represented in physical therapy when clients practice a skill to increase the safety or efficiency of a task. For example, when a person with an above-knee amputation learns to use a prosthesis, the slow transition from taking a few uncoordinated steps to walking smoothly across the floor represents the associative stage. In essence, the client needs practice time to enhance her or his performance of a skill. Group therapy sessions and home exercise programs can be cost-effective methods for maximizing practice time of clients in the associative stage of learning.

The autonomous stage of learning is described as the *automatic stage*. Relative to the first two stages, performance in this stage requires very little attention and information processing. After several years of practice, my current driving style characterizes the autonomous stage. Recently, I was changing the radio station, holding a conversation with another adult, and monitoring children in the back seat while driving. In a physical therapy setting, the autonomous stage of practice is probably most apparent when clients are trying to unlearn compensatory or inefficient strategies for producing movement. For example, the techniques of forced use[5] and constraint-induced facilitation[6] were designed to discourage persons with long-term hemiparesis from performing activities with their least-impaired upper limb (an autonomous activity), and encourage performance of activities with their most-impaired upper limb (a cognitive activity).

At least two views can explain the development of the autonomous stage. One view states that during practice, performers learn to recognize critical aspects of their environment. Automaticity occurs because performers attend to a critical subset and ignore noncritical subsets of original information.[7] Therefore, automaticity occurs due to a reduction in the amount of original information processing. An alternative view states that the amount of information processing remains constant, whereas the speed of processing increases.[8] This view is most often explained by taking several sequential segments of an action and putting them together to form a larger unit; this is termed *chunking*. An example would be taking several individual letters and putting them together to form a word. Learners are thought to process the word as a whole unit, and not as individual letters. Processing a whole unit is thought to take less time than processing each component separately. Thus, by putting information into larger units, information processing is faster and automaticity occurs.

Error Detection

The capability to detect errors is another process that is thought to develop with learning. Error-detection capabilities are thought to require memory of sensory feedback from previously performed actions. Adams, in his 1971 closed-loop theory of learning, argued that performers accumulate memories of sensory feedback associated with each previously performed motor outcome. Storage of a memory for every action performed is termed an *exemplar memory*. Adams called these exemplar memories *perceptual traces*.[9]

Schmidt, in his 1975 schema theory of learning, argued that performers develop a recognition schema during practice.[10] These schema consist of a memory of initial environmental conditions, sensory feedback, and motor outcomes. In contrast to Adams' theory, in which every action is stored in memory, Schmidt suggests information from individual actions is kept only long enough

Table 11-3 Summary of Theories of Motor Learning

Adams' theory
- Focuses on slow, positioning tasks.
- Sensory feedback is required for movement (now known to be false).
- Exemplar (or individual) sensory and motor memories are stored each time an action is performed.
- Enhancing sensory feedback will enhance learning.
- Errors will always interfere with learning (now known to be false).
- Emphasizes practicing tasks to be performed at a later time (termed *specificity of learning*).

Schmidt's theory
- Focuses on fast, timing tasks.
- Defines a class of tasks as actions having identical relative timing and amplitude.
- Generalized sensory and motor memories are stored for a class of tasks.
- Novice actions should be performed as well as practiced actions within the same class of tasks.
- Errors can enhance learning.
- Emphasizes benefits of practicing several variations of a class of tasks (termed *variability in practice*).

Newell's theory
- Emphasizes performer, task, and environment constraints and relationships.
- Emphasizes relationships between sensory (perceptual) cues and motor (action) strategies.
- Emphasizes relationships between sensory and motor processes.

---

to develop or update a *generalized* memory. (See Table 11-3 and Appendix 11-A for summaries of Adams', Schmidt's, and Newell's theories of motor learning.)

In summary, Adams states that a memory is stored for every action that is performed, whereas Schmidt states that only a few generalized memories are stored. For example, in the functional task of transferring from a chair to standing, Adams' theory suggests that a sensory memory trace would be stored for each transfer that is attempted. Schmidt's theory suggests that only one sensory memory would be stored, and this memory would be a composite memory of all previous chair-to-standing transfers.

Regardless of whether exemplar (perceptual traces) or generalized (schema) memories are stored, Adams' and Schmidt's theories argue that error detection is possible due to the development of sensory feedback memories. The memories that enable error detection are thought to be used differently for slow-positioning and fast-timing tasks.

In slow-positioning tasks, sensory feedback is used to guide the action to its endpoint. Thus, performers move until feedback from the present action matches the memory of sensory feedback for the desired action. In fast-timing tasks, performers are unable to use sensory feedback to alter an action on-line, or during an action. In such tasks, sensory feedback is used to detect errors after the action has ended.[11]

Reaching for a cup while reading the newspaper is an example of a slow-positioning task. People will often reach toward the general direction of a cup, then use shoulder abduction and adduction until the hand hits the cup. They will then grasp the cup and bring it to their lips. Because sensory feedback is used during production of such an action, people are unable to determine the ultimate accuracy of their movements.

Trying to catch a glass of juice that is falling off a table is an example of a fast-timing task. A movement such as this is too fast for sensory feedback to be used during the movement. Sensory feedback can be used only after the movement to determine the accuracy of the action—that is, the person is holding the glass or looking at a puddle on the floor.

Several practice variables are thought to enhance the development of error-detection processes. These include allowing performers time to think about an action before feedback is provided by a therapist, asking performers to estimate their own errors before feedback is provided, and withholding therapist feedback on some practice trials (especially near the end of practice). Several studies demonstrate that increasing the amount or quality of sensory feedback during practice enhances performance. Expert coaches are thought to stress the development of error detection with the idea that if performers learn error detection, they will learn to evaluate their own performances, and can then continue to practice without the presence of a therapist or coach. For more detail on the effects of practice variables on error detection, see Swinnen et al.[12]

Motor Memories

In addition to storing generalized memories of sensory information, Schmidt[10] proposed that performers store generalized memories of motor information. He named this process the *recall schema*. This memory includes an abstraction or generalization of initial conditions, response specifications (time and amount of muscle activity used), and outcomes. In contrast, Adams[9] suggested that exemplar memories of individual actions are retained. An example of the difference between the two models can be seen with the functional task of chair-to-stand transfers. For this task, schema models suggest that only one generalized motor memory of chair-to-stand transfers is stored, and this memory is a composite of all previous attempts at this transfer. On the other hand, exemplar models suggest that motor traces from all previous chair-to-stand transfers are stored in memory. Results from several studies, however, have led many motor behaviorists to believe that exemplar and generalized memories are stored in memory.[13]

Forgetting and Retrieval Practice

A main goal of practice is to strengthen sensory and motor memories, or to retard forgetting. Forgetting has been hypothesized to occur because of trace decay and interference. *Trace decay* is considered a passive process in which a memory is simply weakened with time. *Interference* is an active process in which memories of different tasks disrupt one another. Little evidence exists to support task interference in motor learning. Thus, most forgetting is thought to occur secondary to trace decay, with the amount forgotten being dependent on the type of task. For example, forgetting is minimal for continuous tasks, such as bicycle riding, walking, running, ice skating, and skiing, and is more prevalent in discrete tasks, such as performing transfers, locking a wheelchair, removing foot rests, and bed mobility.

Ideally, performers will develop strong sensory and motor memories for actions during practice. To be successful in performing a task, however, performers must be able to retrieve those memories from long-term memory. Thus, a goal of practice is learning to retrieve information from long-term memory.[14] For example, if I ask you to solve the following math problems—multiply four times three, five times six, seven times two, and four times three—you will most likely have to retrieve all the answers from long-term memory. However, if I ask you to solve the following math problems—multiply four times three, four times three, and four times three—you can probably supply answers for the second and third questions using short-term memory without having to retrieve answers from long-term memory. Similar scenarios are present in physical therapy. For example, clients with left hemiparesis often forget to use their right arm to assist moving the left arm during transfers. When these clients are asked to perform the tasks roll from supine to right sidelying and back to supine, roll from supine to right sidelying and back to supine, and roll from supine to right sidelying and back to supine on sequential trials, they are not required to retrieve items from long-term memory on each trial. In contrast, if the tasks are presented in the sequence roll from supine to right sidelying, transfer from right sidelying to sitting, and transfer from sitting to left sidelying, clients would likely retrieve information from long-term memory on every trial.

Retrieval practice can be enhanced by switching the tasks performers practice on a trial-by-trial basis (termed *random* or *serial practice*), instead of using drills or practicing the same task on sequential trials (termed *blocked practice*). Blocked and random practice conditions have been studied under the label of *contextual interference* or *practice schedule*, which is discussed later in this chapter.

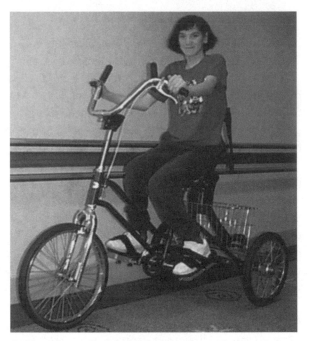

Figure 11-2   Child with cerebral palsy learning to ride a tricycle.

Focusing on Actions, Not Movements

Many motor behaviorists argue that memories for movements focus on task goals.[15] There is little evidence that performers store and retrieve memories for individual segments of an action (e.g., extend the elbow, open the fingers, close the fingers, then grasp an object), without regard for the task goal or the environment. This principle suggests that patients should practice tasks or actions, not individual movements. For example, Figure 11-2 shows a child with cerebral palsy learning to ride a tricycle. The therapy goal is to enhance interlimb coordination between her legs. During practice, the therapist and child focus on an outcome goal (moving the tricycle as fast as possible), and not on the movements of interlimb coordination.

Learning to Exploit Biomechanics

Increased consistency in kinematics and coordination also occurs with practice. Performers are thought to learn to take advantage of the passive inertia properties of muscles, joints, and limbs.[15,16] With practice, performers demonstrate increased speed and decreased energy costs because they have learned to optimize the peripheral sensory and motor requirements of the task.

Physical therapists and physical therapist assistants should be able to help clients exploit biomechanics to achieve a goal. For example, therapists most often teach a force-control strategy for sit-to-stand transfers. Although this strategy is relatively safe, a momentum strategy is more efficient. Shumway-Cook and Woollacott[17] advocate that clients be allowed to explore several strategies for transfers to have choices available. When clients seek safety over efficiency, they may choose a force-control strategy. When efficiency is the primary goal, a momentum strategy may be chosen.

Gentile's Task Taxonomy

What processes are critical for a particular task? Gentile attempted to answer this question by classifying tasks.[18] Her hypothesis was that the sensory, motor, and cognitive demands of a task are dependent on task goals, and environmental and performer contexts.

Table 11-4 lists Gentile's taxonomy of tasks. The rows are classified into one of four environmental contexts. In the first two categories, termed *stationary*, the environment is stable while the task is being performed. In the last two categories, termed *motion*, the environment is moving while the task is being performed. In the first and third categories, termed *no intertrial variability*, the environment remains constant from trial to trial. In the second and fourth categories, termed *intertrial variability*, the environment changes from trial to trial. Examples of tasks in each category are as follows:

1. Getting out of bed at home, brushing your hair, and propelling a wheelchair in the downstairs hallway are examples of a stationary environment with no intertrial variability (i.e., the environment is stationary, and does not change from one repetition to the next).
2. Propelling a wheelchair throughout the house on hardwood floors, carpet, and throw rugs; drinking from a glass or a mug; or walking with a cane, walker, or holding on to a wall are examples of stationary tasks with intertrial variability (i.e., the environment is stationary, yet it may change from trial to trial).
3. Stepping onto a moving walkway at airports, selecting food off of a cafeteria conveyor belt, or walking through a revolving door at the front of a hospital are examples of a motion environment with no intertrial variability (i.e., the environment is moving, but the movement does not change from trial to trial).
4. Maintaining balance on a moving bus, walking in a crowded mall, and catching a falling cup of juice are examples of a motion environment with intertrial variability (i.e., the environment is moving, and the movement changes between trials).

Table 11-4 Gentile's Taxonomy of Tasks

Performer context

			Body stability No manipulation	Body stability Manipulation	Body transport No manipulation	Body transport Manipulation
Environmental context	Stationary No intertrial variability		Closed Consistent Motionless Body stability	Closed Consistent Motionless Body stability	Closed Consistent Motionless Body transport	Closed Consistent Motionless Body transport
	Stationary Intertrial variability		Variable Motionless Body stability	Variable Motionless Body stability	Variable Motionless Body transport	Variable Motionless Body transport
	Motion No intertrial variability		Consistent Motion Body stability	Consistent Motion Body stability	Consistent Motion Body transport	Consistent Motion Body transport
	Motion Intertrial variability		Open Variable Motion Body stability	Open Variable Motion Body stability	Open Variable Motion Body transport	Open Variable Motion Body transport

Source: Adapted from AM Gentile. Skill Acquisition: Action, Movement and Neuromotor Processes. In J Carr, R Shepard, J Gordon, et al. (eds), Movement Science: Foundations for Physical Therapy Rehabilitation (2nd ed). Rockville, MD: Aspen Press, 2000.

As shown in the top of Table 11-4, tasks with little or no variation that are performed in a stable environment are termed *closed tasks*. These tasks require consistent patterns of movement and can be done automatically (or with little attention). Tasks that vary with each repetition, or that are performed in a changing environment are termed *open tasks* (see Table 11-4). These tasks require attention and a relatively high amount of information processing. Examples of functional closed-skill tasks are climbing a familiar flight of stairs and transferring from a wheelchair to a therapy mat. Examples of functional open-skill tasks are walking down a crowded corridor and maintaining balance while standing on a moving bus.

With the columns, Gentile separates tasks into one of four performer contexts. In the two categories on the left, termed *body stability*, the person focuses on maintaining a posture. In the two categories on the right, termed *body transport*, the person focuses on transporting himself or herself to another location. In the first and third categories, termed *no manipulation*, the person focuses on one task (e.g., holding a posture, or transporting herself or himself to another location). In the second and fourth categories, termed *manipulation*, the person is required to perform two tasks simultaneously (e.g., holding a posture and manipulating an object, or transporting himself or herself to another location while manipulating an object). Examples of tasks in each category are as follows:

1. Maintaining a sitting or standing posture is an example of body stability without manipulation.
2. Drinking from a cup while sitting and opening a kitchen cabinet while standing are examples of body stability with manipulation.
3. Walking and propelling a wheelchair with two feet are examples of body transport without manipulation.
4. Walking and talking simultaneously or carrying a cup of hot coffee from the stove to the kitchen table is an example of body transport with manipulation.

How does Gentile's taxonomy relate to physical therapy? Tasks frequently performed in physical therapy can be placed into one of Gentile's categories. Then these categories of tasks can be used to (1) understand the processes required for different physical therapy tasks, (2) evaluate the processes that a client is successful and unsuccessful at, (3) design an efficient exercise program based on a person's impairments and the tasks he or she would like to perform, and (4) educate clients and families on categories of tasks and processes that are safe and unsafe for clients to perform.

Variables That Influence Skill Learning

Considerable research effort within the fields of psychology, kinesiology, physiology, and engineering have focused on variables that influence skill learning. Information in this section is based on the premise that findings from experiments in these fields can be generalized to clinical populations. Although this generalization is probably most often correct, generalizing findings from experiments on normal populations to findings of clinical populations should be done with caution.

At least three weaknesses are revealed when attempting to generalize findings from motor learning experiments to real-world tasks, including those tasks performed in clinical environments. First, the majority of motor learning experiments tend to use single-joint or single-limb actions. These tasks are relatively simple compared to multiple-joint, multiple-limb actions that coaches and therapists attempt to help clients learn or relearn. Second, tasks and environments in most motor learning studies have been held constant. Thus, there is very little motor learning research under conditions with changing tasks or environments. Studies using changing tasks, environments, or both have typically focused on motor control mechanisms and not motor learning effects. Third, the majority of motor learning studies have focused on persons without cognitive, affective, or physical impairments (i.e., a normal population). Very few studies have focused on motor learning in therapeutic environments.

The few motor learning studies performed with clinical populations, however, suggest that the principles of motor learning are similar for populations with and without physical impairments.[19,20] Several therapists with expertise in motor learning have made the assumption that motor learning principles and results from experiments of motor learning provide a theoretical basis and suggestions for therapeutic interventions used by therapists.[21–23] Further research focusing on persons with physical impairments is needed to confirm the effectiveness of motor learning variables in therapeutic settings.

The purpose of this section is to provide readers with information on how to apply motor learning principles to clinical situations. As shown in Table 11-5, prepractice and practice variables are covered. This section is intended to be solely a summary of variables found to influence learning. For a more comprehensive review, readers should see Schmidt[1] or Magill.[24]

Prepractice Variables

Therapists can manipulate several motor learning variables even before practice begins. These prepractice variables include motivation, goal setting, ensuring that clients understand task goals, modeling, and demonstrations. Clients and their families should be included in goal formation. Goals should be motivating and challenging, yet clients should be able to learn to achieve the set goals. Goals should be objective and measurable (e.g., walk independently without losing balance for 80 meters in 1 minute). The goal "do the best you can" should be avoided, as it has been shown to be less effective for learning than objective, measurable goals. Goals should also be on the action or task level (e.g., walk up the steps). Performers should not be asked to perform motions (e.g., bend your hip and knee).

Before beginning practice, or in the early stages of practice, therapists should ensure that performers understand task goals and strategies for

Table 11-5 Variables That Influence Motor Learning

Prepractice variables
Goal setting
Understanding task goals
Understanding critical sensory cues and motor strategies
Modeling, demonstration
Practice variables
Amount of practice
Rate of improvement and over practice
Frequency of feedback (100% or reduced frequency of KR)
Scheduling of feedback (faded, bandwidth, or summary KR)
Timing of feedback (instantaneous or delayed KR)
Types of feedback (KR or KP)
Videotape feedback
Discovery, learning, and guidance
Variability in practice (several variations of a task)
Contextual interference effects (random, serial, and blocked practice effects)
Part- and whole-task practice
Speed-accuracy trade-off
Audience effects

KP = knowledge of performance; KR = knowledge of results.

achieving a task. Therapists should alert performers to critical sensory information and changes in sensory information. Motor strategies should be suggested by modeling or demonstrating tasks to performers. Modeling, or demonstrations, can be achieved by watching other clients learn a task, having a therapist model the desired action, or viewing oneself on videotape.

Practice Variables

Amount of Practice and Rate of Improvement

The amount of practice and the amount learned are often directly related. Therefore, therapists should take great pains to maximize practice. This can be achieved by increasing the amount of practice performed in a therapy session or by giving clients a HEP to practice outside of therapy sessions.

Research on constraint-induced therapy stresses the importance of practice for persons post stroke.[5,6] In several studies of constraint-induced therapy, patients are encouraged to use their involved arm for 90% of waking hours, and patients practice specific skills for 6–8 hours a day. Because practice is the most important variable for learning, therapists can no longer be the sole provider of direct intervention. A work group at the National Center for Medical Rehabilitation Research has recommended that family members, volunteers, or other lay persons be used to supplement treatment.[25]

An issue that has long been of interest to therapists and companies that provide financial compensation for therapeutic interventions is the rate of performance improvement. For almost every task, rate of improvement is directly related to the amount left to improve.[26] Thus, clients, therapists, and third-party payers should expect to see a decrease in the rate of improvement as the number of completed therapy sessions increases. This decreased rate of improvement may account for why several third-party payers terminate payment for services after a set number of clinic visits, or when a client has learned to perform a functional task.

However, therapists and third-party payers should also consider the learning effects of continued practice after a goal has been achieved. Continuation of practice after a criterion level of performance has been reached is termed *over learning* or *over practice*. Over practice is expensive, but the effects of over practice are thought to retard forgetting. In a classic study, Melnick had performers practice a balance task on an unstable surface in which the goal criterion was to maintain standing balance for at least 28 seconds.[27] Four practice conditions were used: subjects in the criterion condition (C) received no further practice after they reached the criterion goal; in the C-50%, C-100%, and C-200% conditions, performers practiced 50%, 100%, and 200% more trials, respectively, after they reached the criterion goal. Each subject participated in a retention session 1 week or 1 month after practice. The balance time on the first retention trial and the number of retention trials required to reach 28 seconds of standing balance were used as measures of amount learned.

Results of both retention trials were similar. The average time to achieve standing balance during the first retention trial was reliably longer for groups with over practice than for the C group. In addition, the average number of trials required to reach 28 seconds of standing balance were reliably less for the C-200% group than the criterion group. These results suggest that practice conditions that include over practice are more effective for learning than conditions in which performers practice until they reach a criterion goal. These beneficial learning effects are thought to be especially potent when, after some time interval without practice, the first attempt at a response is critical, such as to avoid falls or accidents. To balance the costs and benefits of practice beyond criterion levels, Magill[24] suggests that performers practice 100% beyond criterion levels.

In summary, the amount learned is usually directly related to the amount of practice. Therefore, clients should be encouraged to increase their practice time by using HEPs or by participating in group practice sessions. These extended practice sessions should be especially beneficial for safety and for generalizing skills to novel situations.

Augmented Feedback

Secondary to the amount of practice, information feedback is often considered to be the most important variable influencing skill learning.[28,29] Information feedback, presented before, during, or after an action, is information that informs performers about the correctness or effectiveness of an action. Intrinsic information feedback that is inherent in a task is provided by sensory systems, whereas extrinsic information feedback, which is not readily available in a task, is termed *augmented information*. A type of augmented information that has been studied extensively is knowledge of results (KR). *KR* is defined as extrinsic, postresponse information about the relationship between an action and a predetermined goal. Examples of KR occur when performers are told that their actions are too fast or too long, meaning that they need to decrease their speed or move a shorter distance, respectively, to achieve a goal.

Investigators have altered numerous variables, including the amount, temporal location, or the precision of KR, or any combination of these, in attempts to understand the principles of augmented feedback. The study of frequency and scheduling of information feedback has received a relatively large research effort.

Frequency of KR is most often studied by having several groups of performers practice the same number of actions, in which one group receives KR after every action and other groups receive KR less frequently.[30,31] Winstein and Schmidt[31] compared 100%-KR and 50%-KR practice conditions. In the 100%-KR condition, augmented feedback was presented after every practice action, whereas in the 50%-KR condition, augmented feedback was presented after 50% of the practice trials. After two practice sessions on 2 consecutive days, performers in both groups participated in retention sessions 10 minutes and 24 hours after the end of the second practice session. Performance during the practice sessions was similar for both groups. The 50%-KR group, however, demonstrated slightly smaller errors than the 100%-KR group on the 10-minute retention session, and significantly smaller errors on the 24-hour retention session. This result suggests that withholding augmented feedback on some practice trials is more beneficial for learning than providing augmented feedback on every practice trial.

Several schedules can be used to withhold augmented feedback after some practice actions. Winstein and Schmidt[31] and Ho and Shea,[30] in their studies of KR frequency, presented augmented feedback frequently early in each practice session and less often as the practice session continued. This is termed a *faded feedback schedule*. Because frequency and scheduling of feedback were manipulated, these experimental designs confounded the effects of feedback frequency and scheduling. To study the effects of feedback scheduling independent of feedback frequency, Nicholson and Schmidt[32] compared three 50%-KR practice conditions: (1) constant, (2) faded, and (3) reverse-faded. The constant condition feedback was presented on odd-numbered practice trials and withheld on even-numbered practice trials. In the faded condition, feedback was presented frequently early in practice and less often as practice continued. In the reverse-faded condition, feedback was presented seldom early in practice and frequently late in practice. The task and number of practice and retention trials were identical to the Winstein and Schmidt experiment.[31] During practice and in the 10-minute retention session, there were no reliable group performance differences. However, group differences in performance emerged during the 24-hour retention session, in which gradually increasing the frequency of feedback across practice degraded performance and gradually decreasing the frequency of feedback across practice enhanced it. These results suggest that a faded feedback schedule is more effective for skill learning than a constant feedback schedule or a reverse-faded feedback schedule.

Similar results have been found using bandwidth feedback during practice. In bandwidth feedback conditions, precise quantitative feedback is presented when performance lies outside a bandwidth of correctness surrounding a target, and withheld when performance is within a bandwidth of correctness. Because errors are typically large early in practice, performance is frequently outside the bandwidth of correctness, resulting in frequent feedback. As practice continues, errors typically become smaller, resulting in performances within the bandwidth of correctness, so feedback is frequently withheld. Relative to practice with feedback on every trial, practice with bandwidth feedback is beneficial for learning.[33,34]

Augmented feedback can be presented instantaneously after completing an action, or it can be delayed by some time interval. Swinnen et al.[12] had subjects practice for 2 days using instantaneous- or delayed-feedback conditions. In the instantaneous-feedback condition, KR was presented 290 milliseconds after performers completed an action: In the delayed-feedback condition, KR was presented 3.2 seconds after performers completed an action. Relative to practice with instantaneous augmented feedback, withholding KR for as little as 3.2 seconds after completing an action enhanced performance during long-term retention sessions even after 4 months without practice. These results suggest that delaying the presentation of augmented feedback for a few seconds after each practice action is more effective for learning than providing feedback instantaneously after each practice action.

Closely related to KR is knowledge of performance (KP). *KP* is defined as extrinsic feedback providing kinematic information about an action. An example of KP occurs when performers are told that they lack full knee extension in the terminal swing phase of gait. KP has been shown to have performance and learning effects similar to KR, suggesting that the principles of KR and other forms of extrinsic feedback are similar.

In summary, findings from several studies suggest that practice conditions with augmented extrinsic feedback withheld on some trials and delayed for a few seconds after an action are more effective for learning than practice conditions with frequent feedback, or those with feedback presented instantaneously after an action. There are several possible explanations for these findings.[35,36] One reason is that when feedback is presented instantaneously on every practice trial, performers are discouraged (or possibly prevented) from attending to their own sensory feedback and developing a strong relationship between sensory feedback and action outcomes. After all, why should performers expend energy to attend to sensory feedback when the consequences of actions (i.e., KR) are provided by someone else? A second explanation is that frequent augmented feedback discourages retrieval practice. Because frequent feedback provides solutions for correcting subsequent actions, performers have no need to retrieve their own solutions from long-term memory. A third possible explanation is that frequent augmented feedback late in practice may encourage performers to alter their actions based primarily on random variability or neuromuscular "noise" due to unstable neuromuscular processes.[37] Thus, frequent augmented feedback late in practice is less effective for learning than practice with feedback withheld on some trials.

The learning effects of frequent, immediate, augmented feedback have not been incorporated into equipment designs that are often found in therapeutic settings. In fact, just the opposite is true. Manufacturers often boast that their equipment has the capability to provide immediate, frequent feedback. Therapists need to be wary that this frequent, immediate feedback may enhance performance during therapy but may be ineffective for long-term retention.

Video Feedback

In 1976, Rothstein and Arnold published a review on the effects of videotape feedback.[38] Critical variables for effective videotape feedback were skill level and the use of verbal cues. Advanced performers benefited from videotape feedback, regardless of the provision of verbal cues. In contrast, to be effective for learning, novice performers needed verbal cues to focus their attention to pertinent information on the videotape.

Because therapy usually focuses on early stages of skill learning, videotape replay can be an effective method for learning. Videotape feedback can provide understandable information about correct, as well as efficient, movement kinematics. However, to optimize learning, therapists should focus a client's attention on critical aspects of the videotape. Similar to augmented feedback, videotape feedback should be provided frequently early in practice and less often as practice continues.

Videotape replay was used during therapy for David, the client with cerebral palsy who was described at the beginning of this chapter. During the terminal swing phase of gait, David lacked full knee extension, which resulted in a flexed knee on initial contact, a shortened stride length, and reduced gait velocity and function. I filmed a sagittal view (left and right sides) of David walking, and then David and I watched his video, as well as a video of an individual without any known physical impairments. We watched the videos at regular speed (60 frames per second), and at slow speeds focusing on the knee joint in terminal swing and initial contact. David was able to see and understand how a lack of full knee extension in terminal swing interfered with stride length and velocity. He then was able to provide his own solution for this problem.

Discovery Learning and Guidance

Discovery learning consists of providing performers with a challenging yet achievable problem and encouraging them to discover their own solutions. Guidance, usually considered the opposite of discovery learning, consists of verbal guidance, physical guidance, or both, used to achieve the goal with minimal, if any, errors.

In 1983, Hagman[39] examined the effects of guidance versus discovery learning. Compared to practice with discovery conditions, practice with guidance conditions demonstrated reliably large errors on a 24-hour retention session. Similar results have been found in children and older adult performers, suggesting that discovery practice is more effective for retention than guidance practice conditions, regardless of the performer's age.

Winstein and colleagues[40] compared the effects of physical guidance and frequent KR on skill learning. Practice with physical guidance on every trial (frequent KR) resulted in small errors during acquisition and large errors during retention. This suggests that frequent on-target performance, achieved via physical guidance, is detrimental to learning. Although frequent augmented feedback and guidance should be avoided, the effects of physical guidance appear to be especially ineffective for learning.

David, the client described previously, provided a good example of discovery learning when we were working on increasing knee extension in terminal swing. After David watched videotapes of himself and an individual without physical impairments, he attempted to recognize the perceptual differences when his knee was extended and slightly flexed in terminal swing. He would perform approximately five gait cycles in the view of a video camera, and then he would try and identify what cycles had correct and incorrect knee positioning. Then he watched the videotapes to receive feedback. David was determined to have correct knee positioning regardless of his footwear; thus, he performed this activity with sneakers, loafers, and cowboy boots. He discovered relationships between sensory feedback and knee positioning, and between weight and heel height of shoes and knee positioning.

Variability in Practice

Variability in practice refers to practice with several different versions of a task; specifically, at least two different overall time durations, overall force amplitudes, or both. *Constant practice* refers to practice with solely one version of a task—that is, one overall duration and amplitude. Schmidt's schema theory states that, relative to constant practice of a criterion speed, variability in practice enhances the learning of a criterion speed by allowing rule formation.[10] Studies using adult performers show mixed support for Schmidt's hypothesis. Studies using children performers, however, consistently show that practice variability is more effective for learning a criterion speed than practicing solely the criterion speed. In addition, variable practice usually results in more effective performance during transfer sessions when performers are practicing novel speeds, regardless of the performers' ages. These effects have been found in laboratory and real-world tasks, including badminton and forearm tennis serves, suggesting that practicing a task at several speeds enhances learning of the task goal and learning to generalize the task to a new goal. For a review of practice variability, see Shapiro and Schmidt.[41]

Functional tasks practiced in therapy often have several, not one, criterion speed. For example, my average gait speed in candlelit restaurants is different from my average gait speed in shopping malls. Based on results from studies of variability in practice, therapists should encourage clients to practice several speeds of functional tasks, using multiple strategies in multiple environments.

Practice Schedule or Contextual Interference

During a typical therapy session, several tasks are practiced. Often, several trials of one task are practiced before initiating practice of a second task. This scheduling is termed *blocked practice*. An alternative way to schedule practice is to practice different tasks on consecutive trials. This scheduling is termed *random practice*. Studies of blocked and random practice conditions have been termed *contextual interference paradigms*. Contextual interference effects are closely related to forgetting and retrieval practice, which was presented earlier in this chapter.

Results from several studies on contextual interference demonstrate that blocked practice is more effective than random practice for acquisition of a task, blocked and random practice produce equivalent performance on blocked retention tests, and random practice is more effective for performance on random retention tests than blocked practice.[42] These results suggest that, relative to practicing the same task over and over, intermingling different tasks throughout practice is beneficial for learning. These results have been generalized to several real-world tasks, including verbal learning, badminton serves, and wiring diagram tasks used in industry.

Contextual-interference effects are attributed to storage of more elaborate memory patterns[42,43] and retrieval practice[14] associated with random practice conditions. It is interesting to note that no major theory of motor learning can explain the effects of contextual interference on performance and learning. However, Magill and Hall provide an extensive review of contextual interference effects.[44]

Part- and Whole-Task Practice

To optimize learning, should functional tasks be taught as a whole or should individual segments of a task be taught separately and then combined to form a whole action? The answer to this dilemma is task dependent.[45]

When the task to be learned is the timing between segments, then whole-task practice enhances learning. For example, when learning to shift gears in an automobile, it is easy to learn to depress the clutch and to move the gear stick from one gear to another. The difficult part of the task is the coordination of depressing the clutch while changing gears. Because coordination (or timing) is the item to be learned, practice sessions should focus on the whole task. Coordination of segments is often the focus of continuous tasks, such as walking, swimming, and driving, suggesting that whole-task practice should be performed for these actions. Physical therapy tasks in which whole-task practice is recommended include wheelchair wheelies and momentum transfers.

When the task to be learned is information processing rather than coordination, part-task practice should be more beneficial for learning than whole-task practice. For example, the task of going from home to a downtown therapy location requires strategies for understanding spatial directions. The focus is on learning how to solve a maze of streets, and then making appropriate left and right turns to arrive at the location. Because information processing is the item to be learned, the focus of practice should be on learning segments of the task (e.g., directions from my house to the freeway, directions for freeway intersections, and directions from the freeway exit to the therapy setting). Information processing is often the focus of serial tasks, including floor-to-stand transfers and assembly line activities. Part-task practice should be used for these activities. Part-task practice is also efficient when a task consists of difficult and relatively simple segments. In such situations, performers can concentrate on difficult segments without needing to repeat the relatively simple segments of a task.

Speed-Accuracy Trade-Off

Physical therapy goals often include criteria for increased accuracy and speed when performing functional tasks. However, increasing speed usually results in decreased spatial accuracy, which is termed *speed-accuracy trade-off*. Because speed and accuracy are inversely related, therapists may choose to work on speed or accuracy during a therapy session. Bobath[46] argues that therapy interventions should focus on accuracy, and speed should be increased only after accuracy has been achieved. However, several lines of research suggest that when accuracy and speed are important components of a task, both should be emphasized early in practice.

In one experiment, performers practiced the criterion speed throughout practice (60 repetitions of a task per minute), or the practice speed was gradually increased across practice (beginning at 10 repetitions per minute and increasing to 60 repetitions per minute). Practicing the criterion speed throughout practice was more effective for learning a 60-repetitions-per-minute action than gradually increasing movement speed across practice.[47]

Malouin et al. and Richards et al.[48,49] reported on the use of an intensive gait-training program in clients with acute cerebrovascular accidents. Their program included speed training (via the use of a treadmill), and accuracy training (via the use of a limb-load monitor). Results from their studies demonstrated that an intensive gait-training program can be tolerated by clients with acute stroke, and that it is more effective for enhancing gait function than a conventional gait-training program.

These findings suggest that, in contrast to traditional approaches used in neurorehabilitation in which accuracy is acquired before working on developing speed, therapists should focus on increased accuracy and speed beginning on the first day of therapy.

Audience Effects

The presence or absence of an audience can have dramatic effects on performance.[50] When a skill is well learned and an audience has little evaluation potential, performance is usually enhanced by an audience. When a skill is poorly learned or the audience has a relatively large evaluation potential, or both, performance is usually degraded by an audience. For example, although I am a novice singer, I enjoy singing. My best singing performances occur when I have the house to myself and I am in the shower. At a recent business party, to my surprise, the host announced that I was going to sing a song for the guests. I was very embarrassed and nervous, and during the performance my voice cracked several times. The audience interfered with my novice singing capabilities. Similar scenarios occur in physical therapy when therapists ask clients to demonstrate motor skills in the presence of their families. For example, imagine a 55-year-old man poststroke who is an inpatient in a rehabilitation setting. He has successfully accomplished the tasks of bed mobility and sit-to-stand transfers, and is just beginning to take a few steps with close supervision for balance and safety. His wife is healthy, but she is concerned that she may not be able to care for her husband at home. She is concerned that if he lost his balance she would be unable to catch him, and, therefore, she is considering long-term institutional care. To help the wife make an educated decision about placement, you invite her to observe her husband practicing in physical therapy. Her husband performs bed mobility and supine-to-sit transfers faultlessly, and his wife smiles and relaxes. Then, as he attempts to transfer from sit-to-stand, he loses his balance and falls back onto the mat. His wife becomes tense, sits on the edge of her chair, and starts offering verbal and nonverbal suggestions (e.g., "be careful"). The client attempts another sit-to-stand transfer, but this time his movements are guarded and tense. He is successful with his transfer, but he decides he is too uncomfortable to take any steps. One explanation for this scenario is that the client's performance degraded because sit-to-stand transfers and gait were poorly learned tasks and his wife had evaluation potential. I am not suggesting that families be excluded from therapy sessions, but rather that therapists evaluate and consciously manipulate the effects of audiences on performance.

Special Considerations for Children and Older Adults

Adult, pediatric, and older adult populations use the same processes for learning, suggesting that variables that influence learning are similar for all three populations. The differences in learning between these populations appear to be in the rate of learning and in the strategies chosen to perform tasks.

Children and older adults demonstrate relatively long reaction and movement times when performing tasks, and the duration of their responses is exaggerated further when they are required to make choices. Most learning specialists suggest that neither immaturity nor aging of the sensory and motor systems is the primary cause of slower reaction and movement times. Rather, slowness of central information processing degrades sensory-motor control in pediatric and older adult populations.[51] In essence, these populations take longer than average to make decisions. Motor learning principles suggest that therapists and coaches should encourage central information processing by requiring clients to make decisions (i.e., to problem solve) during practice, and to increase the duration of time provided to make decisions.

The previous section of this chapter on variables that influence skill learning suggested several variables that therapists can manipulate to encourage problem solving. In addition, for older adults, imagery has been found to be almost as effective as physical practice, suggesting that mental and physical practice should be used with older adults.[52] For children, variability in practice has been shown to be more effective for learning than constant practice, suggesting that children should practice several variations of a task.[41] Unfamiliar units of measure and very precise feedback can be confusing for children and degrade learning, and thus, should be avoided.

Summary

Motor learning principles provide a theoretical basis for physical therapy interventions. Many motor learning variables are under the control of therapists and can easily be incorporated into therapeutic settings. A challenge for therapists is to test the generalization of motor learning principles to actions performed by persons with physical dysfunction.

Several lines of research suggest that errors are not detrimental to learning. Practice conditions that allow a drift in performance away from the task goal (e.g., withholding augmented feedback on some trials, random practice, and discovery learning) enhance performance on long-term retention tests. These findings suggest that compared with practice conditions that prevent errors, practice conditions that allow some errors enhance learning. One explanation for these findings is that practice conditions with errors force performers to engage in processes that enhance their learning.

A common trend that emerges from the guidance, KR, and contextual interference literature is that practice conditions that encourage (or possibly force) performers to engage in sensory encoding and retrieval processes are more effective for learning than practice conditions that frequently provide solutions. Possibly, a therapist's role is to provide several tasks, several variations of each task, and several environments that encourage information processing. Information processing should be enhanced by providing occasional, not frequent, guidance or KR, or by intermingling tasks throughout the therapy session, rather than completing one task before beginning practice on a second task. Certainly, drills in which performers repeat the same movement over and over to memorize a normal movement pattern should be avoided.

At least three major themes emerge from motor learning studies. First, temporary and permanent effects of variables can have remarkably different effects on performance. Second, learning is process specific: Performers remember processes, not specific movement patterns. Third, practice conditions that encourage (or possibly force) performers to process information or engage in sensory encoding and memory retrieval processes are more effective for learning than practice conditions that provide frequent solutions.

References

1. Schmidt RA. Motor Control and Learning: A Behavioral Emphasis (2nd ed). Champaign, IL: Human Kinetics, 1988.
2. Resnick MB, Eyler FD, Nelson RM, et al. Developmental intervention for low birth weight infants: improved early developmental outcome. Pediatrics 1987;80:68.
3. Turnbill JD. Early intervention for children with or at risk of cerebral palsy. Am J Dis Child 1993;147:54.
4. Fitts PM, Posner MI. Human Performance. Belmont, CA: Brooks/Cole, 1967.
5. van der lee JH, Wagenaar RC, Lankhorst GJ, et al. Forced use of the upper extremity in chronic stroke patients. Stroke 1989;30:2369–2375.
6. Kunkel A, Kopp B, Muller G, et al. Constraint-induced movement therapy for motor recovery in chronic stroke patients. Arch Phys Med Rehabil 1993;74:347.
7. Schmidt RA. The Acquisition of Skill: Some Modifications to the Perception-Action Relationship Through Practice. In H Heuer, AF Sanders (eds), Perspectives on Perception and Action. Hillsdale, NJ: Erlbaum, 1987;77.
8. Keele SW. Attention and Human Performance. Pacific Palisades, CA: Goodyear, 1973.
9. Adams JA. A closed-loop theory of motor learning. J Mot Behav 1971;3:111.
10. Schmidt RA. A schema theory of discrete motor skill learning. Psychol Rev 1975;82:225.
11. Schmidt RA, White JL. Evidence for an error detection mechanism in motor skills: a test of Adams' closed-loop theory. J Mot Behav 1972;4:143.

12. Swinnen S, Schmidt RA, Nicholson DE, et al. Information feedback for skill learning: instantaneous knowledge of results degrades skill learning. J Exp Psychol Learn Mem Cogn 1990;16:706.
13. Lee TD, Hiroth TT. Encoding specificity principle in motor short-term memory for movement extent. J Mot Behav 1980;12:63.
14. Lee TD, Magill RA. The locus of contextual interference in motor-skill acquisition. J Exp Psychol Learn Mem Cogn 1983;9:730.
15. Bernstein N. The coordination and regulation of movements. Oxford, UK: Pergamon Press, 1967.
16. Kelso JAS, Holt KG, Kugler PN, et al. On the Concept of Coordinative Structures as Dissipative Structures. II. Empirical Lines of Convergence. In GE Stelmach, J Requin (eds), Tutorials in Motor Behavior. Amsterdam: North-Holland, 1980;49.
17. Shumway-Cook A, Woollacott M. Motor Control: Theory and Practical Application (2nd ed). Baltimore: Lippincott Wilkins, 2001.
18. Gentile AM. Skill Acquisition: Action, Movement and Neuromotor Processes. In J Carr, R Shepherd, J Gordon, et al. (eds), Movement Science: Foundations for Physical Therapy in Rehabilitation (2nd ed). Rockville, MD: Aspen Press, 2000.
19. Swanson LR, Lee TD. Effects of aging and schedules of knowledge of results on motor learning. Gerontology 1992;47:406.
20. Merians A, Winstein C, Sullivan K, et al. Effects of feedback for motor skill learning in older healthy subjects and individuals post-stroke. Neurol Rep 1995;19:23.
21. Winstein CJ. Designing Practice for Motor Learning: Clinical Implications. In MJ Lister (ed), Contemporary Management of Motor Control Problems. Proceedings of the II Step Conference. Alexandria, VA: Foundation for Physical Therapy, 1991.
22. Crutchfield CA, Barnes MR. Motor Control and Learning in Rehabilitation. Atlanta: Stokesville Publishing, 1993.
23. Montgomery PC, Connolly BH. Motor Control and Physical Therapy: Theoretical Framework and Practical Applications. Hixson, TN: Chattanooga Group, 1991.
24. Magill RA. Motor Learning: Concepts and Applications (6th ed). Dubuque, IA: McGraw-Hill, 2001.
25. Fuher MJ, Keith RA. Facilitating patient learning during medical rehabilitation: a research agenda. Am J Phys Med Rehabil 1998;78:557–561.
26. Newell A, Rosenbloom PS. Mechanisms of Skill Acquisition and the Law of Practice. In JR Anderson (ed), Cognitive Skills and Their Acquisition. Hillsdale, NJ: Erlbaum, 1981;1.

27. Melnick MJ. Effects of over learning on the retention of a gross motor skill. Res Q Exerc Sport 1971;42:60.

28. Bilodeau IM. Information Feedback. In EA Bilodeau (ed), Acquisition of Skill. New York: Academic, 1969;255.

29. Newell KM. Knowledge of Results and Motor Learning. In J Keough, RS Hutton (eds), Exercise Sport Science Review. Santa Barbara, CA: Journal of Publishing Affiliates, 1976;195.

30. Ho L, Shea JB. Effects of relative frequency of knowledge of results on retention of a motor skill. Percept Mot Skills 1978;46:859.

31. Winstein CJ, Schmidt RA. Reduced frequency of knowledge of results enhances motor-skill learning. J Exp Psychol Learn Mem Cogn 1990;16: 677.

32. Nicholson DE, Schmidt RA. Scheduling Information Feedback to Enhance Training Effectiveness. Proceedings of the Human Factors Society 35th Annual Meeting. Santa Monica, CA: Human Factors Society, 1991;1400.

33. Sherwood DE. Effect of bandwidth knowledge of results on movement consistency. Percept Mot Skills 1988;66:535.

34. Lee TD, White MA, Carnahan H. On the role of knowledge of results in motor learning: exploring the guidance hypothesis. J Mot Behav 1990;22: 191.

35. Salmoni AW, Schmidt RA, Walter CB. Knowledge of results and motor learning. A review and critical reappraisal. Psychol Bull 1984; 95:355.

36. Schmidt RA. Frequent Augmented Feedback Can Degrade Learning: Evidence and Interpretations. In GE Stelmach, J Requin (eds), Tutorials in Motor Neuroscience. Dordrecht, Germany: Kluwer Academic Publishers, 1991;59.

37. Nicholson DE. Information Feedback Disrupts Performance Stability [Ph.D. dissertation.] University of California, Los Angeles, 1992.

38. Rothstein AL, Arnold RK. Bridging the gap: application of research on videotape feedback and bowling. Mot Skills: Theory Pract 1976;1:35.

39. Hagman JD. Presentation- and test-trial effects on acquisition and retention of distance and location. J Exp Psychol Learn Mem Cogn 1983;9:334.

40. Winstein CJ, Pohl PS, Lewthwaite R. Effects of physical guidance and knowledge of results on motor learning: support for the guidance hypothesis. Res Q Exerc Sport 1994;65:316.

41. Shapiro DC, Schmidt RA. The Schema Theory: Recent Evidence and Developmental Implications. In JAS Kelso, JE Clark (eds), The Development of Movement Control and Coordination. New York: Wiley, 1982; 113.

42. Shea JB, Morgan RL. Contextual interference effects on the acquisition, retention, and transfer of a motor skill. J Exp Psychol Hum Learn 1979;5:179.

43. Shea JB, Zimny ST. Context Effects in Memory and Learning of Movement Information. In RA Magill (ed), Memory and Control of Action. Amsterdam: North-Holland, 1983;345.

44. Magill RA, Hall KG. A review of the contextual interference effect in motor skill acquisition. Hum Move Sci 1990;9:241.

45. Naylor J, Briggs G. Effects of task complexity and task organization on the relative efficiency of part and whole training methods. J Exp Psychol 1963;65:217.

46. Bobath B. Adult Hemiplegia: Evaluation and Treatment (3rd ed). Oxford, UK: Heinemann Medical Books, 1990.

47. Sage GH, Hornak JE. Progressive speed practice in learning a continuous motor skill. Res Q Exerc Sport 1978;49:190.

48. Malouin F, Potvin M, Prevost J, et al. Use of an intensive task-oriented gait training program in a series of patients with acute cerebrovascular accidents. Phys Ther 1992;72:781.

49. Richards CL, Malouin F, Wood-Dauphinee, et al. Task-specific physical therapy for optimization of gait recovery in acute stroke patients. Arch Phys Med Rehabil 1993;74:612.

50. Singer RN. Effect of an audience on performance of a motor task. J Mot Behav 1970;2:88.

51. Welford AT. Motor Performance. In G Barren, K Schaiek (eds), Handbook of the Psychology of Aging. New York: van Nostrand Reinhold, 1977;3.

52. Surberg PR. Aging and effect of physical-mental practice upon acquisition and retention of a motor skill. J Gerontol 1976;31:64.

Annotated Bibliography

Campbell SK. Proceedings of the consensus conference on efficacy of physical therapy in the management of cerebral palsy. Pediatr Phys Ther 1990;2:121. This publication is based on a conference, sponsored by the American Physical Therapy Association Pediatric Section, in New Orleans in 1990. Theoretical and clinical articles related to efficacy of physical therapy interventions in children with cerebral palsy were written on several topics, including rate of motor development, improving postural control, neurophysiology and motor control theories, promoting family functioning and functional independence, the role of the physical therapist in family stress and coping, and physicians' beliefs in the efficacy of physical therapy.

Carr HJ, Shepherd RB, Gordon J, et al. Movement Science: Foundations for Physical Therapy in Rehabilitation (2nd ed). Rockville, MD: Aspen Press, 2000. This book was designed to demonstrate how basic science principles from the field of neuromotor control and learning could be applied to physical therapy practice. It includes chapters on assumptions underlying physical therapy interventions, Carr and Shepherd's motor learning model, skill acquisition, and recovery of function after brain injury.

Harrow AJ. A Taxonomy of the Psychomotor Domain. New York: David McKay, 1972. Educators in classroom and clinical situations use Bloom's taxonomy to develop cognitive and affective objectives, practice activities, and evaluation items. Harrow developed a taxonomy for psychomotor skills that can be used in classroom and clinic situations. His taxonomy consists of seven hierarchical levels: (1) perception, (2) set, (3) response, (4) mechanism, (5) complex overt response, (6) adaptation, and (7) origination.

Lister MJ (ed). Contemporary Management of Motor Control Problems. Proceedings of the II Step Conference. Alexandria, VA: Foundation for Physical Therapy, 1991. This publication is based on a conference, sponsored by the American Physical Therapy Association Neurology and Pediatric Sections and the Foundation for Physical Therapy, in Norman, Oklahoma, in 1990. Twenty-eight papers focus on new information in the field of motor control, development and learning, issues that challenge current physical therapy approaches, and suggestions for how motor control, development, and learning issues can be integrated into physical therapy practice.

Magill RA. Motor Learning: Concepts and Applications (6th ed). Dubuque, IA: McGraw-Hill, 2001. This book was designed for an undergraduate course in motor learning. It includes chapters on motor learning principles for several types of tasks, performers, and environments. It focuses on performance and learning effects of several variables while providing a brief theoretical explanation of motor learning phenomena.

Schmidt RA. Motor Control and Learning: A Behavioral Emphasis (3rd ed). Champaign, IL: Human Kinetics, 1999. This book was designed for a graduate course in motor learning. It includes sections on motor behavior and control and motor learning and memory. It contains hundreds of references to motor behavior research and literature. It is essentially an encyclopedia for the field of motor behavior.

Winstein CJ, Knecht HG. Movement Science. Alexandria, VA: American Physical Therapy Association, 1991. This publication consists of 24 contributions published in the December 1990 and January 1991 special issues of *Physical Therapy*. The contributions present current research in the field of movement science and provide suggestions for clinical application and for application in physical therapy programs.

Theories of Motor Learning

In this appendix, three well-known theories of motor learning (by Adams, Schmidt, and Newell) are briefly described, and suggestions are given for their application to physical therapy practice. The assumptions and predictions of these theories can also be found in Table 11-3.

Adams' Closed-Loop Theory

In 1971, Adams published a closed-loop theory of motor learning.[1] Adams proposed that memory consists of perceptual and memory traces. The memory trace is used to select the direction of movement and to initiate an action. The perceptual trace, consisting of sensory feedback for an intended action, serves as a reference of correctness and is developed during practice. Any mismatch between ongoing sensory feedback and the perceptual trace is detected as error. Adams hypothesized that performers continue to move until ongoing sensory feedback matches the stored perceptual trace. This theory predicts that sensory feedback is a requirement for movement and learning, learning is directly related to the strength of the perceptual trace, practice without errors strengthens the perceptual trace and enhances learning, practice with errors weakens the perceptual trace and degrades learning, and previously practiced actions are performed better than unpracticed actions (termed *specificity of practice and learning*).

A strength of Adams' theory is its predictions for slow, positioning actions. A weakness of the theory is that it is unable to account for movement and conditioned learning without sensory feedback. In 1968, Taub and Berman[2] demonstrated that conditioned learning can occur in primates after deafferentation. Additional research has revealed several other weaknesses of Adams' theory. For example, practicing several variations of a task by changing the overall amplitude or duration (termed *variable practice*) is at least as effective, or more effective, for learning in children than practicing one variation of a task (termed *constant practice*).

There are at least three ways that Adams' theory might relate to physical therapy. First, it outlines the processes used for producing slow movements. Physical therapists can use these steps when educating clients to perform slow actions. Second, because this theory stresses the benefits of making sensory feedback more accurate, or more apparent to performers, it advocates the use of many facilitation techniques, visualization, and biofeedback. Third, this theory argues for specificity of practice and learning. Clients should practice the tasks they want to perform after discharge, and they should practice them in an environment that is as similar as possible to the post-therapy environment.

Schmidt's Schema Theory

In 1975, Schmidt[3] published an open-loop theory of motor learning, in which performers learn schema and motor programs during practice. Schmidt argued that instead of storing information for every practiced action, performers store generalized rules about a class of actions. Schmidt proposed that a generalized motor program and two memory templates are stored: (1) a recognition (sensory) schema to evaluate actions, and (2) a recall (motor) schema to produce actions. The generalized motor program is described in vague terms. Schmidt stated that it consists of a central framework of a task without specifics. Recognition and recall schemes were described in the chapter section Processes of Learning.

The recognition and recall schemes are modified and updated based on outcome feedback. Any variables that strengthen the recognition and recall schemes should enhance learning; thus, errors in practice should enhance, not hinder, learning. Because traces of individual trials are not stored, this theory predicts that novel actions will be performed as accurately as practiced movements within the same class of actions. Variations within the same class of actions occurs by altering the overall duration or amplitude of a movement.

Strengths of Schmidt's theory are its attention to fast, timing actions and its prediction of variability in practice effects, which are discussed in the chapter section Variables That Influence Skill Learning. Variability in practice effects seems to be especially beneficial for learning in children, because children have less practice than adults. Because adults have a large amount of practice, they may have experienced variable practice before coming to an experimental situation. Weaknesses of Schmidt's theory are its failure to explain how generalized motor programs are developed and to account for novel strategies for actions when performers are given new constraints or new environments.

What does Schmidt's theory have to do with physical therapy? First, Schmidt outlined the processes used to perform fast, timing actions. Physical therapists can use these steps when educating clients to perform fast actions. Second, Schmidt's theory supports the idea that clients should practice several versions of a task. For example, instead of practicing gait training on one surface at a single speed (which may be all that a client in a nursing home is required to perform), clients should practice walking on several surfaces (e.g., tile, carpet, grass, cement, and gravel) at several speeds (e.g., slow, self-chosen, and maximal). Third, Schmidt argued that errors can enhance learning. Thus, clients should be allowed to make errors so that they can distinguish between correct and incorrect perceptual feedback and motor actions to achieve a goal.

Newell's Theory

In 1991, Newell[4] suggested that instead of learning motor programs, practice leads to a stronger coupling between perception and action. Newell argued that learning consists of developing optimal strategies to solve an action problem for a given task and environmental constraints. Newell defined two workspaces—*perceptual* and *motor*. During learning, performers explore their workspaces to identify critical perceptual cues and motor strategies for performing efficient actions.

Because Newell's theory is relatively new, few studies have been performed to test it. Its strength is in its focus on the relationship between sensory and motor processes. The major weakness is that it is essentially an untested theory. Physical therapists can apply this theory by helping clients understand the critical perceptual cues and motor strategies of a task.

Please refer to the annotated bibliography and references at the end of this chapter for more information regarding these and other theories of motor learning.

References

1. Adams JA. A closed-loop theory of motor learning. J Mot Behav 1971;3:111.
2. Taub E, Berman AJ. Movement and Learning in the Absence of Sensory Feedback. In SJ Freedman (ed), The Neuropsychology of Spatially Oriented Behavior. Homewood, IL: Dorsey Press, 1968.
3. Schmidt RA. A schema theory of discrete motor skill learning. Psychol Rev 1975;82:225.
4. Newell KM. Motor skill acquisition. Annu Rev Psychol 1991;42:213.

12

Educational Materials for Use in Patient Home Education Programs

Paul Ogbonna

Mrs. Tyrell was discharged home 3 days after surgery for a right total hip replacement and given a home exercise program (HEP). This patient was confused about how to use her quad cane and had many questions and concerns. "On which side of the body should I hold my cane?" "Does the right or left foot move out first?" "How much weight should I put on the side of my surgery?" She complained, "All the exercises are painful when I perform them." The family requested a home health agency to send a physical therapist and advised Mrs. Tyrell to stop further exercises or walking until a physical therapist came. It took several days before the therapist was able to evaluate the patient, due to the delay in going through complicated insurance procedures for authorizing a home care visit. Mrs. Tyrell started to experience physical complications as a result of poor HEP instructions and delayed follow-up physical therapy services. She was finally evaluated, taught an appropriate HEP, and placed on three times per week intensive therapy (with supervision). Both Mrs. Tyrell and her family were relieved and happy.

Many patients risk not progressing, or even injuring themselves when performing exercises incorrectly due to poor HEP instructions. It is the responsibility of the physical therapist and physical therapist assistant to ensure that patients are properly instructed on what types of exercise are good and safe to perform and how, when, and for what duration during each session.

One of the problems facing therapists is finding time to construct well-written and well-directed home exercise programs for the patient under their care. Home exercise programs are an essential extension of clinic-based therapy. These programs may be performed at home, work or in any place appropriate for the patient. Home exercises also enable patients to be active participants in their care and therapy. Home exercise programs should, therefore, be precise and clearly written in a simple language, easy to understand language, with appropriate and plain diagrams.[1]

Chapter Objectives

After completing this chapter, the reader will be able to

1. Define the components of a patient/family home education program and discuss the importance of designing programs that are responsive to the individual needs of each patient and his or her family.
2. Give examples of home programs that include the use of personalized exercises, videos, exercise cards, and instruction sheets.
3. Describe different ways of using the Internet to support physical therapy home education programs.
4. Identify how to assess, evaluate, and use online exercise programs available through the Internet.
5. Discuss cultural barriers in using prepackaged home programs with patients and families in home settings.

Benefits of Home Exercise Programs

Home exercise and home education programs are part of the continuation of physical therapy treatment. They provide patients with a guide to continue at home what they were doing at the clinic under supervision of the therapist. Participating in a home program can increase patients' confidence and boost self-esteem by teaching them to participate in their

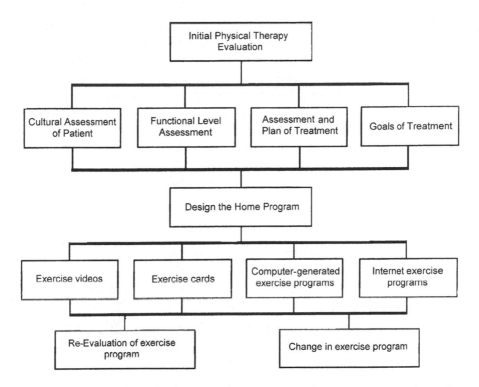

Figure 12-1 Guidelines for designing home patient education programs from the first to last stage.

own recovery. Patients realize all is not lost after a disability, and that with hard work they can regain many of their functional skills.

In addition, there are many different types of exercise programs and resources available to therapists so that less time is spent writing and editing instructions. This allows therapists to increase productivity by devoting more time to treatment, care, and patient management.

Creating a Home Education Program

Patient Assessment

The first step in designing a patient HEP is assessment (Figure 12-1). Patient functional status, patient/family education evaluation, and cultural considerations are assessed and considered in designing the program. Patients' functional status can be evaluated by the physical therapist using basic tests for range of motion, muscle strength, balancing, posture, and gait patterns. A comprehensive assessment may be needed for some patients, due to complex problems and their home care needs. Two assessment instruments that may be used are the Comprehensive Assessment and Referral Evaluation, which assesses physical, mental, social, nutritional, and economic aspects, and the Multidimensional Functional Assessment Questionnaire, which measures mental health, physical health, and activities of daily living function.[2]

Chapter 8 presents many ideas about patient education, including a section on creating HEPs. Chapters 9 and 10 present techniques on how to assess patient receptivity to change and how to facilitate health behavior changes. The information in those chapters will help you understand the context within which educational materials presented in this chapter might be used.

Knowledge and Skill Levels

Assess the patient's current understanding of his or her illness by asking simple opening questions, such as: "How are you feeling today?" "What did the doctor tell you about your illness?" "What are your problems?" "Do you understand the diagnosis for your condition?" Establish trust with the patient by being an active listener. Ask: "What impact has this problem had on your life?" "What are the characteristics of the problem?" "What do you want to be able to do that you can't do now?"

Learning Barriers

Identify barriers to learning. Common barriers are fatigue, pain, language, cognitive/sensory impairment, age, culture, conflict with values, and anxiety. Questions that may help you to understand the patient's barriers to learning are: "Do you have a primary language other than English?" "Where does it hurt when you move your body?" "Is it all right to give you some home exercise programs?" "Do you think you will have any problems in performing these exercises at home?"

A major learning barrier may be culture. Bates and Plog, cited by Samovar and Porter in *Communication Between Cultures*,[3] define *culture* as the following:

> Culture is a system of shared beliefs, values, customs, behaviors, and artifacts that the members of the society use to cope with their world and with one another, and that are transmitted from generation to generation through learning. This definition includes not only patterns of behavior but also patterns of thought (shared meanings that the members of society attach to various phenomena, natural and intellectual, including religion and ideologies), artifacts (tools, pottery, houses,

machines, works of art), and the culturally transmitted skills and technique used to make artifacts.[3]

For example, in some cultures, illness is viewed as a result of a sin committed by the patient or a member of the family. In other cultures, illness is regarded as a punishment for evils committed in present or past lives. There is no doubt that culture is a very sensitive issue and may affect care and rehabilitation.

> Consider patient cultural characteristics when providing care. Identify their cultural beliefs and respect them. Treat each patient as an individual. Avoid stereotypes. Consider other factors that may affect care: age, gender, family, socioeconomic factors. Endeavor to learn about the patient's cultural beliefs and attitudes towards health care and providing care.[4]

Mukai states, "Create an atmosphere of trust and respect, and encourage openness to discuss problems."[5] Thus, ask the patient such questions as: "What customs, traditions, or practices are important to you?" "Would you prefer a family member be involved in your care?" "What religion do you identify yourself with?" "Are there any other things about your customs you would like me to know that would affect the way the treatment should be planned?" Answers to these questions should help the physical therapist know and understand the patient's cultural background and how this may impact care.

In summary, physical therapists should conduct a cultural assessment to provide an outline of patients' cultural background, either during initial evaluation or before designing the home education program. Cultural awareness and understanding will help all health care providers increase competence and improve patient care outcomes.

Identifying Patients' Learning Preferences

There are different methods of teaching or presenting HEPs, including handouts, audio-visuals, demonstrations, family involvement, and verbal, group, or individual discussion. The physical therapist should try to find out the learning preferences of the patient. Ask the patient: "Do you prefer reading materials, videos, demonstrations, or a combination of one or two of these techniques?" Be ready to show examples: Bring a relevant video exercise tape, handouts, and some portable exercise equipment for demonstration. In the past, for many physical therapists and physical therapist assistants, creating and designing HEPs for patients was a frustrating and difficult task. For example, positions and exercises had to be found in a textbook, professional magazine, or from some other source; photocopied; cut; pasted and provided to patients, along with specific instructions, cautionary notes, stick figures, and so forth.

Types of Educational Materials used in Creating Home Exercise Programs

Computers

Today, physical therapists and physical therapy assistants can use computers to create and design HEPs for their patients. Because information technology has improved, HEPs can be designed with a click of a mouse. With the use of laptops, providers can have access to any exercise program, even in a client's home. Computer programs help physical therapy clinicians provide quality custom-generated exercises with instructions and illustrations.[6] The instructions can be printed in different languages, such as Spanish and French, to respond to the needs of a diverse patient population. One of the advantages of computer-generated exercise programs is that the products look professional. The exercise program along with names of the clinic, the physical therapist, and the patient can be viewed, edited, printed, and saved in the computer. Thus, a computer-based home program can be reviewed and upgraded accordingly by therapists as the treatment progresses. Examples of these programs include www.physiotools.com, Exercise Pro (BioEx Systems, Inc., Austin, TX), and Visual Health Information (VHI; Tacoma, WA).

Exercise Pro is one of the computer programs that help physical therapists create their own home exercises immediately in a clear, concise, and professionally illustrated manner[7] (Figure 12-2).

> There are over 1,500 exercises for you to create individual home programs or you may select from the many pre-defined protocols. Each exercise has professional illustrations to help increase understanding. Choose weights, tubing, canes, balls, and many more devices for each exercise. Increase picture and text size for clients with poor eyesight. Exercise Pro also includes educational text such as diabetic foot care, crutch training, body mechanics, etc. Exercise Pro allows you to view exercises in English, and print in Spanish. It also has report capabilities.[7]

Professionally Illustrated Cards

Professionally illustrated cards can help physical therapists recall the basics of what they learned in school.

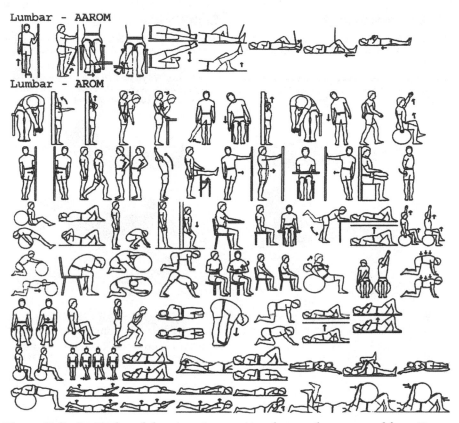

Figure 12-2 Examples of therapeutic exercises that can be generated from Exercise Pro 2. Lumbar active-assistance range of motion (AAROM) and lumbar assistance range of motion (AROM). (Reprinted with permission from BioEx Systems Inc., Austin, TX.)

- Teach simple exercises to patients that they can remember and easily perform at home.
- Start with one or two exercises, monitor performance, and encourage compliance.
- Gradually change or increase the number of exercises to avoid boredom, and steadily progress the patient.

It is important that the illustrated cards be clearly labeled with specific instructions on frequency, number of times the exercise should be repeated, and the level of intensity (Figure 12-3). Remember to include instructions for exercise progression, if needed. Again, do not over-prescribe exercise programs for patients.

☐ **PRONE PRESS-UP**

1 Lie on your stomach with your feet slightly apart. Rest your forehead on the floor. Relax your stomach and back muscles.

2 Keeping your neck straight, push yourself up on your forearms. **Hold for _____ seconds,** then slowly lie back down. **Repeat _____ times.**

☐ **PARTIAL CURL-UP**

1 Lie on your back with both knees bent, your feet flat on the floor, and your hands crossed over your chest.

2 Looking at the ceiling, tighten your stomach muscles, and slowly lift your shoulder blades off the floor—no higher than 30 degrees. **Hold for _____ seconds,** then slowly lie back down. **Repeat _____ times.**

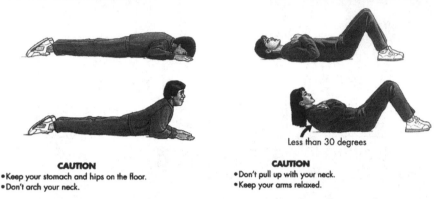

Less than 30 degrees

CAUTION
• Keep your stomach and hips on the floor.
• Don't arch your neck.

CAUTION
• Don't pull up with your neck.
• Keep your arms relaxed.

Figure 12-3 Example of professionally illustrated cards for home exercises. Prone press-up and partial curl-up with instructions on frequency, number of times, and level of intensity of exercise. (Reprinted with permission from Krames Communications, San Bruno, CA.)

Physical therapists also can create sharp and professional-looking home exercises with simple, easy-to-use exercise kits available in the market today. Computerized card collections are available to every therapist who can use a computer. For example, the Adult Home Exercise Program for Rehabilitation was developed by the author and the staff of the department of physical therapy at the University of Texas Medical Branch in Galveston, Texas.[8] These exercise cards are well organized according to the diagnosis or condition of the patient, and easily can be followed by patients and their family members (Figure 12-4). The computer-generated exercise cards are reproducible and frequently used in adult rehabilitation centers.

Another set of professionally illustrated exercise cards are by VHI.[9] These computer-generated cards are well organized into different categories: aquatic exercise, exercises and rehabilitation, balance and vestibular activities, complete fitness, assisted exercise and rehabilitation, activities of daily living, geriatric exercise and rehabilitation, early development, functional activity and exercise, pediatric functional activity and exercise, amputee lower extremity rehabilitation, cardiac rehabilitation, body

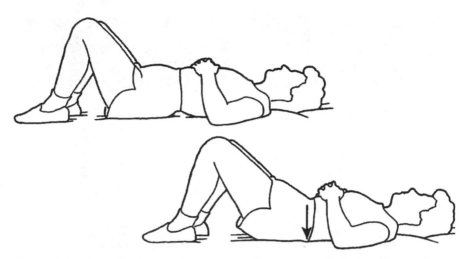

Figure 12-4 Example of computer-generated exercise cards for home exercise program. Lower back—flexion exercise (pelvic tilt). Exercise card has space for special instructions for the patient. (Reprinted with permission from Therapy Skill Builders, Tucson, AZ.)

mechanic resource library, communication flip chart, and others (Figure 12-5).

According to the handbook published by VHI, this comprehensive collection features

- Therapeutic interventions to teach compensations or adaptations for postural stability in a variety of situations.
- Exercises to enhance static and dynamic postural stability in a variety of reduced and conflicting sensory environments.
- A wide variety of exercises related to functional activities.
- Comprehensive eye exercises in varying functional postures for increasing gaze stabilization and oculomotor control.
- A wide variety of exercise progressions, from easy to advanced.
- The resources to address patients' needs at all stages of rehabilitation.[9]

Video Exercise Tapes

Another form of home exercises often used by physical therapists is videotape exercises. "The main advantage to videotapes is that they provide a visual, real-time depiction how a movement position, transfer or stretch should be executed. The patient can stop and rewind the video to clarify any unclear points."[6] Exercise videos are becoming popular among

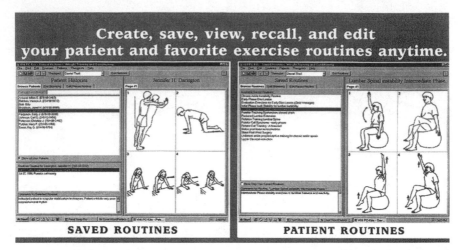

Figure 12-5 Physical therapists can create, save, view, recall, and edit their patients' home and favorite exercise routines anytime with their computers. (Reprinted with permission from Visual Health Information, Tacoma, WA.)

patients and prescribing therapists today. This trend was stimulated by the popularity of "lose weight quick," "tone your muscles," "work out," "keep fit," "stretch," and "aerobic" exercise videos available in the supermarket. Physical therapists should be careful when recommending some of these unprofessionally produced exercise videos to their patients due to liability concerns. Patients do ask their physical therapists whether these exercise videos are good for them. It would be advisable to have a small library of videos you could certify as safe and effective for patients to use. Physical therapists can preview most of these videos in the rehabilitation department of hospitals and clinic libraries.

Internet

The Internet is regarded as one of the greatest communication breakthroughs in human information technology history. The information super highway is now speeding the health care industry along. Many patients and their families are becoming savvy about the wealth of the health-related information now available through the Internet. Physical therapists and physical therapist assistants must be prepared to keep up with this ever-changing, high-technology information system.

There is no doubt about the explosion of health care information on the Web. "According to the Cyber Dialogue, a leading Internet consumer relationship management company, 34.7 million American adults this year will

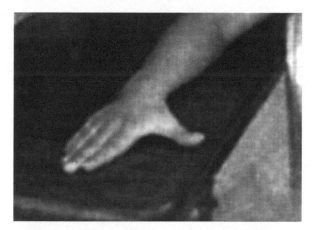

Figure 12-6   Example of exercise video for active wrist extension. (Reprinted with permission from PeakCare, Inc., Englewood, CO.)

search for information by navigating more than 17,000 health-related Web sites."[10] By 2005, 88.5 million adults will use the World Wide Web to find health care data, shop for health products, and communicate with payers and providers through online channels. In a recent study by Chang,[11] a survey of Internet Health Usage by Patients conducted by the Find/SVP Emerging Technologies Research Group, 36% of the general Internet user population falls into a group that shares the characteristic of being active and heavy consumers of health and medical information online. Approximately 80% of the surveyed users expressed some interest in accessing health and medical information online.[11]

One company that provides Internet user exercises is PeakCare Systems,[12] which has developed systematic exercise videos that both providers and patients can order from the Internet. The videos and software programs are specifically designed to be directed and supervised exclusively by licensed health care professionals. There are various exercises organized according to medical specialty (e.g., orthopedic, geriatric, and pediatric) (Figure 12-6). The PeakCare tapes and programs make it easy for physical therapists to design exercise programs unique to each patient.

> The multimedia flexibility of the World Wide Web has proven itself a very attractive way of presenting information to an audience seeking a specific type of information. The web can support multimedia presentations, medical image libraries, online textbooks, patient/practitioner information files, interactive programs, and numerous other applications.[11]

According to Chang, "The Medical Internet now features on-line journals (both exclusive and electronic versions of print editions), electronic networks, news services, continuing education classes, clinical practice guidelines, patient education handouts, drug databases, discussion forums, image and video clip libraries, and interactive programs among others."[11]

Evaluating the Quality of Online Programs

One of the problems that may face physical therapists and physical therapist assistants is the ability to evaluate the quality of online programs. There may be concerns about the veracity of information, accuracy, readability, and timeliness of Web site content. Other concerns are over misinformation or useless information. Today many organizations, such as Health on the Net, Hi-Ethics, and the American Medical Association, are developing guidelines to help patients and health care practitioners determine quality health care information, content objectives, and reliability. In assessing different Internet-based exercise programs and other health care–related Web sites, the following guidelines may be of help. Look for

- Credibility (source of information, currency, relevance)
- Content (accuracy, original sources, disclaimers, and peer review)
- Disclosure (purpose of site, profiling of the site's purpose and background)
- Link (selection, architecture, content, back linkages, and description)
- Design (accessibility, organization, internal search engine)
- Interactivity (mechanism for feedback, chat rooms, tailoring of information)
- Caveats (alert information)[11]

Physical therapists and physical therapist assistants also can rely on most professional journals that feature yearly summaries of companies that manufacture or sell different exercise software, computer programs, and the services that they provide. For physical therapy–related Web sites, there are no ratings about which Web sites are the best. We have to keep ourselves and our patients surfing to be up to date with the fast-changing information super highway.

Liability Concerns

Physical therapists and physical therapist assistants should be aware of other issues raised by the explosion of the use of the Internet today. There are concerns about privacy, confidentiality, quality assurance, professionalism, liability, and responsible practice. However, some institutions and groups, such as Hi-Ethics, e-Health Initiative, the American Medical Association and Health on the Net, have moved to assist in reducing the falsehood and manipulation of different e-companies.[11] Be aware of the litigious society in which we operate, and take precautions. Always instruct the patient that none of the exercise programs should be performed without recommendation and direction of a health care provider. Remember that all companies that designed and produced these exercise programs have their own disclaimers carefully worded and printed on the video covers, on the Internet, or in exercise program handbooks. These disclaimers protect the producers, physical therapists, and physical therapist assistants from liability implications. Here is an example of a disclaimer on an exercise video titled "60-Plus Aging Well: A Celebration. Stretch and Sway," produced by the Somerset County Office on Aging Health Program.[13]

> Before beginning any exercise program consult your physician. Remember not all exercises may be suitable for everyone. The creators, producers, participants and distributors of this program disclaim any liability in connection with the exercises or advice contained herein.

Summary

Educational materials for therapists to use with patients and families are readily available, including professionally illustrated cards, exercise videotapes, and the Internet. It is up to the physical therapists and physical therapist assistants to carefully assess patients physically, cognitively, and culturally, as well as assessing their learning style preferences to select the most effective form of teaching material for both patients and families.

References

1. Ogbonna P. Systems providers professional exercise sheets. Advance for Physical Therapists and Physical Therapist Assistants 1998;33.
2. Arsonson M, Shiffman JK. Clinical Assessment in Home Care. In LW Kaye (ed). New Developments in Home Care Services for the Elderly: Innovation Policy, Program and Practice. New York: The Harworth Press, 1995;213–312.

3. Samovar LA, Porter RE. Communications Between Cultures (2nd ed). Belmont, CA: Wadsworth Publishing, 1995;47.
4. Developing Cultural Competencies. Deerfield, MA: Channing L. Bete, 1998. Center for Cross-Cultural Health. http://www.crosshealth.com.
5. Mukai CPS W. Chinese perspectives. Geriatric Nursing 1999;18–22.
6. Bassett J. Customizing a home program. Advance for Physical Therapists and Physical Therapist Assistants 2000;11–12.
7. User's Guide to Exercise Pro 2. BioEx Systems, Inc., Austin, TX, 1997.
8. Bezner J. The Adult Home Exercise for Rehabilitation. Tucson, AZ: Therapy Skill Builders, 1989.
9. PC-Kits Tutorial. Visual Health Information, Tacoma, WA, 1999.
10. Brooks B. Don't get blown away by the e-health explosion. Nursing Spectrum 2000;9(20):10–11.
11. Chang S. Do Healthcare Providers Need the Internet? An Introduction to Cyber Space for the Medical Professional. 1999; http://hyperlinked.com/mednet/fulltext.html.
12. PeakCare, Inc. PeakCare Systems and PeakCare Professional Products. Englewood, CO. http://www.peakcare.com.
13. 60-Plus Aging Well: A Celebration. Stretch and Sway. Somerset, NJ: Somerset County Board of Chosen Freeholders, Somerset County Office on Aging.

Annotated Bibliography

Muse T. Modifying Exercise Programs to Fit Your Patient's Medication Is Critical. Advance for Physical Therapists and Physical Therapist Assistants 2001;March 12:9–10. This article emphasizes the importance of proper history taking to find out what type of medication patients are using. This information influences the types of exercises and workouts. The article lists some advice to therapists on monitoring medications and exercises. It classifies common prescriptions, their interactions, and how they affect the cardiovascular system.
Julia M (ed). Multicultural Awareness in the Healthcare Profession. Boston: Allyn & Bacon, 1996. A great book for cultural awareness in the health care professions. There are 9 chapters dealing with cultural beliefs, concepts, and attitudes within different cultural groups in the United States. This is a must read for all health care professionals working in home, hospital, school, and other settings.
Witting P. Patient Education: A Healthcare Professional Guide. Philadelphia: Lippincott Williams & Wilkins, 1998. Patients today are participating actively in the management of their health care. They demand to be

informed and educated. This book is well organized by body systems and contains numerous illustrations. It explains to professionals not only what to teach, but also how to teach and assess patient learning needs. It contains 12 chapters with appendices and suggested readings. This book is highly recommended for therapists when designing home education programs for patients.

Doak CC, Doak LG, Root JH. Teaching Patients with Low Literacy Skills. Philadelphia: JB Lippincott, 1996. This book contains 10 chapters well written by experienced husband and wife authors. The book covers a variety of topics, ranging from applying theory in pictures, assessment of materials, the comprehension process, and visuals and how to use them, to teaching with theory and learning verification and variation of materials. The book is highly recommended for all health care professionals.

13

Community Health Education: Evolving Opportunities for Physical Therapists

Julie Gahimer and
David M. Morris

The Tone Your Bones (TYB) Program is a community health education program that has been conducted at the University of Alabama at Birmingham since 1998. The purpose of the TYB Program is to facilitate changes in diet, movement patterns, balance, and physical activity behaviors in community-dwelling persons with osteoporosis or osteopenia. This multi-disciplinary program involves physical therapy, medicine, and nutrition. Participants attend two 90-minute sessions each week for 4 weeks (eight sessions total). The initial 15 minutes of the program involves discussion of a specific topic related to management of osteoporosis. Subsequently, participants perform 15 minutes of warm-up exercise. During this time, instructors discuss performing functional movements in a safe manner (i.e., avoid spinal flexion and rotation during lifting). Next, participants spend 30 minutes practicing functional movement patterns using a neutral spine posture. Participants then perform exercises designed to improve muscle strength, posture, and balance for 20 minutes. Finally, participants do 10 minutes of cool-down exercises. The program has been modified from its original format based on input from participants. For example, a 2 days per week for 4 weeks format replaced the former 1 day per week for 8 weeks format, because participants lost interest during the long breaks between sessions. Short-term evaluation of the program suggests that it is successful in improving strength, flexibility, balance, and health status from the first to the eighth session. Long-term evaluation to examine the impact of the program on reducing the incidence of fractures in participants is planned. Also, plans are underway to implement similar programs in retirement centers and assisted living facilities.

Chapter Objectives

After completing this chapter, the reader will be able to

1. Discuss the role(s) of the physical therapy professional as a community health educator and opportunities that may exist for community health education in her or his current practice setting.
2. Understand the language and focus of community health education.
3. Describe selected theoretical models of designing and evaluating community health education programs.
4. Use strategies to assist physical therapists to develop as effective community health educators.
5. Give examples of community health education programs relevant to physical therapy practice.

Contemporary Health Care Focus: Community Health Care and Prevention

A shift in the focus of the health care delivery system has occurred as a result of our rapidly evolving society. Changes in population characteristics, lifestyles, environmental factors, and health disorders have altered the leading causes of death and illness. Concerns of government policy makers about the growing cost of health care have prompted restructuring and reorientation of the system toward one that focuses on community and health promotion. In 1987, Wallack proposed that "Personal health and well-being are gaining priority on the American Agenda. A renewed interest in health promotion has been facilitated by the need to contain health care costs, a realization of the limits of medicine in preventing illness, and a deeply rooted societal ethic of personal responsibility for individual health."[1(p923)]

As health promotion has evolved, it has become increasingly aimed at the community level. One driving force behind this move is the development of Healthy People 2000 and Healthy People 2010, the disease prevention agendas for the United States.[2,3] Healthy People 2000 has as its origin the 1979 Surgeon General's Report,[4] also called Healthy People, which stated that the nation's health strategy must emphasize the prevention of disease. Released in 1990, Healthy People 2000 is a comprehensive agenda with 319 objectives organized into 22 priority areas to accomplish three overarching goals: (1) increase years of healthy life, (2) reduce disparities in health among different population groups, and (3) achieve access to preventative health services. This consensus document was developed with comments from more than 10,000 individuals and organizations. Since the document was published, 47 states, the District of Columbia, and Guam have developed their own Healthy People plans. By 1995, 8% of the Healthy People 2000 goals had been met, and significant progress has been made toward another 40% of the goals. Despite its success, a recent report by Francis highlighted the lack of progress of Healthy People 2000 toward physical activity and fitness goals.[5] Francis reported that only 1 of 13 physical activity and fitness objectives had been met or exceeded in 1999. Although progress toward five other objectives has been made, three are actually further from attainment. These figures should be of particular concern to physical therapy professionals.

Healthy People 2010 is well underway. After an inaugural planning meeting in 1997, input has been received from numerous parties by way of focus group sessions, public meetings, and a Healthy People 2010 Web site. This new document is greatly influenced by factors such as changing demographics, advances in preventive therapies, and new technologies. The 2010 framework has two overarching goals: to increase years of healthy life, and to eliminate (as opposed to reduce) health disparities. These goals will be supported by four enabling goals: promoting healthy behaviors, protecting health, achieving access to quality health care, and strengthening community prevention. New areas of focus include disability, people with low income, race and ethnicity, chronic diseases, and public health infrastructure. As a member of the Healthy People Consortium, the American Physical Therapy Association was instrumental in helping to develop the Health People 2010 objectives. This input is evidenced by the inclusion of a new focus area related to arthritis, osteoporosis, and chronic low back pain. The Healthy People documents are helpful to community health educators in two ways. First, they draw attention to priority needs and problems. Second, they can serve as a benchmark or standard of comparison for a target community with regard to the performance of the entire nation.

Another example of the move toward a community focus in health education comes from the Healthy Cities[6] concept. Healthy Cities is a community problem-solving process for health promotion that has been implemented worldwide. The Healthy Cities concept was developed in Canada and Europe during the mid-1980s. A Healthy City is defined as "one that is continually creating and improving those physical and social environments and strengthening those community resources which enable people to mutually support each other in performing all the functions of life and achieving their maximum potential."[6(p299)] The process involves establishing a broad-based structure for Healthy Cities, encouraging community participation, assessing community needs, establishing priorities and strategic plans, soliciting political support, taking local action, and evaluating progress. Critical to the Healthy Cities concept is the active role of local government in the process. The focus is not confined to one or more health problems, but "is intended to build health into decision-making processes of local governments, community organizations, and businesses, to develop a broad range of strategies to address the broad social, environmental and economic determinants of health."[6(p300)] Examples of Healthy Cities projects (also called Healthy Communities) are prevalent in the health promotion literature. These descriptions can assist community health educators by providing examples of a variety of community participation strategies to promote health.

Community Health Education and Health Care Practitioners

Although promoting more healthy lifestyles in the community is not the primary concern of all physical therapists, such health education and promotion principles are increasingly apparent in the day-to-day practices of many rehabilitation practitioners. The purpose of this chapter is to familiarize physical therapists with concepts of community health education to improve their ability to integrate these concepts into current physical therapy practice, leading to improved outcomes for all physical therapy clients.

Helvie[7] identified the difference between hospital and community health practices in nursing. This contrast has been adapted for physical therapists (Table 13-1).

In nursing education, alternative settings are used for community health nursing clinical rotations. These sites include public health agencies, Visiting Nurse Association and other home health agencies, schools, adult day care senior centers, neighborhood clinics, occupational health centers, social service clubs for boys and girls, hospices, homeless shelters, child day care centers, and day care centers for special needs children. Examples for physical therapy students are scarce, but they are becoming more common.

When referring to occupational therapists, Baum and Law point out that, due to changes in the health care system, practitioners must focus on the long-term health needs of clients so that clients can develop healthy behaviors and thus minimize the health care costs associated with disabling conditions.[8,9] Doing so requires a shift in thinking from a biomedical to a sociomedical framework and taking an active role in building healthy communities.

Table 13-1 Differences in Clinic-Based Physical Therapy and Community-Based Physical Therapy

	Clinic-based	*Community-based*
Unit of service	Individual focused; hospitalized patient.	Community groups and subgroups specific to age, health problem, condition, or setting.
Activity focus	Treatment of disease, short-term intervention for restoration of health.	Multiple focuses: health promotion, screenings, rehabilitation, and consideration given to socioeconomic and cultural factors that affect health conditions.
Range and variability of work	Works with disease classifications, acutely ill patients.	Works with entire spectrum of health and illness, all settings, all ages.
Boundaries of service	One institution, treatment, and recovery.	All institutions (e.g., schools, industries).
Coordination	Within the institution.	Between a variety of medical and nonmedical personnel.
Legal and medical authority	Institutional policy and state practice acts; always under medical care; diagnosis and treatment orders from referring physician provide framework for care.	Health officer, health regulations and laws, and political jurisdiction; frequently no medical diagnosis from referring physician; services obtained through multiple public agencies.
Autonomy	Physician is medical authority; workload regulated by admissions.	Medical management and authority shared by multiple professionals.
Family and patient autonomy	Individual autonomy of patient is restricted and must fit into institutional routine.	Complete autonomy and control.
Predictability of events	Treatment of patient in one time and place.	Interplay of home environment; social, physical, and emotional climate; cultural background.

A recent Pew Health Professions Commission Report[10] states that "most of the nation's educational programs remain oriented to prepare individuals for yesterday's health care system." The Commission proposed the characteristics and needs of the health care system of the early twenty-first century that clearly speak to promoting health at a community level. They include

- Incorporating the multiple determinants of health into clinical care
- Improving access to health care for those with unmet health needs
- Partnering with communities in health care decisions

- Rigorously practicing preventive care
- Integrating population-based care and services into practice
- Working in interdisciplinary teams
- Ensuring that care balances individual, professional, system, and societal needs
- Being advocates for public policy that promotes and protects the health of the public

Physical Therapist's Role in Community Health

Community health in physical therapy is not a new idea, but a revisited one. In 1970,[11] Helen Blood wrote about developing community health content for physical therapy curricula. However, over the ensuing years, physical therapists have concentrated primarily on curative approaches for the individual, with little attention paid to community health and prevention. Although providing care for individuals and their families is an important aspect of physical therapy practice, increasing emphasis is now being placed on working with groups to influence the health of the entire community. Three specific documents published in recent years outline the most current approaches to preparing physical therapists for practice: the *Guide to Physical Therapist Practice*,[12] the Commission on Accreditation in Physical Therapy Education accreditation criteria,[13] and the *Normative Model of Physical Therapist Professional Education*.[14] Each advocates curricular content addressing health promotion and disease prevention. The *Guide to Physical Therapist Practice* provides specific examples of screening, prevention, and wellness activities performed by physical therapists (Table 13-2).

Within the Evaluative Criteria for Accreditation of Education Programs for the Preparation of Physical Therapists document, Standard 3.8.3.34 states that "programs must provide evidence that they provide learning experiences in which students consider the promotion of optimal health by providing information on wellness, disease, impairment, functional limitations, disability and health risks related to age, gender, culture and lifestyle."[13(p33)] Thus, physical therapists have a clear and mandated role in the community health focus on health promotion and disease prevention.

Language and Focus of Community Health Education

For readers unfamiliar with the language of community health education, common terms and definitions are listed in Table 13-3. In addition, Table 13-4 contains a list of the 10 principles of effective health education proposed by Freudenberg et al.[15] These principles are designed to build

Table 13-2 Health Promotion and Disease Prevention Content from the *Guide to Physical Therapist Practice*

Screening activities:
  Identification of lifestyle factors that may lead to increased risk for serious
    health problems
  Identification of elderly individuals in a community center or nursing home
    who are at high risk for falls
  Identification of workplace risk factors

Prevention and wellness activities:
  Identification of workplace risk factors
  Back schools
  Workplace redesign
  Strengthening, stretching, and endurance exercise programs
  Postural training to prevent and treat low back pain
  Exercise programs, including weight bearing and weight training, for those at
    risk of osteoporosis
  Exercise training, gait training, and balance and coordination activities for those
    older adults at risk for falls
  Exercise programs, cardiovascular conditioning, and instruction in ADL and
    IADL to prevent dysfunction for women who are pregnant
  Broad-based consumer education and advocacy programs to prevent problems

Community settings:
  Schools
  Hospices
  Corporate or industrial health centers
  Industrial, workplace, or other occupational environments
  Athletic facilities, fitness centers, and sports training facilities

---

ADL = activities of daily living; IADL = instrumental activities of daily living.
Source: Adapted from the Guide to Physical Therapist Practice (2nd ed). Phys Ther
2000;81:31–102.

the capacity and guide the actions of individuals and communities to promote health and prevent disease. Note that a key element in these principles is active participation from the target audience in planning, implementing, and maintaining health programs. Reviewing these principles gives therapists a sense of the skills needed to engage in community health education.

Theoretical and Conceptual Tools of Community Health Education

The following section addresses selected theories and concepts that physical therapists, as health educators, will find useful when working with people at the community level. In Chapters 9 and 10, models of intrapersonal health behavior are presented, including the Health Belief

Table 13-3   Operational Definitions Related to Health Education

---

Health promotion—any combination of educational, organizational, economic, or environmental supports for behavior change conducive to health.[a]

Health promotion and disease prevention—"the aggregate of all purposeful activities designed to improve personal and public health through a combination of strategies, including the competent implementation of behavioral change strategies, health education, health protection measures, risk factor detection, health enhancement, and health maintenance."[b]

Community health education—the application of a variety of methods for education and mobilization of community members in actions for resolving health issues and problems that affect the community. Examples of methods include group process, mass media campaigns, strategic planning and skills training with community organizations, and advocacy initiatives related to legislation and policymaking.[b]

Community health educator—a person who works with the community in promoting capacity and action targeted to health problems.

---

[a]Adapted from Green LW, Kreuter MW. Health Promotion Planning: An Educational and Ecological Approach (3rd ed). Mountain View, CA: Mayfield Publishing Co., 1999.

[b]Adapted from D Breckon, JR Harvey, RB Lancaster. Community Health Education: Settings, Roles, and Skills for the 21st Century (4th ed). Gaithersburg, MD: Aspen, 1998.

Model, the Transtheoretical Model of Change, and the Patient-Practitioner Collaborative Model. Community health education programs target the health behavior of groups of people. However, interpersonal health behavior models are critical for predicting and influencing health behavior at both the individual and community level. Concepts and theories presented here include social cognitive theory, communication theory, social market-

Table 13-4   Principles of Effective Health Education

---

1. Tailor to a specific population within a particular setting
2. Involve the participants in planning, implementation, and evaluation
3. Integrate efforts aimed at changing individuals, social and physical environment, communities, and policies
4. Link participants' concerns about health to broader life concerns and to a vision of a better society
5. Use existing resources within the environment
6. Build on the strengths found among participants and their communities
7. Advocate for the resources and policy changes needed to achieve the desired health objectives
8. Prepare participants to become leaders
9. Support the diffusion of innovation to a wider population
10. Seek to institutionalize successful components and to replicate them in other settings

---

ing, and the health promotion planning model PRECEDE-PROCEED (PRE-CEDE = predisposing, reinforcing, and enabling causes in educational diagnosis and evaluation; PROCEED = policy, regulatory, and organizational constructs in educational and environmental development).

Social Cognitive Theory

The Social Cognitive Theory (SCT) is a particularly useful model for understanding health behavior at the interpersonal level.[16] A primary tenet of SCT states that health behavior is a dynamic interaction between three factors: behavior, personal factors (including cognitions), and environmental influences. This interaction is referred to as *reciprocal determinism*. This theory, originally called *Social Learning Theory*, can be traced back to Millard and Dollard's explanation of modeling behaviors in animals and humans.[17] This theory was particularly influential in the field of health education, as it integrated previously disparate concepts from cognitive, emotional, and behavioral perspectives of health behavior. The major concepts of SCT and implications for community health interventions are outlined in Table 13-5.

One example of applying SCT to physical therapy community health education can be illustrated in planning an exercise program for clients after myocardial infarction. After exploring each of the SCT constructs as it relates to the target population, program elements can be modified to optimize participation. For example, family members and significant others can be invited to participate in an exercise session. This opportunity to experience the exercises should improve their understanding of the program and lead to optimal environmental support. A buddy system—in which phone calls are made between patients who are "buddies" responsible for calling and supporting one another—may be incorporated into the program as an element of observational learning. Self-efficacy can also be heightened with one-to-one sessions with a personal trainer early in the program, in which participants receive personalized instruction and positive reinforcement.

Communication Theory

Substantial time, effort, and resources are applied to developing health education programs. Often, much less attention is given to dissemination of the message throughout the target community. Health educators working at the community level must incorporate effective communication strategies into program development and implementation. Concepts from McGuire's Communication/Persuasion Matrix can be helpful in exploring this area of study.[18]

Table 13-5 Major Concepts of Social Cognitive Theory and Implications for Intervention Strategies

Concept	Definition	Implications
Environment	Factors physically external to the person	Provide opportunities and social support
Situation	Person's perception of the environment	Correct misperceptions and promote healthful norms
Behavioral capability	Knowledge and skill to perform a given behavior	Promote mastery learning through skills training
Expectations	Anticipatory outcomes of a behavior	Model positive outcomes of healthful behavior
Expectancies	Values that the person places on a given outcome, incentives	Present outcomes of change that have functional meaning
Self-control	Personal regulation of goal-directed behavior or performance	Provide opportunities for self-monitoring, goal setting, problem solving, and self-reward
Observational learning	Behavioral acquisition that occurs by watching the actions and outcomes of others' behavior	Include credible role models of the targeted behavior
Reinforcements	Responses to a person's behavior that increase or decrease the likelihood of reoccurrence	Promote self-initiated rewards and incentives
Self-efficacy	The person's confidence in performing a particular behavior	Approach behavioral change in small steps to ensure success, seek specificity about the change sought
Emotional coping responses	Strategies or tactics that are used by a person to deal with emotional stimuli	Provide training in problem solving and stress management; include opportunities to practice skills in emotionally arousing situations
Reciprocal determinism	Dynamic interaction of the person, the behavior, and the environment in which the behavior is performed	Consider multiple avenues to behavioral change, including environmental, skill, and personal change

McGuire's Communication/Persuasion Matrix is a useful model to explain and plan public communication campaigns. This model identifies both input and output variables that influence how persuasive communication occurs. Input variables are the independent variables and persuasive messages that can be manipulated. Categories of input variables include source factors, message factors, channel factors, receiver factors, and destination factors. Table 13-6 describes each type of input variable and provides examples of using them to promote an arthritis exercise program.

Output variables are successive response substeps required if a communication is to be effective. For example, the target group must be exposed to a message, attend to it, like it to the extent that group members become interested, comprehend the message, and so on, until they have consolidated the message into their everyday behavior (Table 13-7). The output variables, or substeps, provide a useful checklist for developing and evaluating a communication effort. Communication campaigns may direct efforts that stop too early along the communication chain or skip important output variables, rendering the effort ineffective.

An example of an effective communication campaign is a series of full-page advertisements developed by the American Physical Therapy Association to educate women, ages 35–54 years, with children, about the role of physical therapists in health care. The black-and-white photographs are artistically designed and contain clever, thought-provoking text that readily engages the observer. One such advertisement displays a young girl in a slumped sitting posture typical of her age (Figure 13-1). The text briefly discusses the development of poor posture across a lifetime and its painful consequences. The advertisement goes on to describe the role of physical therapy in alleviating and preventing postural pain as well as how readers can learn more about physical therapy. The advertisements appeared in such women's magazines as *Ladies Home Journal*, *Essence*, and *Better Homes and Gardens*. Each advertisement contained a coupon, toll-free number, and Web site address for further information. Large posters were also created of the advertisements to allow physical therapists to reinforce the messages in their facilities.

Social Marketing

To change the health behavior of a community group, a large audience must not only receive the message, but also must be convinced of its need. Social marketing goes beyond communication theory, as it also incorporates principles of program planning, implementation, refining, and evaluation. The goal of social marketing is to increase the acceptability of ideas or practices through examining a target group and subsequently selecting and using the most effective communication strategies for that group.[19] Social marketing is distinguished from commercial marketing in that the latter is focused on profit and organizational change. Instead, social marketing is focused on benefiting the target audience through behavior change. Another key concept of social market-

Table 13-6   Example of Persuasive Communication Input Variables Used to
Promote an Arthritis Exercise Program

Input variable	Definition	Example
Source factors	Characteristics of the perceived communicator to whom the message is attributed. Examples include credibility, attractiveness, and power.	Using a celebrity with personal experience to promote an idea (e.g., an actor who has arthritis).
Message factors	Characteristics of the message, including delivery style, types of appeals, inclusions and omissions, organization of the message, and quantitative aspects such as length and repetition.	Focus message on benefits of exercise for persons with arthritis (i.e., weight control, better endurance, and fewer medical complications). Use short, succinct, and lively information segments.
Channel factors	Media that send persuasive messages, including variables such as audio vs. visual vs. both, written vs. spoken word, verbal vs. nonverbal messages, and vocal vs. visual nonverbal cues.	Televised public service announcements could be used. They may be scheduled during persuasive daytime programming or other times, when the target audience is most likely to watch television.
Receiver factors	Audience characteristics, including capacity variables such as age, education, and intelligence; demographic variables, such as gender and ethnicity; and personality, lifestyle, and psychographic variables.	The target audience for an arthritis exercise group is an older adult population. All input variables should consider characteristics of this group (e.g., possibly unfamiliar with exercise principles, has conservative values).
Destination factors	The type of behavior for which the communication is aimed, such as immediate vs. long-term change, influencing a specific change or whole ideological system, or changing an existing belief vs. conferring resistance against subsequent attacks.	The goal of this communication is long-term change. Therefore, the focus is on outcomes of the program rather than on specific exercises.

Source: Adapted from McGuire WJ. Theoretical foundations of campaigns. In Rice RE, Atkin CK (eds). Public Communication Campaigns. Newbury Park, CA: Sage Publications,1981:43–65.

Table 13-7 Features of Communication/Persuasion Process

Phase in the process	Supporting features
Exposure ↓	Access or exposure to communication
Attention ↓	Attending to and becoming interested in the topic
Comprehension ↓	Learning about the topic ("learning what") Skill acquisition ("learning how")
Belief ↓	Attitude change from direct persuasion
Decision ↓	Decision making, public commitment
Learning	Demonstration and guided practice with feedback and continued confidence building

Source: Adapted from Green LW, McAlister AM. Macro-intervention to support health behavior: some theoretical perspectives and practical reflections. Health Education Quarterly 1984;11:323–329.

ing is that the target audience has a primary role in the process, making it consumer driven. One such model of social marketing is the Marketing Process Model proposed by Novelli.[20] This model includes the following six stages:

1. *Marketing analysis (planning and strategy)*—this analysis takes place at four levels by exploring the mandates and goals of the organization delivering the program, the target consumer, the resources available to the organization delivering the program, and the competitors of the program planned.
2. *Planning (selecting channels and materials)*—at this stage, the program's structure and organization are established. Activities include setting program objectives, segmenting the target audience, and proposing an action plan.
3. *Developing, testing, and refining plan elements*—involves pilot testing program elements and refining them as a result. This "pretesting phase" is a distinguishing characteristic of social marketing.
4. *Implementation*—at this stage, the program begins. Concurrently, process evaluation is used to examine whether the program elements are carried out as intended.
5. *Assessing effectiveness*—this stage involves systemic examination of how well the program is meeting its objectives.
6. *Feedback to stage 1 (feedback to refine program)*—as program deficits or shortcomings are identified, this feedback process allows for program modifications to improve effectiveness and enhance outcomes.

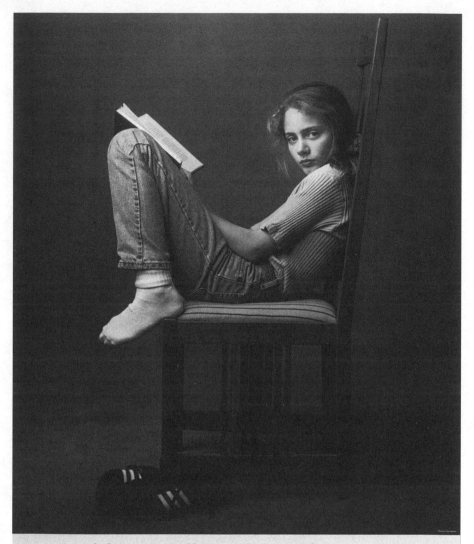

Figure 13-1   American Physical Therapy Association communication campaign poster: "Girl in Chair."

Table 13-8   Examples of Health Education Media Channels

Computer (Internet)

Television and radio (public service announcements, news coverage, feature presentations, consultations)

Posters (billboards, buses and trucks, public facilities)

Brochures and flyers (inserts in utility bills, health care facilities, workplaces)

Resource materials (guidelines, school curriculum materials, reprints, and resource directories)

Presentations (community groups, health care facilities)

Workshops

Counseling and testing

Newspapers (feature stories, news coverage, advertisements)

Newsletters and journals (organization newsletters, health problem updates)

A social marketing approach has been applied to numerous community health projects, including the Pawtucket Heart Health Program and the Stanford Five City Project; both of these are aimed at improving cardiovascular status in target audiences.[21] Using the media is a great way to reach a large number of people effectively. Health messages can be disseminated and promoted through a variety of health education media channels (Table 13-8).

PRECEDE-PROCEED

Typically, health educators identify a target audience, explore their health problems, and attempt to "fix" the problems through the development of a health education program. Many obstacles can interfere with this process if the program is not well planned. Several program planning models have been proposed for health promotion programs, including the PRECEDE-PROCEED model.[22] This model is not a theory, as it does not attempt to predict or explain the relationship among factors thought to be associated with an outcome of interest. Instead, the model provides a structure for the application of theories related to health promotion and disease prevention to optimize the selection and implementation of intervention strategies.

The PRECEDE-PROCEED model is said to "begin at the end," as it focuses on the outcome of interest first and works backward to determine how best to achieve it. The planning process described in PRECEDE-PROCEED subscribes to the principle of participation. This principle states that, by allowing members of a target group to define their own high-priority problems and goals and provide their ideas for solutions to health problems, the likelihood of achieving change is dramatically enhanced. The model consists of nine phases in the planning and implementation process. Phases 1 and 2 involve epidemiologic and social diagnosis, respectively, and determination of the health problems to be addressed. Phase 3, behavioral diagnosis, identifies behaviors leading to the health problems intended for influence. Educational diagnosis, Phase 4, examines three types of contributors to problem behaviors: predisposing factors (antecedents that provide a rationale or motivation for a behavior), reinforcing factors (elements that appear subsequent to the behavior that provide continuing reward or reinforcement of the behavior), and enabling factors (antecedents that enable or allow a motivation to be realized). Phase 5, administrative and policy diagnosis, identifies policies, resources, and circumstances prevailing in a program's organizational context that could facilitate or hinder program implementation. Phase 6 concerns program implementation. Finally, Phases 7–9 address evaluation of the program, including process, impact, and outcome evaluation. Examples of successful applications of the PRECEDE-PROCEED model to health education program planning can be found throughout the health promotion literature.

One example of using the PRECEDE-PROCEED model for patient community education can be illustrated by applications made to the Tone Your Bones program described in the opening scenario in this chapter[23] (Table 13-9).

Program Evaluation Principles

At least six different forms of program evaluation are frequently discussed in the community health education literature.[22] Process, impact, and outcome evaluation are critical steps of the PRECEDE-PROCEED planning model previously discussed.

Formative evaluations produce data and information during the development phase of a program and can be used to explore the feasibility of implementing a program. The process allows program developers to assess barriers to implementing a new program and modify the program structure before costly mistakes are made. A frequently used technique for formative evaluation involves pilot testing a message with a focus group.

Process evaluation is designed to document the degree to which program procedures were conducted according to the written plan. This approach strives to prevent the occurrence of making a conclusion that a program is ineffective, whereas, in fact, the program was never really implemented as designed. Particular objects of interest include program inputs, implementation activities, and stakeholder reactions. Examples of process evaluation methods include quantitative periodic surveys, audits, and counts of services

Table 13-9   Application of the PRECEDE-PROCEED Model to the Tone Your Bones Program[23]

PRECEDE-PROCEED phases	*Sample findings*
Phase 1 (Social Diagnosis): Assess social and quality of life concerns of population.	• Fear of losing independence owing to a fracture. • Fear of pain associated with a fracture. • Desire to avoid spinal deformity. • Desire for community participation.
Phase 2 (Epidemiologic Diagnosis): Identify specific health problems that are relevant to quality-of-life concerns.	• Falls more likely lead to fractures in persons with osteoporosis. • Fractures lead to disability and often death (20% of individuals who experience a hip fracture die within 1 year; an additional 25% are placed in extended care facilities).
Phase 3 (Behavioral Diagnosis): Identify the specific health-related behaviors that are causally linked to the health problems. Select the most important one(s) based on importance (relevance to changing the health problem) and changeability.	• Improving nutrition. • Regularly and appropriately exercising. • Using proper body mechanics during functional movements.
Phase 4 (Educational Diagnosis): Identify the predisposing, enabling, and reinforcing factors relevant to the prioritized behavior(s), and select the most important ones based on their importance and changeability. (Note that this example only shows factors relevant to engaging in regular physical activity.)	*Predisposing factors:* • Perceived health status. • Knowledge of effects of inactivity. • Beliefs in benefits of physical activity and value placed on these beneficial outcomes. • Belief that it is possible to affect health and quality-of-life outcomes. • Perceived barriers or negative consequences (fear of injury or disease flare, costs, inconvenience). • Belief that important others (e.g., doctor, therapist, family, peers) want person to exercise and be motivated to comply with those opinions. • Exercise self-efficacy. • Current exercise level or status (intention to exercise; stage of change). • Knowledge of appropriate exercise prescription (type, frequency, intensity, duration); precautions for exercise. *Enabling factors:* • Availability and convenience of exercise facilities. • Transportation. • Skill in performing physical activity in safe manner.

Table 13-9 *continued*

PRECEDE-PROCEED phases	Sample findings
	• Time management and pacing skills. *Reinforcing factors*: • Perceived improvement in symptoms, functional ability, psychosocial status, and other intrinsic rewards. • Negative consequences of exercising.
Phase 5 (Administrative or Organizational Diagnosis): Assess organizational, administrative, managerial, and policy factors that can support or inhibit a program.	• Initial funding was grant supported. • Publicity (e.g., newspaper or magazine articles, local news spots) means good visibility for university. • Stakeholders have expectation of program being continued. • Administration appears supportive of program.
Phase 6: Program Development and Implementation	—
Phase 7: Evaluation	• Process evaluations resulted in program changes (e.g., change in format from 1 to 2 times per week). • Impact evaluation suggested that the program was effective in improving strength, flexibility, balance, and health status. • Outcome evaluation of effect on incidence of fracture is planned.

rendered. Information gathered during process evaluation is often used immediately to modify the program. An example of process evaluation used with physical therapy community health education can be illustrated with an example of a community health fair. As the program activities occur, program administrators may "float" through the crowd and observe interactions between program personnel and target group members. Administrators' abilities to evaluate the interactions could be enhanced by using checklists of activities that the program personnel are trained to carry out. Also, they may conduct face-to-face interviews with a sample of program participants to gain insight into the immediate effects of the educational efforts.

Impact evaluation is designed to explore the intervention efficacy or effectiveness in producing midterm (i.e., 12–24 months) cognitive, belief, skill, and behavioral changes for the target population. Exploration of predisposing, enabling, and reinforcing factors (discussed earlier) is particularly important with this sort of evaluation.

In contrast, outcome evaluation explores the long-term effects of an intervention. Objects of interest in this type of evaluation include health status, quality-of-life indicators, mortality, morbidity, and social indicators (i.e., employment, independent living).

Economically based evaluation methods are also important to justify program expenses. Cost-effectiveness analysis explores the relationship between intervention cost (input) and the program output. Thus, it is a ratio of cost per unit of impact. The objective of the evaluator is to determine whether an intervention has produced a change, either positive or negative, from baseline. Examples might include increased adherence, reduced days missed from work, increased use of services, or decreased injuries on the job. Cost-benefit analysis extends this evaluation to explore the relationship between intervention program cost and program health outcomes, expressed in monetary benefits. It is a ratio of costs per unit of economic benefit and net economic benefit. This form of evaluation usually compares two or more alternatives (i.e., experimental program and control program).

Community Health Education: Strategies Used by Physical Therapists

McKenzie and Smeltzer[24] have described many strategies and interventions for implementing health education activities. Physical therapists may not readily see their role as community health educator. However, many therapists already use educational strategies to improve the overall health of their clients.

Physical therapists can use communication activities, such as hosting a series of health-related announcements sponsored by local radio or television stations, or distributing pamphlets or brochures and displaying posters developed by the American Physical Therapy Association or other health organizations on prevention and health promotion. In addition, therapists can develop patient education materials that communicate their message in a client-friendly manner to facilitate program adherence. These communication efforts can be extended through more formal community educational activities, including presentation of workshops, seminars, or lectures to church groups, local businesses, foundations, organizations for older adults, retirement communities, corporations, schools, or service organizations.

Physical therapists can also incorporate behavior modification techniques into their practices. Examples may include increasing awareness of physical activity by having individuals keep logs, journals, or diaries, and having a system of rewards or reinforcement. Incentives in the form of rewards can include social reinforcers, such as praise, public recognition, encouragement, and personal letters, or material reinforcers, such as certificates, pins, towels, preferred or free parking, and discounts to local health clubs. Monetary reinforcers, such as tokens, coupons, raffles, points redeemable for some merchandise, and gift certificates, can also be used.

Therapists can be instrumental in environmental change activities. They can become involved in local, social, economic, political, and physical aspects of the "environment." These activities may assist in decision making for provisions of exercise opportunities for the community (e.g., the development of walking trails), helping in the design of community facilities to make them accessible for the disabled, addressing transportation issues in a community, or providing listings of accessible gyms and health clubs.

Therapists can be active in community advocacy, organizational culture, and social activities by attending planning board committee meetings; being a part of letter-writing campaigns directed toward key decision makers about community health–related issues; conducting personal visits to educate and lobby key legislators; incorporating a fitness and wellness mentality among persons in corporations, schools, and nonprofit groups; and participation in health fairs. Social activities—including developing support groups, facilitating after-hours exercise groups (in hospitals, outpatient settings, or apartment complexes for older adults), offering ongoing e-mail for persons post-discharge (for continuity of care), and creating buddy systems for persons dealing with the same dysfunction—can be effective and easy to implement.

Physical therapists can also be involved in health status evaluation activities, such as conducting Health Risk Appraisals (HRAs) and fitness screenings at health clubs, community health centers, health care facilities, and schools.

Finally, therapists can actively be involved in technology-delivered activities by using computer-assisted instruction for teaching individuals and by informing individuals of Web site addresses that offer information and Web support groups on health issues and services.

Community Health Education Served by Physical Therapists

In today's health care environment, physical therapists can be creative in exploring a variety of practice settings and opportunities. These may include community settings, such as governmental units, voluntary health agencies, local health departments, and community churches or other faith settings. Mullen et al.[25] discuss the perspective that the delivery settings constitute important dimensions of health education and promotion policy, programs, and research about program needs, feasibility, efficacy, and effectiveness.

In the following sections, we briefly discuss those community health education settings most predominant in the work of physical therapists, including health care settings, schools, corporate settings, settings that serve older adults, settings designed for persons with disabilities, health education centers, health clubs, and support groups.

Health Care Settings

Opportunities for providing community health education in health care settings have grown tremendously. Most hospitals provide health programs for community residents. Woods[26] describes a hospital affiliated physical therapy wellness program named The Total Rehabilitation and Athletic Conditioning Center (TRACC). It is a hospital affiliated physical therapy clinic that also provides the community with health promotion and prevention programs for a variety of health conditions. Physical therapists affiliated with the program are leading the way in efforts to improve the health status of their community. Specific programs include exercise classes, a preventive medicine program, a physical therapy maintenance program, and a work-site rehabilitation and prevention program.

School Settings

School health education is an applied field of study that draws from public health, family life, childhood growth and development, nutrition, psychology, and other disciplines. School health programs involve the school health environment, school health services, and school health instruction. Physical therapists can serve as curriculum consultants, subject matter experts, guest lecturers, initiators, and coordinators. In addition, institutions of higher learning often employ health education specialists to work with students, faculty and staff, and other community work-site programs.[27]

Corporate Settings

The concept of work-site health promotion has grown out of the older industrial medicine and industrial hygiene programs that were concerned with first aid and medical care; environmental hazards, such as toxic components and noise; and safety programs that stressed accident prevention.

Many work-site and corporate health promotion programs encompass educational, organizational, and environmental activities designed to support the healthy behavior of employees. These programs exist under the names of *work-site health promotion, employee wellness programs,* and *employee assistance programs.* Financial incentives and disincentives for employee involvement are often incorporated into these programs.

Corporate on-site physical therapy is an evolving trend. Physical therapists have had a presence in more traditionally "blue collar" industrial sites for many years. These are sites in which people are more inclined to have back problems due to manual labor. Newer, developing programs are unique in that they are geared to the more "white collar" environment. Wynn[28] describes an on-site physical therapy program developed at CIGNA Corporation, a health care insurance and financial services organization headquartered in Philadelphia. Its goal is to have a healthy and productive workforce. Hank Balavender, a therapist involved in the development of this program, states, "My advice to physical therapists who may be interested in pursuing a similar program is to establish a relationship with a company and become an educational resource. Take the opportunity to educate not only the employees, but the employers as well, on the benefits of physical therapy."[28(p70)]

Settings That Serve Older Adults

Health promotion is often overlooked in relation to the elderly and is even more overlooked with persons who are institutionalized. Most health promotion programs directed toward the elderly tend to focus on isolated individuals as their target population. Minkler[29] proposes that health promotion could potentially play a significant role in improving the health and quality of life of nursing home residents. Many persons remain in these facilities for several years and could benefit greatly from group health promotion interventions. The benefits would be that they could maintain functional independence and a higher quality of life, and be less of a physical burden on the staff.

Minkler states that several major changes must take place if this concept is to take hold in the long-term care environment, including overcoming the "youth bias" inherent in many conventional health promotion efforts, seeing the frail elderly as legitimate health promotion recipients, developing alternative and adequately funded settings for the many frail elders who would be better served in less-intense care environments, and decreasing the dependency that long-term-care settings facilitate. Specific interventions for nursing home settings might include teaching self-management skills, providing supportive networks that stress health maintenance and health promotion, and providing an environment committed to encouraging independence (Figure 13-2).

Holly, quoted in an article by Woods,[30] describes an innovative program in which he brings assistive technology to the nursing home environment and fitness training to the retirement community. He reports,

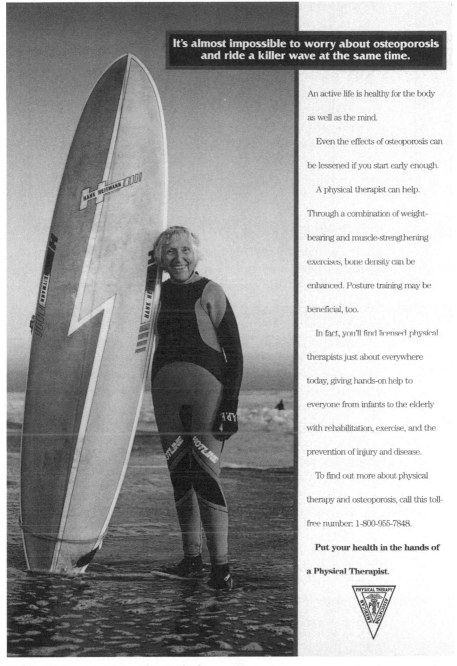

It's almost impossible to worry about osteoporosis and ride a killer wave at the same time.

An active life is healthy for the body as well as the mind.

Even the effects of osteoporosis can be lessened if you start early enough.

A physical therapist can help. Through a combination of weight-bearing and muscle-strengthening exercises, bone density can be enhanced. Posture training may be beneficial, too.

In fact, you'll find licensed physical therapists just about everywhere today, giving hands-on help to everyone from infants to the elderly with rehabilitation, exercise, and the prevention of injury and disease.

To find out more about physical therapy and osteoporosis, call this toll-free number: 1-800-955-7848.

Put your health in the hands of a Physical Therapist.

Figure 13-2   American Physical Therapy Association communication campaign poster: "Surfer."

In some respects, managed care, with its limited number of visits, is closing out opportunities for physical therapists. But with its emphasis on cost containment, there are just as many opportunities in the area of prevention programs opening up. With managed care companies looking for more economical ways to deliver health care, prevention programs are beginning to get the attention of many companies. Physical therapists are well positioned. We can go into the retirement communities and skilled nursing facilities and design programs to increase strength and prevent greater loss of bone mineral density that will inevitably lead to hip fractures.[31(p58–59)]

Settings Designed for Persons with Disabilities

Like the frail elderly and those in long-term care settings, persons with disabilities have been largely overlooked and rarely included in health promotion research and intervention programs. Almost all of the research in the area of health promotion has involved persons without disabilities. Consequently, we know little about the needs and outcomes related to these interventions.

In recent years, rehabilitation services have declined dramatically. Patients are much more likely to be discharged from inpatient settings with much rehabilitation to be done on their own, outside the traditional setting. Opportunities exist for health promotion and disease prevention for this specific, often neglected, population to enhance and maintain their functional independence.[31,32]

There continues to be an increased interest in health promotion behaviors among persons with chronic and disabling conditions. The purposes of health promotion programs for the disabled include reduction of secondary conditions (e.g., obesity, hypertension, pressure ulcers), maintenance of functional independence, provisions for leisure and recreational enjoyment, and enhancement of overall quality of life.

Rimmer[31,32] describes a program funded by the Centers for Disease Control and Prevention, Office of Disability and Health, that is a comprehensive health promotion program for stroke survivors. He notes that, aside from regular medical visits, stroke survivors have limited opportunities for improving or maintaining their health after rehabilitation. They often return to an unhealthy lifestyle after their injury, which increases the risk for secondary conditions and another stroke. This program includes three major components: exercise, nutrition, and health behavior. Rehabilitation (physical and occupational therapy, speech-language pathology, and rehabilitation engineering) is interwoven into the program.

Health Education Centers

Physical therapists can become involved in community centers for health education. Centers have traditionally been used to provide programming for elementary students. Health education centers are usually privately funded, non-profit organizations that approach health education in a multimedia fashion, with the goal of being educational as well as entertaining.

In 1996, there were 25 stand-alone health education centers. Many of these centers remain idle during the summer months. An opportunity exists to use the health education centers to provide health education to populations in a community during the summer months. By broadening the population base that is served by these centers to include both school children and community adults, the centers will be more efficiently used.

Physical therapists can play a role in community health education centers by developing cooperative agreements between local health departments, medical facilities, fitness centers, voluntary agencies, and religious organizations; facilitating the development of a health education resource library; initiating new community-oriented and outreach programs; participating in health education research; and assisting centers to serve as locations for patient education.[33]

Health Clubs

A growing number of physical therapy practices are combining traditional rehabilitation services with nonclinical fitness offerings to make use of a fully-equipped gym and the expertise of a physical therapist. Advantages of such programs include patients' or clients' progression from their rehabilitation into a fitness program located in a familiar environment. In addition, they have more access to equipment and amenities that they would not have in most private practices, including exercise and weight equipment, a pool, an indoor running track, and basketball and racquetball courts.[34] Therapists in these settings can, for example, conduct complimentary seminars or clinics on sports injuries, provide free consultations and health screenings, and write articles for the club newsletter. Sample programs include a pelvic floor rehabilitation program, a prenatal and postpartum pregnancy program, a postsurgical breast cancer program, a lymphedema program, an osteoporosis fracture prevention program, and a home health program.[35]

McManus[36] describes a group program that she developed for persons with chronic pain, illness, and stress-related medical conditions. The program includes stretching and strengthening, proper posture, mind-body awareness, the importance of pacing, and how attitudes influence health.

Support Groups

Patient support groups are becoming more popular. Some groups operate out of facilities such as hospitals or clinics, whereas others are sponsored by national health care organizations. In some instances, groups are organized by individuals with disabilities or disorders, or by their families. Examples in the physical therapy literature include the involvement of physical therapists in support groups for people who have experienced stroke; people with arthritis, breast cancer, or hemophilia; and people who have undergone heart transplants.

Therapists can become involved in these support groups even if on a consultant basis. Support groups can be an excellent resource for encouraging patients to stick to their home program, providing continued education for a particular condition, and assisting in meeting rehabilitation goals begun in the clinic.[37]

Funding Issues

Seeking funds to support community health education efforts can be a challenge. This is especially true because insurance companies rarely cover preventive services. Many times, those most in need of services are the least likely to be able to afford to pay for them privately. Physical therapists can seek opportunities to obtain funds from external funding sources through grants and other fund-raising endeavors.[38]

Millions of dollars are available through grants and contracts from both governmental agencies (for more information on the Internet, see http://www.nih.gov) and private foundations (e.g., the American Heart Association, the Multiple Sclerosis Society, or the Arthritis Foundation). Religious and related charities are the most popular recipients of these funds. Health-related programs usually receive the second-largest sum. Although dollar amounts fluctuate each year, large sums of money are available and often go unclaimed. These funding sources often prefer to support projects that include some sort of partnership with community agencies. Physical therapists could greatly enhance the services they are able to provide through such partnerships.

Summary and Future Directions in Community Health

Changes in the health care delivery system have challenged physical therapists, like other health professionals, to explore new ways to deliver and enhance their services. Strategies to promote health in the general public have been developed and described. Beckon et al.[27(p348)] state that

... health education will continue to flourish well into the new millennium if professional preparation, practice and research keep up with the pace of change. Trends for the new millennium will require more leadership training and policy development, more education of the public, more training and retraining of public health professionals, and more attention to priorities established by the citizenry. More collaboration networks will emerge, promoting practice that works at fostering accountability.

Teaching community health education principles to physical therapists will enhance the delivery of their services and allow new employment opportunities. Refer to the Appendices following this chapter for further information on what physical therapy educational programs could teach about community health, as well as a list of health care organizations from which physical therapists can seek additional information or with which they can become affiliated.

References

1. Wallack L, Winkleby M. Primary prevention: a new look at basic concepts. Soc Sci Med 1987;25(8):923–930.
2. National Health Promotion and Disease Prevention Objectives. Healthy People 2000: Summary Report. Washington, DC: U.S. Department of Health and Human Services, GPO, 1992.
3. National Health Promotion and Disease Prevention Objectives. Healthy People 2010 Web site. Available at: http://www.health.gov/healthypeople. Accessed: November 23, 2001.
4. U.S. Dept. of Health, Education, and Welfare, Public Health Service. Healthy People: The Surgeon General's Report on Health Promotion and Disease Prevention. Washington, DC: U.S. Department of Health and Human Services, GPO, 1979.
5. Francis KT. Status of the Year 2000 Health Goals for Physical Activity and Fitness. Phys Ther 1999;79(4):405–414.
6. Flynn BC. Healthy cities: toward worldwide health and promotion. Annu Rev Public Health 1996;17:299–309.
7. Helvie C. Community Health Nursing: Theory and Process. Philadelphia: Harper & Row, 1981.
8. Baum C, Law M. Community health: a responsibility, an opportunity and a fit for occupational therapy. Am J Occup Ther 1998;52(1):8–10.
9. Baum CM, Law M. Occupational therapy practice: focusing on occupational performance. Am J Occup Ther 1997;51:277–288.

10. O'Neil EH and the Pew Commission for the Health Professions. Recreating Professional Practice for a New Century. San Francisco: Pew Health Professions Commission, 1998.
11. Blood H. Developing community health content in a physical therapy curriculum. Phys Ther 1970;50:1226–1238.
12. Guide to physical therapist practice (2nd ed). Phys Ther 2001;81:31–102.
13. Evaluative Criteria for Accreditation of Education Programs for the Preparation of Physical Therapists. Commission on Accreditation in Physical Therapy Education. Alexandria, VA: American Physical Therapy Association, 1998.
14. Normative Model of Physical Therapist Professional Education, Version 2000. Alexandria, VA: American Physical Therapy Association, 2000.
15. Freudenberg N, Eng E, Flay B, et al. Strengthening individual and community capacity to prevent disease and promote health: in search of relevant theories and principles. Health Educ Q 1995;22(3):290–306.
16. Baranowski T, Perry CL, Parcel GS. How Individuals, Environments, and Health Behavior Interact: Social Cognitive Theory. In K Glanz, FM Lewis, BK Rimer (eds), Health Behavior and Health Education: Theory, Research, and Practice (2nd ed). San Francisco: Jossey-Bass, 1997.
17. Miller NE, Dollard J. Social Learning and Imitation. New Haven, CT: Yale University Press, 1941.
18. McGuire WJ. Theoretical foundations of campaigns. In Rice RE, Atkin CK (eds). Public Communication Campaigns. Newbury Park, CA: Sage Publications,1981:43–65.
19. Lefebvre RC, Rochlin L. Social marketing. In Glanz K, Frances ML, Rimer BK (eds). Health Behavior and Health Education. San Francisco: Jossey-Bass, 1997.
20. Novelli WD. Developing Marketing Programs. In Fredrickson LW, Solomon L, Brehony K (eds), Marketing Health Behavior. New York: Plenum, 1984.
21. Lefebvre RC, Flora JA. Social marketing and public health interventions. Health Educ Q 1988;15(3):299–315.
22. Green LW, Kreuter MW. Health Promotion Planning: An Educational and Ecological Approach (3rd ed). Mountain View, CA: Mayfield Publishing Co., 1999.
23. Peel C, Lein D, Kitchens B. Tone your bones program for preventing fractures as a result of osteoporosis. J Phys Ther Educ 2001;15(2):23–28.
24. McKenzie JF, Smeltzer JL. Planning, Implementing, and Evaluating Health Promotion Programs (3rd ed). Boston: Allyn & Bacon, 2001:20–26.
25. Mullen PD, Evans D, Forster J. Settings as an important dimension in health education/promotion policy, programs, and research. Health Educ Q 1995;22(3):329–345.

26. Woods EN. Facility profile, making TRACCs toward a healthier community. PT Mag June 1995;3(6):40–52.
27. Breckon D, Harvey JR, Lancaster RB. Community Health Education: Settings, Roles, and Skills for the 21st Century (4th ed). Gaithersburg, MD: Aspen, 1998.
28. Wynn K. Setting corporate trends with on-site PT. PT Mag July 1996:66–71.
29. Minkler M. Health promotion in long-term care: a contradiction in terms? Health Educ Q 1984;11(1):77–89.
30. Woods EN. Innovative programs in geriatrics. PT Mag May 1995:58–63.
31. Rimmer JH, Hedman. G. A health promotion program for stroke survivors. Top Stroke Rehabil 1998;5(2):30–44.
32. Rimmer JH. Health promotion for people with disabilities: the emerging paradigm shift from disability prevention to prevention of secondary conditions. Phys Ther 1999;79:495–502.
33. Clark JK, Clark SE, Sauter M. Expanding the role of community centers for health education. J Health Educ 1996;27(4):253–256.
34. Fausnaught M. Building a practice: niches in fitness and aquatics. PT Mag March 2000:30–35.
35. Mangano JH, Dawson T. Under one roof. PT Mag Dec 1999:28–33.
36. McManus C. Movement with awareness: The Wellness Program. PT Mag March 2000:36–43.
37. Parascandola M. Patient support groups. PT Mag May 1999:34–41.
38. Bauer DG. The "How To" Grants Manual: Successful Grantseeking Techniques for Obtaining Public and Private Grants (3rd ed). Phoenix: American Council on Education and the Onyx Press, 1995.

Annotated Bibliography

Breckon D, Harvey JR, Lancaster RB. **Community Health Education: Settings, Roles, and Skills for the 21st Century (4th ed).** Gaithersburg, MD: Aspen, 1998. Breckon and colleagues describe current and future perspectives in practice and professional preparation of health educators. They address aspects of choosing a setting, specifics of entering the profession, and aspects regarding mobility in the profession. The text encompasses the specific aspects of program planning, applying principles of learning, primary prevention and intervention strategies, group dynamics, public relations and marketing, working with the media, using educational methods and materials, developing printed materials, grant application, and community fund raising. Specifics on healthy communities; health departments and other tax-supported agencies; traditional and emerging voluntary health organizations; medical settings;

work-site health promotion and employee assistance programs; school health; college, university, and professional organizations; and faith community settings are described. Physical therapy is not directly referred to anywhere in the book; however, many of the chapters discuss concepts pertinent to the practice of physical therapy.

Glanz K, Lewis FM, Rimer BK, eds. Health Behavior and Health Education: Theory, Research, and Practice (2nd ed). San Francisco: Jossey-Bass, 1997. The editors of this textbook set out to present theoretical constructs and principles of health behaviors and health education in an accessible and practical manner, rather than the abstract, lofty way they are often delivered. The book includes contributions by many of the leaders in the field of health behavior and education. Descriptions of the theories and concepts are enhanced by chapters that describe the strengths and weaknesses of each and practical examples of the theories put into practice. The book is particularly well suited for individuals who know little about the topic. As such, it would be a useful reference for physical therapists and physical therapist assistant education programs.

Green LW, Kreuter MW. Health Promotion Planning: An Educational and Ecological Approach (3rd ed). Mountain View, CA: Mayfield Publishing Co., 1999. A classic text in the area of health promotion. This third edition of the book reflects the ongoing development of the PRECEDE-PROCEED model for health promotion. One of the strengths of the PRECEDE-PROCEED model is the structure and guidance it provides to health professionals in thinking more broadly about the planning, implementation, and evaluation of a health promotion program. The book is an excellent reference text for physical therapists. The authors provide clear examples of applied theories, practical strategies, and tools for planning and implementing a program, as well as a number of examples of programs. The Evaluation and Accountability component and the reference list are exceptionally well done. For any therapist considering seeking grant funding for a health promotion program, this book is a must.

Areas of Responsibility for Entry-Level Health Care Practitioners and Suggested Topics for Physical Therapy Curricula

Entry-level responsibility areas	Curricular topics
Assessing individual and community needs for health education	Health behavior theory Program planning models (PRECEDE-PROCEED, PATCH)
Planning effective health education programs	Health behavior theory Program planning models (PRECEDE-PROCEED, PATCH)
Implementing health education programs	Program planning models (PRECEDE-PROCEED, PATCH) Communication theory Funding health education programs
Evaluating effectiveness of health education programs	Program evaluation (formative, implementation process, outcome, cost-effectiveness)
Coordinating provision of health education services	All concepts
Acting as a resource person in health education	All concepts
Communicating health and health education needs, concerns, and resources	Communication theory

PATCH = planned approach to community health; PRECEDE = predisposing, reinforcing, and enabling causes in educational diagnosis and evaluation; PROCEED = policy, regulatory, and organizational constructs in educational and environmental development.

B

Organizations and Resources for Community Health Education

American Association for Health Education
American Public Health Association
American School Health Association
American Society for Health Care Education and Training
Association of State and Territorial Directors of Health Promotion and Public Health Education
Association for Worksite Health Promotion
International Union for Health Promotion and Health Education
National Council for the Education of Health Professionals in Health Promotion
National Wellness Association
Resource Guide For National Health Organizations Applicable to Health Education/ Disease Prevention for Physical Therapists
Society for Public Health Education
Society of State Directors of Health, Physical Education, and Recreation
Wellness Councils of America

C

Community Health Organizations with Which Physical Therapists May Become Affiliated

Administration on Aging
Alzheimer's Association
American Alliance for Health, Physical Education, Recreation and Dance
American Association of Cardiovascular and Pulmonary Rehabilitation
American Association for Respiratory Care
American Association for World Health
American Chiropractic Association
American College of Preventative Medicine
American College of Sports Medicine
American Diabetes Association
American Institute for Preventative Medicine
American Journal of Health Promotion/Wellness Councils of America
American Occupational Therapy Association
American Physical Therapy Association
American Public Health Association
American Running and Fitness Association
Aquatic Exercise Association
Aquatic Therapy and Rehabilitation Institute
Associated Bodywork and Massage Professionals
Association for Worksite Health Promotion
Health Information Resource Center
Medical Fitness Association
National Association for Home Care
National Athletic Trainers Association
National Center for Health Education
National Osteoporosis Foundation
National Rehabilitation Awareness Foundation

National Strength and Conditioning Association
National Stroke Association
President's Council on Physical Fitness and Sports
Society for Public Health Education
U.S. President's Committee on Employment of People with Disabilities
Youth Fitness Coalition

14

Postprofessional Clinical Residency Education

Carol Jo Tichenor and
Jeanne M. Davidson

When I came to the residency program, I wanted to learn many different examination and treatment techniques so that I would have a large "bag of tricks" to use with my patients. Day after day over a year, I had the opportunity to work with my clinical supervisors. They challenged me to "think on my feet" and to respond to the emerging data from the patient. I learned how to conduct a focused examination; systematically prioritize problems for the difficult, multifactorial patient; justify a treatment plan; and reassess the effects of treatment. Although I came to the residency program to advance my skills and knowledge within a clinical specialty area, I also became a "generalist." I strengthened my patient management skills in a manner that would impact all types of patients. I learned how to listen to my patients and understand their perception of the disease or dysfunction, so that I could better judge their readiness to learn and their ability to change in response to my recommendations. Doing so has changed the manner in which I listen and communicate in my professional, as well as personal, life. The changes from the manner in which I originally practiced physical therapy are far beyond my initial expectations. After this year of intensive clinical supervision and didactic education, I believe that I have gained the tools that will enable me to continue to grow throughout the rest of my career. I am confident that I am prepared to meet the rapid changes in service delivery models that are happening in physical therapy and throughout health care.

Chapter Objectives

After completing this chapter, the reader will be able to

1. Discuss the history and philosophy of residency education.
2. Identify key components of residency curricula.
3. Describe various residency teaching strategies to facilitate the development of efficient, systematic clinical reasoning skills and provide a rationale for their use.
4. Identify resources that can be used in the design of residency curricula.

Clinical Residency Today

Our country is undergoing health care changes unlike any in the history of medicine, and we, as physical therapists, are facing one of the most difficult job markets in the history of our profession. Many physical therapists are concerned about the loss of jobs, decrease in benefits, stasis in salaries, and loss of support for continuing education from employers. All health care professions are faced with the challenge to develop service delivery models that preserve quality while providing cost-effective, clinically effective, accessible, consumer-oriented care. Physical therapists are being asked to seriously re-examine their paradigm of practice. How can the patient's needs be addressed in fewer visits? Is there a role for more group intervention to decrease costs? Are there any practitioners with musculoskeletal backgrounds who can serve patients in conjunction with, or in place of, the physical therapist? Are there new venues to which physical therapists can expand practice? Some physical therapists respond to these challenges by becoming paralyzed, unable and unwilling to change their paradigm of practice. Others respond by seeking clinical and academic education that will enable them to be more effective and efficient in their examination and treatment skills. The preceding sketch outlines the advanced patient management and communication skills that some physical therapists seek to stay competitive in the current health care environment.

In their desire to attain advanced skills in examination and treatment, some therapists seek postprofessional master's degree studies or clinical doctorates in physical therapy (DPTs), but emphasis on *advanced clinical training* is highly variable in many existing programs. Others turn to the continuing education market. Physical therapists, frustrated by a piecemeal approach to weekend continuing education courses, are rethinking their professional goals to establish sound, cohesive, professional plans for themselves—plans that will have a major impact on their level of clinical competence over time.[1] Postprofessional clinical residency education can assist physical therapists to achieve advanced clinical competence. This chapter focuses on the curriculum components and teaching strategies for an orthopedic manual physical therapy (OMPT) residency program or an orthopedic physical therapy residency program. Several curricular components overlap in these two clinical specialty areas. The concepts presented are also applicable to many other advanced clinical specialty areas within physical therapy, as well as to aspects of physical therapy professional curricula. The educational principles and teaching strategies presented in this chapter and the resources outlined in Appendix 14-A can assist educational institutions and health care organizations in the design of residency curricula. Potential applicants to residency programs may also use the concepts in this chapter to determine whether the scope and intensity of residency education meet their career objectives.

What Is a Residency Program?

The American Physical Therapy Association (APTA) Committee for Clinical Residency and Fellowship Program Credentialing proposes the following definition of clinical residencies[2(p16)]:

> A clinical residency is a planned program of postprofessional clinical education that is designed to significantly advance the graduate's preparation as a provider of patient care services beyond entry level expectations in a defined area of clinical practice. The program combines the opportunities for ongoing clinical supervision and mentoring, with a theoretical basis for advanced practice and scientific inquiry. A clinical residency program is not synonymous with the terms "clinical internship" or "clinical fellowship."

In addition to medicine, which has had ambulatory care residencies since the early 1870s,[3] podiatry,[4] optometry,[5] and psychology[6] are among the many professions that have recognized the knowledge, clinical competence, and confidence that can be attained through residency education for entry into the profession and for specialization. Each of these professions has established an accreditation process for clinical residencies. For physical therapy, the concept of residency training dates back to the 1960s, with the development of the University Affiliated Programs that incorporated formalized, interdisciplinary, long-term training in pediatrics.[7] In the late 1970s, the lack of opportunities for advanced training in manual therapy in the United States led some American physical therapists to travel to such countries as Norway and Australia to receive long-term mentoring and advanced course work.[1] Over the years, a limited number of orthopedic, pediatric, and sports physical therapy residency programs have also developed in various parts of the United States.[1]

In 1993, the American Academy of Orthopedic Manual Physical Therapists (AAOMPT) created the Standards for Orthopaedic Manual Physical Therapy Residency Education[8] and a formal recognition process to assess OMPT programs. These standards were updated in 1999.[9] APTA developed a credentialing process for postprofessional clinical residencies in 1998 and for fellowship programs in 2000.[2] Under the APTA definition, a fellowship program has the same components as a clinical residency, except a fellowship curriculum is in a "focused area of clinical practice, education, or research."[2] A *fellowship* is designed for board-certified, postresidency-prepared, or postdoctoral-educated physical therapists. For the purposes of this chapter, the term *residency* also applies to fellowship programs.

Mission and Philosophy of Residency Education

It is impossible to outline a single residency philosophy that can cross many clinical specialty areas and includes a broad range of part- and full-time models. However, based on our communications with residency programs across the country, key aspects that are common to many current programs can be summarized. Residency education is founded on the premise that the development of advanced clinical practice requires a significant commitment of time and practice over an extended period. It is also based on the tenet that consistent clinical supervision, critique, and feedback are necessary for the development and refinement of advanced evaluation and treatment skills.[9,10] Residency education is committed to the development of a therapist's ability to link theory and practice through the combination of didactic and clinical course work and supervised and unsupervised clinical training. Beyond instruction and refinement of advanced therapeutic techniques, the core of residency curricula is the development of a systematic, clinical reasoning process. Residency programs also seek to educate clinicians who will be able to critically review current literature and will continue to expand the body of knowledge in their specialty through the conduction of clinical research and the publication of case studies. At the foundation of residency curricula is the goal to develop clinicians who will substantially advance the practice of physical therapy and make lasting contributions to their professional communities through teaching, consultation, or both.

Overview of Residency Models

Various part-time and full-time residency models exist in the United States. In a full-time model, residents typically treat patients in the clinic 20–30 hours per week, during which they receive one-on-one or small-group (e.g., one-on-three) supervision from residency faculty. Lecture and laboratory practice in the specialty area are combined with medical lectures, clinical seminars, and course work in the basic and applied sciences (e.g., neurophysiology, anatomy, biomechanics) and in scientific inquiry.

Residency faculty members are generally physical therapy senior clinicians, coordinators, or clinical specialists on staff at the sponsoring institution. Other residency faculty may be private practitioners in the community who come to the residency on a regular basis to provide lectures or laboratory instruction. Residency faculty generally teach the clinical lectures and laboratory sessions, provide clinical supervision, and conduct the examinations. Having one or more faculty members with prior residency experience on staff or as consultants can be valuable in designing all components of the curriculum, particularly the clinical supervision and examination components. Physicians and other non–physical therapy practitioners may provide medical lectures or other clinical seminars. Basic and applied science and research courses may be taught by residency faculty or by academic faculty from an affiliated university. Existing full-time programs generally range from 1 to 3 years.

Part-time models may require the resident to regularly travel to a designated residency clinic during weekdays, evenings, or weekends to provide patient care and to receive one-to-one clinical supervision. Clinical supervision is given during scheduled meeting times with the residency faculty or in blocks of time (e.g., 2- to 3-week intensives or 1 or 2 weekends per month, over several months). The residency faculty may also travel to the practice site of the resident to provide supervision. The curriculum content identified for full-time programs also applies to part-time programs. Part-time residencies are highly variable in duration. Faculty structure is generally the same as that described for the full-time residency.

The AAOMPT requires that programs have a minimum duration of 11 months,[9] and APTA requires that programs have a minimum duration of 9 months and a maximum of 36 months.[2]

In addition to an extended period of clinical supervision, another key component of residency programs is the use of periodic practical examinations. These examinations, or "technique exams," are designed to assess handling skills and are used in combination with clinical examinations with a patient(s) present. The clinical examinations may involve one to three encounters with the same patient. The residency faculty member scores the resident's ability to examine and evaluate a patient, establish a diagnosis, establish a prognosis, implement a plan of care, re-examine the patient, and document all aspects of the plan of care. Through the clinical examination process, the faculty member assesses the resident's ability to respond to emerging data, which result from the resident's examination and interventions. In turn, this process provides the resident with feedback that can assist her or him to achieve a high level of refinement in clinical reasoning and handling skills.

Some residency programs are now using information technology tools for communication (e.g., the Internet) to have residents take online course work for the didactic components of the curriculum and to facilitate communication between the resident and residency faculty member, especially when the two individuals are not within easy traveling distance. Other residency programs are linking to university programs that may have a distance education component. The resident may, for example, travel to the university for course work such as anatomy, which is taught in an intensive format. Doing so enables the resident to fulfill clinical course work and supervision *at the residency program* while also fulfilling additional basic and applied science requirements through a distance education format.

An increasing number of residency programs have established formal university affiliations with physical therapy curricula, whereby graduate credit is granted toward a postprofessional master's or clinical doctorate in physical therapy for completion of all or portions of a residency curriculum. Some residency programs are located within university settings. The collaboration of physical therapy academic faculty and residency faculty can result in tremendous short- and long-term benefits to the curricula of both organizations. Academic faculty bring expertise in teaching and examination methodology, in the basic and applied sciences, and in research to assist the residency program in developing a sound educational framework for the entire curriculum. Residency faculty bring a high level of clinical expertise, which can contribute to the education of the professional and postprofessional students within the physical therapy program and the therapists within the clinical training sites affiliated with the university. The entire clinical community is enriched.

Key Components in the Design of Residency Curricula

The APTA credentialing and AAOMPT recognition processes require residency programs to demonstrate that curricula reflect practice dimensions of a valid and reliable practice analysis.[2,9] Resources for obtaining existing descriptions of advanced clinical practice (DACP) are included within Appendix 14-A at the end of this chapter. The DACP of the specialty area can provide the framework for determining the major curricular components of the program (e.g., examination, evaluation, diagnosis). Practice dimensions of the DACP, which are stated in behavorial terms, can be used to define the performance outcomes of the program and as instructional objectives in individual courses.

The grid presented in Figure 14-1 provides a temporal illustration of the curriculum of a year-long residency program in OMPT. The curriculum components and design can apply to other clinical specialty areas.

The residents are employed by the medical center and receive a salary and reduced benefit package for 12 months. In a typical week, the resident provides 26 hours of patient care in a large outpatient orthopedic setting and receives 5 hours per week of one-on-one supervision.

The program is divided into four teaching modules, which are reflected in Figure 14-1. OMPT clinical lectures and laboratory instruction are presented during a 1-week introductory intensive to establish a foundation for examination and treatment in the clinic. Selected anatomy and biomechanical lectures are also presented during the initial week and during periodic lectures over the first 4 months of the program, from January through April. Clinical course work and laboratory instruction occur approximately two to three weekends each month and cover the major curricular topics shown in Figure 14-1 (e.g., planning the objective examination, re-examination, implementation of plan of care, and medical lectures). Clinical practice in an outpatient clinic and clinical supervision begin the second week of the program and continue throughout the program. Small group tutorials focused on refinement of clinical reasoning concepts, review and critique of the literature, case study review, and handling skills are held approximately every 3 weeks during nonclinic days. Clinical examinations occur at the end of every module.

When the residents begin clinical practice, patient types are scheduled according to the clinical lecture and laboratory instruction within the curriculum. Hence, in Clinical Rotation I, residents primarily see patients with spinal and shoulder complex dysfunctions while they concurrently receive lectures on examination and treatment of spinal and shoulder complex dysfunctions. Clinical Rotation II focuses on patients with hip, knee, foot, and ankle dysfunctions. These patient types are then added to the resident's schedule.

When a joint complex (e.g., hip) is covered, all aspects of hip examination and implementation of a plan of care are covered during lecture and laboratory sessions. During each module, however, while preparing the resident

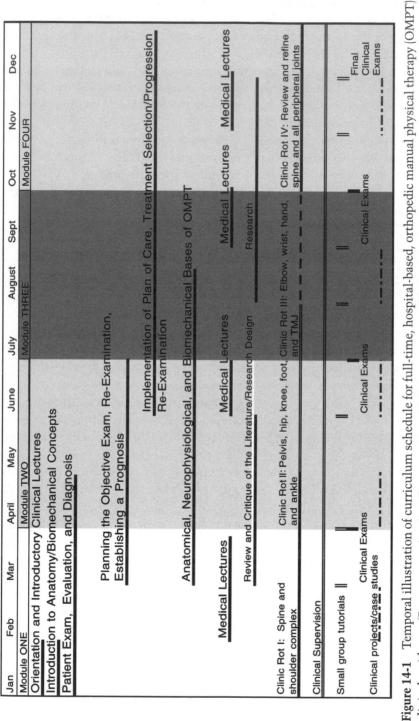

Figure 14-1 Temporal illustration of curriculum schedule for full-time, hospital-based, orthopedic manual physical therapy (OMPT) clinical residency. (Exam = examination; Rot = rotation; TMJ = temporomandibular joint.)

to examine and treat the patient globally, lectures, laboratory, and clinical supervision emphasize the concepts of that module. Thus, lectures on the hip complex emphasize concepts related to planning the objective examination and re-examination, and establishing a prognosis. Similarly, during clinical supervision, the resident is supervised on all aspects of his or her patient care delivery; however, the clinical supervisor will emphasize the concepts that are the focus of each module. When examinations occur at the end of each module, the residency faculty member scores the resident on all aspects of patient care, but points are weighted toward the concepts that are the focus of that module.

Throughout the program, assigned readings and ongoing clinical projects relate to the lectures and laboratory sessions being taught. Course work in anatomy, neurophysiology, and biomechanics is taken online through a university distance learning program or through special lectures provided by academic faculty from affiliating universities. Residency faculty also reinforce the basic and applied science concepts during ongoing lectures.

Laying out the program in a bar graph format allows the program director and faculty to assess the vertical and horizontal relationships between curriculum components. In assessing the horizontal relationships between elements of course work, the faculty need to determine how course material and learning activities are building on one another. For example, initially the resident receives instruction in patient examination, evaluation, and diagnosis, and then progresses to concepts related to establishing a prognosis and implementing a plan of care. When looking at the vertical relationships of the program, the bar graph enables the faculty to determine how different components reinforce each other. For example, lecture concepts are reinforced with tutorial and clinical supervision experiences.

In addition to laying out the temporal sequences via a bar graph approach, the program director and faculty need to consider the relationship of the curriculum components to the DACP for the clinical specialty area and to the methods for evaluation. Table 14-1 provides an example of how the different curriculum components can be organized to show their relationship to the DACP of the clinical specialty area and to the methods for evaluation. This table can provide the program director with an effective method for determining the faculty expertise needed to achieve each program component.

Within Appendix 14-A are descriptions of various standards documents and curriculum resource manuals that are helpful in designing a residency mission and philosophy, in developing a curriculum and program evaluation plan, and in assessing financial considerations and faculty needs in relation to budgetary and curriculum resources.

Table 14-1 Description of Curriculum Components for an Orthopedic Manual Physical Therapy (OMPT) Residency

Curriculum component	Description	Relationship to DACP for OMPT	Time frame	Methods of evaluation
Client interview, history taking, subjective examination concepts	Client interview: subjective examination components, rationale for the questions that are asked, relationship to planning the objective examination, communication strategies, organizing and controlling the interview, interpreting data from the history.	Practice dimensions: examination, evaluation, diagnosis, establishing a prognosis, documentation	Subjective examination concepts are introduced in lectures or labs for every joint complex throughout the program.	Clinical examination with patient present
Treatment selection and progression for patient with spinal dysfunction	Goal setting and identification of OMPT intervention priorities vs. other patient management priorities; planning intervention approach; justifying interventions; identifying indications and contraindications; OMPT reassessment; discussing concepts of treatment selection and progression of OMPT, exercise, ergonomic concepts, and self-mobilization.	Implementation of plan of care, re-examination, documentation	5 hours over first week of program, 4 hours during module II and module IV.	Clinical examination with patient present in modules II, III, and IV Retrospective case study to assess treatment selection and provide rationale during modules III and IV

DACP = descriptions of advanced clinical practice.

Source: Adapted from Guidelines for Curriculum Development for Postprofessional Residencies in Orthopaedic Physical Therapy and Orthopaedic Manual Physical Therapy. La Crosse, WI: APTA, Orthopedic Section, 2000.

Development of Clinical Reasoning in Clinical Residency Education

The greatest challenge of residency education is that curricula focus on the experienced clinician and developing strategies that will enable the practitioner to achieve professional expertise. The progression to advanced clinical practice does not occur in 1, 2, or 3 years of residency training, but rather is based on the development of a clinical reasoning process that occurs over subsequent years of experience and is linked with the concurrent evolution of the clinician's knowledge base.[11] Since the 1980s, various models for clinical reasoning have been researched in the health care professions.[11,12] *Clinical reasoning* is the complex thought process used in the evaluation and management of patients.[13] One physical therapy clinical reasoning model, originally proposed by Maitland,[14,15] was refined by Grant et al.[16] into a more formalized teaching model. The model uses a framework established by Barrows and Tamblyn.[17] It involves the systematic collection of subjective and objective data and the recognition, based on knowledge and experience, of clinical patterns and the variations that may occur. The clinical reasoning process also includes the complex process of identifying, ranking, and re-ranking a working hypothesis to develop an "evolving concept of the patient's problem."[13] This process involves the use of a systematic method for reassessing factors that aggravate or ease the patient's symptoms. Gale and Marsden[18] point out that active interpretation and evaluative thinking processes occur throughout the clinical reasoning process. Factors that influence the effectiveness of clinical reasoning include (1) the presence of a sound knowledge base; (2) how knowledge is stored, retrieved, and refined with repeated use[11,16,19]; (3) experiences, values, and attitudes[20]; and (4) the ability to involve the patient in cooperative decision making.[21,22] Development of these skills is the focus of the clinical supervision process. This development is facilitated as the residency faculty member works collaboratively with the resident with multiple patients over an extended period of time.

Development of experience and its relationship to development of clinical expertise is well described by Benner.[23] Benner uses the Dreyfus model of skill acquisition. This model provides a rationale for selected teaching strategies to enhance the clinical reasoning process during clinical supervision. Benner proposes that, in acquiring and developing skill, the clinician passes through five levels of proficiency: novice, advanced beginner, competent, proficient, and expert. Movement through these five levels of expertise reflects the following changes in four general aspects of skill performance: (1) movement from reliance on abstract principles and rules to use of past concrete experiences as guides; (2) change in the perception and understanding of a situation (i.e., seeing the situation less as a compilation of equally relevant bits of information and more as a complete and complex whole); (3) shift from reliance on analytic, rule-based thinking to intuitive judgment; and (4) passage from a detached observer to an involved and fully engaged participant.

According to Benner, the expert demonstrates "an intuitive grasp of each situation and zeroes in on the accurate region of the problems without wasteful consideration of a large range of unfruitful, alternative diagnoses and solutions. Capturing the descriptions of expert performance is difficult, because the expert operates from a deep understanding of the total situation."[23]

In opposition to Benner, Ruth-Sahd states that the intuitive-based practice of the expert may and should exist at lower levels of proficiency.[24] Over several years of residency teaching, we have observed that the experienced practitioner in a residency program jumps between various levels of proficiency as he or she advances in clinical reasoning skills. This factor can create frustration for the experienced resident and a teaching challenge for the faculty member. Recognition of the importance of varying teaching strategies for the resident enables the faculty to meet the resident's learning needs and the program to achieve its curriculum competencies. Resident learning difficulties and strategies for overcoming these difficulties are discussed later in this chapter.

General Strategies for Linking Academic and Clinical Curriculum Components

As described previously, the works of several authors reinforce the importance of the clinician's ability to effectively use knowledge throughout the clinical reasoning process.[11,16,19] Ongoing critiques of assigned readings from a broad range of peer-reviewed and non–peer-reviewed journals can be integrated with the daily curriculum to expose residents to the problems and pitfalls of scientific literature in an advanced clinical practice area. Repeatedly, residents report that their ability to critique the literature substantially improves their confidence in communicating with other health care professionals as they concurrently develop and refine their clinical skills. Database searching and the demands of evidence-based practice require computer knowledge and skills for both faculty and residents and are valuable curricular components to consider when designing a residency program.

Knowledge from the literature, however, does not always apply to real patients. Of critical importance is facilitating development of the thinking or reflective processes a clinician can use when the textbook knowledge doesn't apply. Schön[25] calls book knowledge "technical rationality" and argues that this knowledge usually does not address the uncertain and frequently complex problems in professional practice. Professionals need to solve the problems of practice by thinking about why something does not work, solving the problem, and consequently adapting their knowledge and skills.

A key characteristic of experts is their superior ability to recognize common clinical presentations, which in turn influences their subsequent clinical reasoning and development of treatment strategies.[13] One method for assisting residents to recognize common clinical presentations is the writing of formal seminar papers that require residents to research and discuss clinical features of relevant pathologies, what is known about the pathology of various syndromes, current medical and physical therapy management, and the efficacy of treatment approaches. These papers can be critiqued in a seminar format with residency peers and can also form the basis of a publication by the resident.

Formalized seminar papers can also be combined with written case studies by the resident. The case study format assists the resident in beginning to organize patient data and justify examination and treatment related to current scientific literature. The patient may be brought into the clinic, with the resident presenting the patient to classmates through a formal or informal demonstration. Benner and Wrubel[26] note that use of case studies can assist residents in achieving a shift in their clinical reasoning processes. They state that the "interaction of the learner's prior knowledge creates experience, a turning point in understanding." Benner and Wrubel[26] and Polanyi[27] point out, however, that many cases are too complex to be transmitted through case exercises or simulations. This is when clinical supervision, the centerpiece of residency education, becomes most valuable. It is not uncommon for residents to easily grasp concepts presented in a lecture, seminar paper, or written case studies, but have significant difficulty synthesizing patient data and making judgments in a clinical setting, where they must quickly recognize clinical patterns, respond to emerging data from the patient, and tailor their examination and treatment to the patient's needs. Ongoing clinical supervision enables the faculty member to challenge the resident to think reflectively and make the connection between book knowledge and live practice.[25,28]

Direct Clinical Supervision and Mentoring: "Reflection-in-Action"

An overview of models for supervision was described in the section Overview of Residency Models. A key consideration in planning supervision schedules is to ensure that there is sufficient time for faculty-resident discussion during and immediately after the patient encounters. At least 30 minutes of discussion time at the end of a 4-hour supervision period has been found useful. The productivity demands of the organization should be evaluated to determine whether the resident has a sufficient caseload in her or his area of specialty and whether there are too few or too many patients to create a good learning environment.

Because the process of supervision takes place in the context of practice, the faculty member and resident are involved in thinking more deeply about the patient. The ongoing supervision model is frequently used in full-time programs, whereas supervision in blocks of time may be used in part-time programs. Other part-time residencies may require the resident to bring in and demonstrate a patient and receive feedback from the faculty and class-mates, or evaluate and treat patients who are on the caseload of the faculty member at the residency clinic on a one-to-one or small-group basis. With these latter supervision strategies, the resident may not have the opportu-nity to receive ongoing supervision throughout the course of the patient's treatment. The resident can maintain contact with the faculty member regarding the progress of his or her caseload through ongoing phone contacts or e-mail discussions.

Clinical supervision of an experienced physical therapist poses complex and sometimes difficult challenges. Many physical therapists come to a resi-dency because of the clinical supervision they will experience; however, work-ing side by side with a clinician or mentor with special expertise sometimes may be threatening, depending on the resident's expectations of the faculty and himself or herself, the resident's performance anxiety, the ability of fac-ulty members to articulate their clinical reasoning process to the resident, and the educational atmosphere of mentorship that the faculty member creates. The resident who is an experienced practitioner brings a much broader base of clinical experience than a physical therapy student brings to a clinical affilia-tion. The experienced resident has also developed some level of self-esteem and self-perception as a professional, which may include a significant level of expertise in selected areas of physical therapy. She or he is being asked to re-think prior clinical reasoning approaches, change old patient interview and examination habits, and identify and refine aspects that are useful and suc-cessful. The resident's ability to make these clinical practice changes depends on flexibility in thinking patterns and willingness to be supervised.

Although residents are adult learners, some are not able to articulate their learning needs, as they have never received this intense level of super-vision before. The clinic coordinator or program director can play a valuable role in ensuring an effective and supportive clinical supervision process by encouraging ongoing feedback between the faculty member and resident and by recognizing the teaching strengths and weaknesses of the faculty member in relation to the resident's learning style.

Tutorial Follow-Up

The value of the clinical supervision process can be enhanced through small group tutorials with other residents, who can provide peer critique of documentation and structured feedback on actual treatment techniques in combination with faculty input. Too often, the resident focuses on practice techniques and devotes insufficient time to perfecting clinical reasoning strategies and patient management skills. Role playing of patient cases during tutorials provides an invaluable avenue for reinforcing interview skills, objective examination schema, and common clinical presentations. Through a combination of skillful clinical supervision and tutorials, the resident comes to realize that wise practice is the integration of all components—medical knowledge, clinical signs and symptoms, clinical techniques, and an understanding of the patient's perspective.

Specific Teaching Strategies to Enhance the Clinical Reasoning Process during Clinical Supervision

The following sections focus on specific teaching strategies to assist the resident to refine interview skills and facilitate the clinical reasoning process through systematic data collection and reassessment. Teaching strategies are derived from the clinical reasoning model developed by Maitland,[14,15] which is described in the section Mission and Philosophy of Residency Education. Teaching methods may be the focus of a faculty-resident discussion during or after initial evaluation and treatment. Common pitfalls of the novice practitioner are described, but the reader should not interpret that these behaviors represent only the less-experienced practitioner. Rather, the term *novice practitioner* will be used in association with learning behaviors through several stages of the practitioner's progression from advanced beginner, to competent, to proficient. A common theme that underlies all strategies is teaching residents to reflect on performance or to continually self-monitor practice, during and after seeing patients. According to Cross,[28] for any experience to have lasting meaning, it must be followed at some appropriate distance by a period of reflection—mere involvement is not enough. Schön[25] refers to these actions as "reflection-in-action" and "reflection-about-action" and views self-correction adaptation processes as essential to the development of expertise.

Developing Patient-Centered Interview Skills

Excellent observation and communication skills are well accepted as attributes of effective health care practitioners. Jensen and her colleagues[29,30] describe the expert clinician's ability to focus on verbal and nonverbal communication with the patient as one of the attributes that differentiates expert from novice clinicians. Benner[31] reports that the effective clinician integrates "the implications of [a patient's] illness and recovery into [her or his] lifestyle" and "most important, captures the patient's readiness to learn." Furthermore, experts strive for collaborative solutions to the patient's problems rather than labeling or blaming the patient. In seeking the best possible care for the patient, experts take seriously the responsibility of advocacy for the patient. Viewing the patient as a trusted source of knowledge begins with the expert's communication to the patient.[31] The expert's data-gathering process begins the moment the patient and therapist meet and includes careful observation of the patient's overall appearance, facial expression, spontaneous postures, and manner of movement. The information gained from these early interactions is used by the expert in recognizing subtle clinical patterns and formulating an initial hypothesis as to the nature of the patient's problems and their relevance to the patient's goals. In addition to role modeling, communication, and observation skills, the manner in which the residency faculty member assists the resident through the subjective examination process will help the resident learn to focus her or his interview skills.

The subjective examination is an interview process whereby data are obtained about the area of a patient's symptoms; the mechanical or nonmechanical behavior of the symptoms; the chronologic history of the patient's complaints; and the possibility of any contraindications or precautions to the ensuing objective examination, treatment, or both. The subjective examination is key to the development of a working clinical hypothesis. During each phase of questioning, the information yielded is grouped into recognizable clinical patterns that support, reject, or modify earlier impressions or observations.[14,15]

The following case study presents a patient with lumbar and lower extremity complaints. It is followed by a discussion of teaching strategies that a residency faculty member could use to guide the resident in his or her clinical reasoning process through the subjective and objective examination and initial treatment planning.

J.T., a 31-year-old male hardware store clerk, presents with complaints of lower back pain and right knee pain. The back pain is at the level of the iliac crest and is distributed in a centralized square area approximately 4 inches wide. He describes the back pain as a deep, constant, dull pain that varies in intensity to a sharp pain at times. He also complains of intermittent stiffness in the same low-back area. The knee pain is in a generalized area around the whole knee and is described as a constant feeling of stiffness with intermittent periods of dull pain in the joint. On observation, the right knee is noted to be swollen and held in slight flexion. The patient states that the lower back is the worst area. He does not believe that the low-back and right knee pains are related—the back pain can be aggravated and eased independent of the knee pain, and vice versa. He does not believe that one symptom affects or causes the other symptom.

The onset of his symptoms occurred 2 nights earlier when he slid into second base during a softball game. He has been prescribed anti-inflammatory medication, given an elastic knee brace, and been put off work for 5 days. He had never had any complaints about his knee or lower back before. He is a physically fit young man who states that he is athletically active year-round. He exercises in the gym three times per week and plays seasonal sports two times per week (e.g., softball, skiing, bicycling, swimming).

Subjective Examination

During a subjective examination, the resident frequently has difficulty obtaining accurate, meaningful data. A common fault lies in the manner in which questions are asked. The resident may be too intent on obtaining the data to fill in the evaluation instead of listening carefully and guiding the patient in telling his or her story. Typical errors include (1) asking biased questions, (2) asking more than one question at a time, (3) making assumptions as to the nature of the patient's problems, (4) failing to allow or make use of the patient's spontaneous comments, (5) repetitively asking questions or pursuing responses that do not yield useful information, or (6) failing to pursue a response in sufficient detail. Table 14-2 provides examples of questions and typical errors made by the novice when interviewing patients regarding areas of symptoms. An alternative questioning style representative of the experienced clinician is also presented in Table 14-2. Maitland[15] summarizes the importance of open-ended questioning, saying, "[T]he patient will tell the therapist what is wrong with him if the therapist will, in fact, listen!" A skillful faculty member can role model an effective, efficient questioning style by rephrasing questions or interjecting a question that facilitates more useful dialogue with the patient. In some cases, when persistent questioning yields no

Table 14-2 Comparison of Questioning Styles of Residents and Experienced Clinicians

Resident questioning	Patient response	Error	Questioning by experienced therapist	Patient response
What is your chief complaint?	What do you mean?	Use of medical jargon	What's the problem that brings you to physical therapy?	I can't move around easily. My back hurts.
Where is your pain?	In my back, mainly.	Biased questions	Where are you having trouble?	In my back, mainly.
Do you mean right in here? (Touching patient's lower back.)	Yes, but over here, too.	Making assumptions; biased questions	Show me where.	(Allows patient to outline area. Clarifies and delineates region if needed.)
Do you have pain in your buttock or down your leg?	No, but my knee also hurts.	Asking more than one question at a time; biased question	Do you have complaints anywhere else?	(Allows patient to answer spontaneously; the therapist then asks about the areas above and below the area in which patient feels pain.) My right knee also hurts.
Describe your pain; is it sharp or dull?	Both.	Asking more than one question at a time; biased question	Describe how your lower back feels.	There's always a dull ache. When I try to bend down, it's stiff, and I get a sharp pain.
Is it constant or intermittent?	Oh, there's always something there.	Use of medical jargon; incomplete data obtained	(Allows spontaneous comments to emerge; then can clarify in more detail.)	

Table 14-3 Examples of Salient Subjective Patient Data and Possible Clinical Interpretations

Interview data	Possible interpretation of symptoms
Lumbar symptoms	
Area of symptoms: central lower-back pain, L4-L5	Possible source: central lying spinal structures
Painful leaning to brush teeth and bending to tie shoes	Painful, limited, or both, in half flexion and full flexion under axial load
Aggravating factors	
Painful with brief periods of sitting and with prolonged standing	Low tolerance for static axial loads in flexion, more so than extension
Painful/stiff rising from chair	Difficulty transitioning to an erect posture
Easing factors	
Lying down with legs extended	Eases with non–weight bearing; with spinal extension bias
Placing hands behind back	Eases with spinal extension biased pressure
Right knee symptoms	
Area of symptoms: whole knee	Multiple sources: tibiofemoral joint and soft tissues surrounding knee
Aggravating factors	
Stiff to walk, go up and down stairs	Difficulty weight bearing in extension and flexion
Easing factors	
Eased by lying down, elevation	Relief with unloading, passive drainage
Eased by ice, Ace wrap	Relief by reducing swelling, supporting joint

useful data, the clinical mentor may urge the resident to "move on" and later explain why the questioning was unnecessary.

Identifying Salient Subjective Information: Pattern Recognition

A key skill in the clinical reasoning process is the ability to identify salient subjective information when there are multiple symptom areas. By *salient,* we mean clinically relevant data (i.e., information pertaining to the provocation of the patient's symptoms or relief of symptoms, pertaining to the patient's current problem, or affecting treatment of the problem). Examples of salient subjective data for the lumbar spine and knee problems presented in the case are summarized in Table 14-3. Subjective data are listed in the left-hand column, and possible interpretations of this initial interview data are listed in the right-hand column. Using this format, the faculty member can assist the resident to identify patterns in the patient's various functional activities that aggravate or ease symptoms. She or he can also assist the resident in determining whether mechanical or non-mechanical factors contribute to the patient's dysfunction.

The faculty member plays a vital role in assisting the resident to identify subjective information that can be used to plan the objective examination and initial treatment. In the clinical reasoning process, this is called *pattern recognition* or *forward reasoning.*[32] For the advanced clinician, the cues presented by the patient in the interview are recognized as fitting with a clinical pattern linked with a hypothesis or diagnosis. Novice practitioners often have difficulty knowing what information to gather from the patient's current status or history and view all data as being of equal value. They also have difficulty prioritizing what data are important to use in further examination and treatment. The residency faculty member may need to selectively intervene, assisting the resident to establish the relationship between symptoms as well as the worst area of symptoms. Determining the relationship between symptoms (e.g., asking, "Does your knee pain increase when your back pain worsens?") helps the resident identify how many separate problem areas the patient may have. Determining the worst problem area enables the resident to prioritize the examination and treatment time during the initial and subsequent treatment sessions. In this case study, the patient reports that the lower back is his most troublesome symptom area. He appears to have two separate problem areas, the low back and knee, and does not think that one symptom affects or causes the other. In this case, the focus for the initial examination should be directed to the lumbar spine with a brief evaluation of the right knee.

Another valuable teaching strategy is having the faculty member document the evaluation concurrently with the resident. The faculty member can role model concise, organized documentation and identify areas in which the resident may have interviewed or tested the patient well but prepared unclear or incorrect written documentation. By writing alternative questions (e.g., "You could have asked the question in the following manner . . .") or additional questions (e.g., "Next time also ask the following . . .") on a photocopy of the resident's written evaluation, the faculty member can also provide specific strategies to help the resident change his or her questioning style.

Objective Examination

The resident needs to continually use data to predict or plan the next step in the process, which is the objective examination. Based on the subjective data, the resident is asked to identify potential joints under

Table 14-4 Structure for Planning an Objective Patient Examination

Joints under the area of SX	*Joints that may refer into the area of SX*	*Contractile tissue under area of SX that must be examined*	*Other structures that must be considered as possible sources*
L4-L5, L5-S1 disk	L3-L4 disk	L4-S1 paraspinals	Neural tension (SLR, prone knee bend)
L4-L5, L5-S1 apo-physeal joints	Right hip	—	—
Right tibiofemoral joint		Right quadriceps	Right knee ligaments
Right patellofemo-ral joint		Right hamstrings	(e.g., collaterals, cru-
		Right gastrocne-	ciates, coronary)
Right superior tibiofibular joint		mius (proximal heads)	Right knee bursae

L = lumbar vertebrae; S = sacral vertebrae; SLR = straight-leg raise; SX = symptoms.
Source: Adapted from forms developed by the School of Physiotherapy, University of South Australia and Curtin University of Technology, Perth, Western Australia.

the area of symptoms, joints that may refer to the area of symptoms, contractile tissues that must be examined under the area of symptoms, and other structures that must be considered as possible sources of symptoms. This thinking process trains the resident to consider all possible contributing factors. Another important aspect of developing systematic clinical reasoning skills is the ability to use hypothesis-guided inquiry, which is also called *backward reasoning*.[31] Too often, novice practitioners consider too few hypotheses in their patient examinations. Doing so can lead to incorrect hypotheses or a delay in determining the patient's major problem areas.[13]

Table 14-4 demonstrates how a clinical training form may be designed to assist the resident in identifying tissues potentially at fault. As noted in Table 14-4, the assessment suggests that there may be a neural tension component contributing to the patient's low-back symptoms. *Adverse neural tissue tension* is a term used to describe any abnormal physiologic or mechanical response from the nervous system that limits the nervous system's normal mobility.[33] The concept of adverse neural tension was originally developed by Elvey[34] and further elaborated on by Butler.[33] Straight-leg raise (SLR) and prone knee-bend tests are among the clinical measures used to assess whether there may be problems with mobility in neural tissues.

Salient subjective information (see Table 14-3) and the plan for the objective examination form (see Table 14-4) are used to develop an initial hypothesis of the patient's problem(s). The preliminary data in Tables 14-3 and 14-4 suggest a possible subacute lumbar derangement syndrome[35] in addition to a right knee problem. According to McKenzie,[35] some of the key features of a lumbar derangement are (1) sudden onset of pain; (2) symptoms that are local, in the midline, or adjacent to the spinal column and may radiate distally in the form of pain, paresthesia, and numbness; and (3) symptoms that may be improved or further irritated after certain repeated movements or the maintenance of certain positions. McKenzie argues that the pain felt with a derangement syndrome may occur as a result of a change in disk shape with malalignment of the intervertebral segment and its related abnormal stresses. This patient's subjective data support the key features of a lumbar derangement. Further refinement of the initial hypothesis of the knee problem will be expected after gathering further objective examination data.

Identifying Salient Objective Information and Correlating Subjective and Objective Information

The next step in the clinical reasoning process is to guide the resident to correlate subjective data with the objective data and to confirm or revise the initial working hypothesis from the subjective data. Selected objective examination findings from the case study are summarized here.

The objective findings at the initial evaluation of the patient J.T. showed limited and painful movements in spinal flexion and extension. There was poor segmental unrolling (movement from the erect position into spinal flexion) at the fourth lumbar through first sacral vertebrae (L4-S1) levels. Side trunk flexion was only slightly limited, and the range was symmetric on the left and right. SLR tests were 70 degrees bilateral and limited by back pain. The neurologic examination was normal. Spinal palpation revealed increased tightness in the lower lumbar paraspinal muscles and restricted passive spinal motion greater at the L4-L5 than the L5-S1 intervertebral segments. The right knee was observed to be swollen and held in slight flexion. Range of motion was limited in flexion to 105 degrees. Knee extension was –5 degrees. Manual muscle tests of the quadriceps and hamstring muscles indicated no presence of muscle weakness (normal). Palpation of the knee joint revealed warmth, tenderness, and effusion surrounding the joint but did not reveal focal areas of pain.

After the objective examination, the clinical mentor guides the resident to analyze the findings and relate the data to the subjective examination. For example, spinal motion is limited and painful in flexion and extension in the sagittal plane, which correlates with J.T.'s complaints of difficulty bending forward to brush his teeth and standing up from a chair. Spinal palpation suggests that muscle tightness and restricted passive movements (centrally directed posterior-anterior and unilateral movements) are greatest at the L4-L5 intervertebral segment, which correlates with the area of complaints identified by the patient.

Knee joint testing reveals limited flexion and extension in a capsular pattern of restriction, suggesting a possible capsulitis of the tibiofemoral joint. According to Cyriax,[36] lesions in the synovial membrane of the knee may result in limitation of movement in a capsular pattern, with greatest limitation in flexion and slight limitation in extension. Preliminary palpation findings during objective examination support this hypothesis. The patient's subjective complaints of difficulty walking on level surfaces and going up and down stairs can be attributed to lack of knee range and intolerance for full extension. A more detailed knee evaluation needs to be performed to assess for other possible structures involved, including knee ligaments, meniscal structures, or the patellofemoral joint.

Prioritizing the Patient's Problems

Assisting the resident in developing the ability to prioritize the patient's problems is a necessary step in helping the resident manage patients with increasingly difficult multifactorial dysfunction. One method for helping the resident organize examination data from a patient with more than one problem area is to use a flow chart. The flow chart organizes the data in a meaningful way by requiring the resident to rank the symptom areas in order of importance. The chart also summarizes the patient's physical problems that may contribute to a limitation in function. The flow chart in Figure 14-2 is an example of conceptual mapping. Conceptual mapping is a strategy for facilitating reflection (i.e., to think about one's thinking and to further analyze one's clinical reasoning processes).[37]

Treatment Selection

All practitioners entering a residency program have had experience selecting and progressing treatment. The challenge for clinical faculty, however, is to guide the resident to select and progress treatment using a systematic clinical reasoning process. Through experience and training in

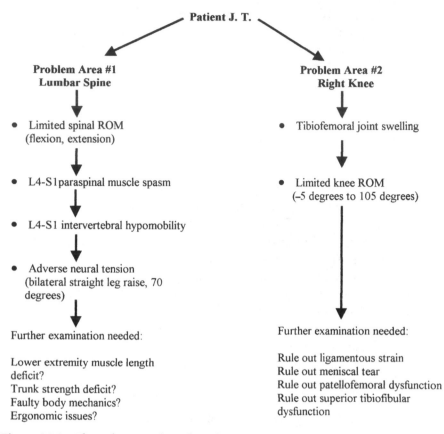

Patient J. T.

Problem Area #1
Lumbar Spine

- Limited spinal ROM
  (flexion, extension)

- L4-S1 paraspinal muscle spasm

- L4-S1 intervertebral hypomobility

- Adverse neural tension
  (bilateral straight leg raise, 70
  degrees)

Further examination needed:

Lower extremity muscle length
deficit?
Trunk strength deficit?
Faulty body mechanics?
Ergonomic issues?

Problem Area #2
Right Knee

- Tibiofemoral joint swelling

- Limited knee ROM
  (–5 degrees to 105 degrees)

Further examination needed:

Rule out ligamentous strain
Rule out meniscal tear
Rule out patellofemoral dysfunction
Rule out superior tibiofibular
dysfunction

Figure 14-2   Flow chart used to identify patient problem areas. (ROM = range of motion.)

advanced techniques in the residency curriculum, the resident has a broader repertoire from which to select a beginning treatment. Some commonly used treatments for J.T., the case study patient, may include joint mobilization; extension exercises; modalities; ergonomic recommendations; and instruction in posture, body mechanics, and home exercise. The specific treatment methods depend on the patient population served; the patient's goals; and the therapist's knowledge base, skill level, and history of successful outcomes.

Having formulated reasonable hypotheses for the sources of the patient's symptoms and prioritized the patient's complaints, the resident can more easily decide where and how to initiate treatment. By using the flow chart of the patient's problems (Figure 14-2), the faculty member can guide the resident to devise a plan of treatment to address each problem area. For example, treatment for lumbar problems may incorporate procedures to increase spinal range of motion. Such procedures may include joint mobilization techniques, such as posterior-anterior pressures over the spinous processes as described by Maitland,[15] repeated extension movements in prone as described by McKenzie for lumbar derangement,[35] or a combination of the two. If paraspinal muscle spasms prevent progress from such treatment techniques, soft-tissue techniques or appropriate modalities may be applied. Restrictions found in SLR may be addressed using neural mobilization techniques described by Butler.[33] The flow chart can be used in a similar fashion to address treatment for the knee. Initial treatment may include the use of ice, instruction in limb elevation, gentle active exercise for the knee and ankle, and application of an external support. The key to the clinical reasoning process is guiding the resident to have the mental discipline to approach treatment planning in this systematic fashion every time a patient is seen. With each new patient, the resident should consider what to do to address each problem; what should be treated on day 1; and what to do if the patient returns feeling better, the same, or worse.

Reassessment

The key to successful treatment of a patient's problem is systematic assessment and reassessment of the symptoms and signs throughout the process of examination and treatment. Through methodical reassessment of the salient subjective and objective data, the resident can (1) detect change in function, (2) reconfirm his or her hypotheses, (3) prove the efficacy of treatment, and (4) consider additional hypotheses or plans for future examination and treatment. The concept of reassessment is a cornerstone of the Maitland[14,15] approach to musculoskeletal examination and treatment.

An example of how the assessment-reassessment process works can be described using the case study presented in this chapter. Key lumbar examination findings include (1) limited spinal motion, (2) paraspinal muscle spasm, (3) segmental hypomobility, and (4) restricted SLR with a possible neural tension component. McKenzie's[35] application of repeated spinal extension movements to reduce lumbar derangement and improve range of motion must be proven beneficial. Before and after application of repeated spinal extension movements, the patient's response to each of these four findings is reassessed. If lumbar spinal motion improves and the paraspinal muscle spasms are decreased, then treatment directed to the muscle spasms (e.g., modalities, soft-tissue techniques) is not necessary. If segmental hypomobility at L4-S1 and restriction in SLR do not fully resolve, however, a treatment plan for joint mobilization may be necessary. If, after applying mobilization techniques to the L4-S1 intervertebral segment, the spinal motion is full range and pain free and SLR improves to within normal limits, then the proposed treatments for SLR neural tissue mobilization are not necessary. Through consistent reassessment of the salient data after each treatment is applied, the value of the technique(s) and whether it (they) should be continued, progressed, or discontinued can be determined.

The clinical reasoning process continues throughout the resident's management of the patient. Assessment and reassessment of the patient's symptoms and signs by using hypothesis-guided inquiry are done throughout the process of examination and treatment. By methodical reassessment of the salient subjective and objective data, the resident can (1) detect change in function, (2) reconfirm her or his hypotheses, (3) prove the efficacy of treatment, and (4) consider additional hypotheses or plans for future examination and treatment.

In summary, the clinical reasoning process with residents uses pattern recognition (forward reasoning) and hypothesis-guided inquiry (backward reasoning). The use of pattern recognition will assist residents in further developing their clinical knowledge base. Hypothesis-guided inquiry is central to the data-gathering process and the interpretation of clinical data used in the evaluation. Clinical teaching in a residency program is a continual reflective process in which residents and faculty further the development and refinement of clinical knowledge.

Formal and Informal Evaluation

Residents are evaluated using a variety of practical and written methods, including special projects such as the seminar papers previously described. Practical examinations with patients may involve performing an entire examination and treatment as faculty score the resident on such factors as (1) thoroughness and accuracy of examination, (2) identification and justification of clinical hypotheses on which the treatment decisions are based, (3) selection and justification of treatment, (4) patient education, (5) time management, (6) treatment progression, and (7) ability to identify and justify the patient's treatment prognosis. Criteria for practical evaluations are established by individual program faculty and are based on the program's graduation competencies and specific course objectives. Efforts should be made to establish intratester and intertester reliability among faculty members for practical examination criteria within a given program. Practical examinations may also involve evaluation of specific patient handling techniques that are performed on faculty. Faculty provide feedback on such areas as accuracy and comfort of patient position, therapist hand position, and therapist body position.

Use of written patient evaluations provides valuable insight into the resident's ability to assess written documentation and plan, progress, and justify treatment. Analysis of written case studies is frequently used to test clinical reasoning skills.

The key component of the evaluation process within a residency program is that faculty have the opportunity to assess the resident on an ongoing basis over an extended period of time. Practical examinations are difficult to compare because of the differences that may exist between patients on any given day. Use of simulated patients, whereby lay persons are trained to enact all aspects of a real case,[38] is emerging as a method of teaching and examination in physical therapy.[39] Evidence studied largely at medical schools shows that the use of simulated patients for educational intervention and examination is reliable and effective.[40]

Summary

Physical therapy describes itself as and prides itself on being a clinical profession, yet the profession has fallen short in making opportunities available for experienced clinicians to receive advanced clinical training. In postprofessional residency education, physical therapists can link theory with clinical practice and receive ongoing clinical supervision over an extended period of time. Postprofessional curricula are directed toward teaching experienced practitioners examination and treatment strategies that will enable them to continually monitor and critique their performance and develop clinical expertise over time. As stated by Rivett and Higgs, "[T]o achieve expertise . . . is to 'rise above mediocrity,' clinicians need to develop and practice relevant strategies to turn their experience into learning."[41]

The physical therapy profession is decades behind other professions in acknowledging the value of residency training for entry into the profession and for specialization. The residency curriculum and teaching strategies presented in this chapter are derived from our knowledge of postprofessional residency programs in OMPT and orthopedic physical therapy throughout the United States. We hope that the ideas in this chapter will stimulate academic and clinical faculty to plan for the addition of extended internships as part of physical therapy professional curricula, the development of residency programs for new graduates, and the expansion of residency programs for experienced clinicians. Health care changes are placing high demands on novice therapists, who must "hit the ground running" after graduating from physical therapy school, and on experienced physical therapists, who must assume new roles with greater responsibility and autonomy. In this new environment, a commitment to clinical residency education is a commitment to clinical excellence. Residency education will be critical for the survival of the physical therapy profession in the twenty-first century.

References

1. Tichenor CJ. Clinical residency: another turning point for our profession? PT Mag 1995;3(1):49.
2. American Physical Therapy Association. Postprofessional Clinical Residency Program Credentialing Application. Alexandria, VA: American Physical Therapy Association, 2000.
3. Stoeckle JD, Leaf A, Grossman JH, Goroll AH. A case history of training outside the hospital and its future. Am J Med 1979;66:1008.
4. Council on Podiatric Medical Education. Standards, Requirements and Guidelines for Approval of Residencies in Podiatric Medicine. Bethesda, MD: American Podiatric Medical Association, 1993.
5. Council on Optometric Education Residency Standards. Accreditation Handbook. St. Louis: American Optometric Association, 1994.
6. American Psychological Association. Accreditation Handbook. Washington, DC: American Psychological Association, 1986.
7. Long TM, Sippel K. A pediatric clinical residency. PT Mag 1995;3(1):57.
8. American Academy of Orthopaedic Manual Physical Therapists. Standards for Orthopaedic Manual Physical Therapy Residency Training. Gulfport, MS: American Academy of Orthopaedic Manual Physical Therapists, 1993.
9. American Academy of Orthopaedic Manual Physical Therapists. Standards for Orthopaedic Manual Physical Therapy Residency Training. Biloxi, MS: American Academy of Orthopaedic Manual Physical Therapists, 1999.
10. American Physical Therapy Association Task Force on Accreditation of Clinical Residencies. Alexandria, VA: American Physical Therapy Association, 1994.
11. Elstein A, Shulman L, Sprafka S. Medical problem solving: a ten-year retrospective study. Eval Health Prof 1990;13:5.
12. Higgs J, Jones M. Clinical Reasoning in the Health Professions. Boston: Butterworth–Heinemann, 1995;35.
13. Jones M. Clinical reasoning in physical therapy. Phys Ther 1992;72:875.
14. Maitland GD. Peripheral Manipulation (3rd ed). Boston: Butterworth, 1977.
15. Maitland GD. Vertebral Manipulation (5th ed). Boston: Butterworth, 1986;1.
16. Grant R, Jones M, Maitland GD. Clinical Decision Making in Upper Quarter Dysfunction. In R Grant (ed), Physical Therapy of the Cervical and Thoracic Spine. New York: Churchill Livingstone, 1988;51.

17. Barrows HS, Tamblyn RM. Problem-Based Learning: An Approach to Medical Education. New York: Springer-Verlag, 1980.
18. Gale J, Marsden P. Clinical problem solving: the beginning of the process. Med Educ 1982;16:22.
19. Grant J, Marsden P. The structure of memorized knowledge in students and clinicians: an explanation for diagnostic expertise. Med Educ 1987;21:92.
20. May BJ, Dennis JK. Teaching Clinical Decision-Making. In J Higgs, M Jones (eds), Clinical Reasoning in the Health Professions. Boston: Butterworth–Heinemann, 1995;301.
21. Higgs J. A programme for developing clinical reasoning skills in graduate physiotherapists. Med Teach 1993;15:195.
22. Payton OD, Nelson CE, Ozer MN. Patient Participation in Program Planning: A Manual for Therapists. Philadelphia: FA Davis, 1990.
23. Benner P. From Novice to Expert: Excellence and Power in Clinical Nursing. Menlo Park, CA: Addison Wesley, 1984.
24. Ruth-Sahd LA. A modification of Benner's hierarchy of clinical practice: the development of clinical intuition in the novice trauma nurse. Holistic Nurse Prac 1993;73:8.
25. Schön DA. The Reflective Practitioner. New York: Basic Books, 1983.
26. Benner P, Wrubel J. Skilled clinical knowledge: the value of perceptual awareness. Nurse Educ 1982;7:11.
27. Polanyi M. Personal Knowledge. London: Rutledge & Kegan Paul, 1958.
28. Cross V. Introducing physiotherapy students to the idea of "reflective practice." Med Teach 1993;15:293.
29. Jensen GM, Gwyer J, Hack LM, Shepard KF. Expertise in Physical Therapy Practice. Boston: Butterworth–Heinemann, 1999.
30. Jensen GM, Gwyer J, Shepard KF, Hack LM. Expert practice in physical therapy. Phys Ther 2000;80(1):28–52.
31. Benner P. Uncovering the knowledge embedded in clinical practice. Image J Nurs Sch 1983;15(2):36.
32. Patel V, Groen G. The General and Specific Nature of Medical Expertise: A Critical Look. In KA Ericsson, J Smith (eds), Toward a General Theory of Expertise. New York: Cambridge University Press, 1991;93.
33. Butler DS. Mobilisation of the Nervous System. London: Churchill Livingstone, 1991.
34. Elvey R. Treatment of arm pain associated with abnormal brachial plexus tension. Aust J Physiother 1986;32:224.
35. McKenzie RA. Mechanical Diagnosis and Therapy for Disorders of the Low Back. In L Twomey, JR Taylor (eds), Physical Therapy of the Low Back (2nd ed). New York: Churchill Livingstone, 1994;171.

36. Cyriax J. Textbook of Orthopaedic Medicine (Vol I). Diagnosis of Soft Tissue Lesions (7th ed). London: Baillière, 1979;81.
37. Tichen A, Higgs J. Facilitating the Use and Generation of Knowledge in Clinical Reasoning. In J Higgs, M Jones (eds), Clinical Reasoning in the Health Professions. Boston: Butterworth–Heinemann, 1995;314.
38. Barrows HS. The Simulated Patient. Springfield, IL: Thomas, 1971.
39. Edwards H, Franke M, McGuiness B. Using Simulated Patients to Teach Clinical Reasoning. In J Higgs, M Jones (eds), Clinical Reasoning in the Health Professions. Boston: Butterworth–Heinemann, 1995;269.
40. Vu NV, Barrows H, Marcy ML, et al. Six years of comprehensive, clinical, performance-based assessment using standardized patients at the Southern Illinois University School of Medicine. Acad Med 1992;67:42.
41. Rivett D, Higgs J. Experience and expertise in clinical reasoning. N Z J Physiother 1995;April:16.

Supplementary Documents to Aid in Developing Residency Curricula

The following documents can be obtained from the American Physical Therapy Association (APTA), 1111 North Fairfax Street, Alexandria, VA 22314-1488. Phone: 703-684-2782, 1-800-999-2782; Fax: 703-684-7343; Web site: http://www.apta.org.

APTA Postprofessional Clinical Residency Program Credentialing Application, 2000. Department of Professional Development. Identifies criteria, forms, and procedures for programs applying for APTA credentialing.

Postprofessional Clinical Residency Program Credentialing Application Resource Manual, 2000. Department of Professional Development. Document includes examples for developing program mission, goals, objectives, performance outcomes, and rationale for organization and sequencing of curriculum components. Document also includes examples of procedures and assessment instruments for evaluating performance of the resident and graduate.

Guide to Physical Therapist Practice, 2000. APTA Service Center, 1-800-999-2782, ext. 3395. Competencies presented in the Guide can be used in establishing program mission, objectives, and outcomes.

A Normative Model for Physical Therapist Professional Education, 2000. APTA Service Center, 1-800-999-2782, ext. 3395. Various matrices presented in this document include primary content area, examples of terminal behavioral objectives, and examples of instructional objectives. These materials can be used to develop residency program objectives and performance outcomes.

Descriptions of Advanced Clinical Practice (DACPs) have been developed for the following specialty areas: cardiopulmonary, geriatrics, orthopedics, neurology, pediatrics, and sports. The DACP defines the practice dimensions and competencies governing advanced clinical practice of a specialty area. Contact the APTA to obtain a copy of the DACP for your specialty area. The competencies defined in each DACP can be used to develop program objectives and performance outcomes.

The following documents may be obtained from the American Academy of Orthopaedic Manual Physical Therapists (AAOMPT), P.O. Box 4777, Biloxi, MS 39535-4777. Phone: 228-392-0028; Fax: 228 392-0666.

Orthopaedic Manual Physical Therapy: A Description of Advanced Clinical Practice, 1998. Practice dimensions and competencies defined in this document can be used to develop program objectives and performance outcomes.

Standards for Orthopaedic Manual Physical Therapy Residency Education, 1999. Document defines criteria for manual therapy residency programs seeking recognition by the AAOMPT. Document also includes minimum standards for duration of residency education, clinical supervision, clinical practical examinations, and non-patient contact hours. Appendix includes examples of program objectives and course syllabi for course work in the applied sciences and manual therapy.

The following document, developed jointly by the Orthopaedic Section, APTA, Inc., and the AAOMPT, can be obtained from either organization.
Orthopaedic Section, APTA, Inc. 2920 East Avenue South, La Crosse, WI 54601-7202. Phone: 1-800-444-3982; Fax: 608-788-3965.
American Academy of Orthopaedic Manual Physical Therapists, P.O. Box 4777, Biloxi, MS 39535-4777. Phone: 228-392-0028; Fax: 228-392-0666.

Guidelines for Curriculum Development for Postprofessional Residencies in Orthopaedic Physical Therapy and Orthopaedic Manual Physical Therapy, 2000. Document includes a comparison of orthopedic versus manual therapy residency curricula; information about developing the mission, philosophy, goals, curriculum, and performance outcomes of a residency; and information about instructional methods, evaluation of program outcomes, residency faculty selection and professional development, and financial considerations for planning a residency.

INDEX